T0263916

Infections in Transplant and Oncology Patients

Guest Editors

KIEREN A. MARR, MD
ARUNA K. SUBRAMANIAN, MD

INFECTIOUS DISEASE CLINICS OF NORTH AMERICA

www.id.theclinics.com

Consulting Editor
ROBERT C. MOELLERING Jr, MD

June 2010 • Volume 24 • Number 2

SAUNDERS an imprint of ELSEVIER, Inc.

W.B. SAUNDERS COMPANY
A Division of Elsevier Inc.
1600 John F. Kennedy Blvd., Suite 1800, Philadelphia, PA 19103-2899.
http://www.theclinics.com

INFECTIOUS DISEASE CLINICS OF NORTH AMERICA Volume 24, Number 2
June 2010 ISSN 0891–5520, ISBN-13: 978-1-4377-1831-7

Editor: Barbara Cohen-Kligerman
Developmental Editor: Theresa Collier

© **2010 Elsevier Inc. All rights reserved.**

This journal and the individual contributions contained in it are protected under copyright by Elsevier, and the following terms and conditions apply to their use:

Photocopying
Single photocopies of single articles may be made for personal use as allowed by national copyright laws. Permission of the Publisher and payment of a fee is required for all other photocopying, including multiple or systematic copying, copying for advertising or promotional purposes, resale, and all forms of document delivery. Special rates are available for educational institutions that wish to make photocopies for non-profit educational classroom use. For information on how to seek permission visit www.elsevier.com/permissions or call: (+44) 1865 843830 (UK)/(+1) 215 239 3804 (USA).

Derivative Works
Subscribers may reproduce tables of contents or prepare lists of articles including abstracts for internal circulation within their institutions. Permission of the Publisher is required for resale or distribution outside the institution. Permission of the Publisher is required for all other derivative works, including compilations and translations (please consult www.elsevier.com/permissions).

Electronic Storage or Usage
Permission of the Publisher is required to store or use electronically any material contained in this journal, including any article or part of an article (please consult www.elsevier.com/permissions). Except as outlined above, no part of this publication may be reproduced, stored in a retrieval system or transmitted in any form or by any means, electronic, mechanical, photocopying, recording or otherwise, without prior written permission of the Publisher.

Notice
No responsibility is assumed by the Publisher for any injury and/or damage to persons or property as a matter of products liability, negligence or otherwise, or from any use or operation of any methods, products, instructions or ideas contained in the material herein. Because of rapid advances in the medical sciences, in particular, independent verification of diagnoses and drug dosages should be made.

Although all advertising material is expected to conform to ethical (medical) standards, inclusion in this publication does not constitute a guarantee or endorsement of the quality or value of such product or of the claims made of it by its manufacturer.

Infectious Disease Clinics of North America (ISSN 0891–5520) is published in March, June, September, and December by Elsevier Inc., 360 Park Avenue South, New York, NY 10010-1710. Periodicals postage paid at New York, NY and additional mailing offices. Subscription prices are $235.00 per year for US individuals, $395.00 per year for US institutions, $118.00 per year for US students, $278.00 per year for Canadian individuals, $489.00 per year for Canadian institutions, $332.00 per year for international individuals, $489.00 per year for international institutions, and $163.00 per year for Canadian and international students. To receive student rate, orders must be accompanied by name of affiliated institution, date of term, and the *signature* of program/residency coordinator on institution letterhead. Orders will be billed at individual rate until proof of status is received. Foreign air speed delivery is included in all *Clinics* subscription prices. All prices are subject to change without notice. **POSTMASTER**: Send address changes to *Infectious Disease Clinics of North America,* Elsevier Health Sciences Division, Subcription Customer Service, 3251 Riverport Lane, Maryland Heights, MO 63043. **Customer Service: 1-800-654-2452 (US). From outside of the US and Canada, call 1-314-447-8871. Fax: 1-314-447-8029. E-mail: JournalsCustomerService-usa@elsevier.com (print support) or JournalsOnlineSupport-usa@elsevier.com (online support).**

Infectious Disease Clinics of North America is also published in Spanish by Editorial Inter-Médica, Junin 917, 1er A 1113, Buenos Aires, Argentina.

Reprints. For copies of 100 or more, of articles in this publication, please contact the Commercial Reprints Department, Elsevier Inc., 360 Park Avenue South, New York, New York 10010-1710. Tel. (212) 633-3812, Fax: (212) 462-1935, E-mail: reprints@elsevier.com.

Infectious Disease Clinics of North America is covered in *MEDLINE/PubMed (Index Medicus), Current Contents/Clinical Medicine, Science Citation Alert, SCISEARCH,* and *Research Alert.*

Printed and bound by CPI Group (UK) Ltd, Croydon, CR0 4YY

Transferred to Digital Print 2011

Contributors

CONSULTING EDITOR

ROBERT C. MOELLERING Jr, MD
Shields Warren-Mallinckrodt Professor of Medical Research, Harvard Medical School; Department of Medicine, Beth Israel Deaconess Medical Center, Boston, Massachusetts

GUEST EDITORS

KIEREN A. MARR, MD
Professor of Medicine and Oncology, Division of Infectious Diseases, Johns Hopkins University School of Medicine, Baltimore, Maryland

ARUNA K. SUBRAMANIAN, MD
Assistant Professor of Medicine, Division of Infectious Diseases, Johns Hopkins University School of Medicine, Baltimore, Maryland

AUTHORS

BARBARA D. ALEXANDER, MD, MHS
Division of Infectious Diseases, Department of Medicine, Duke University Health System, Duke University School of Medicine, Durham, North Carolina

SOWSAN ATABANI, PhD
Department of Infection (Royal Free Campus), University College London; Department of Virology, Royal Free Hampstead NHS Trust, Hampstead, London, United Kingdom

LINDSEY R. BADEN, MD
Assistant Professor of Medicine, Division of Infectious Diseases, Brigham and Women's Hospital; Division of Infectious Diseases, Dana-Farber Cancer Institute; Harvard Medical School, Boston, Massachusetts

EMILY BLUMBERG, MD
Division of Infectious Diseases, Hospital of the University of Pennsylvania, Philadelphia, Pennsylvania

MICHAEL BOECKH, MD
University of Washington, Vaccine and Infectious Disease Institute, Fred Hutchinson Cancer Research Center, Seattle, Washington

EMILIO BOUZA, MD, PhD
Professor and Head of the Department of Clinical Microbiology and Infectious Diseases, Hospital General Universitario Gregorio Marañón; Facultad de Medicina, Universidad Complutense de Madrid, Madrid, Spain

SUNWEN CHOU, MD
Professor, Division of Infectious Diseases, Oregon Health and Science University, Portland, Oregon

ADRIAN EGLI, MD, PhD
Department of Biomedicine, Transplantation Virology, Institute for Medical Microbiology, University of Basel; Department of Medicine, University Hospital Basel, Basel, Switzerland

HERMANN EINSELE, PhD
Department of Medicine, University of Wuerzburg, Wuerzburg, Germany

VINCENT C. EMERY, PhD
Department of Infection (Royal Free Campus), University College London, Hampstead, London, United Kingdom

STACI A. FISCHER, MD
Associate Professor, Division of Infectious Diseases, The Warren Alpert Medical School of Brown University, Providence, Rhode Island

JAY A. FISHMAN, MD
Professor of Medicine, Harvard Medical School; Director, Transplant Infectious Disease and Compromised Host Program; Associate Director, Transplant Center; Division of Infectious Disease, Massachusetts General Hospital, Harvard Medical School, Boston, Massachusetts

MICHAEL GREEN, MD, MPH
Professor, Department of Pediatrics and Surgery, Children's Hospital of Pittsburgh, Pittsburgh, Pennsylvania

MORGAN HAKKI, MD
Division of Infectious Diseases, Oregon Health and Science University, Portland, Oregon

TANZINA HAQUE, PhD
Department of Virology, Royal Free Hampstead NHS Trust, Hampstead, London, United Kingdom

ILKKA HELANTERÄ, MD, PhD
Transplant Unit Research Laboratory, Transplantation and Liver Surgery Clinic; Department of Medicine, Division of Nephrology, Helsinki University Hospital, and University of Helsinki, Helsinki, Finland

JOHN W. HIEMENZ, MD
Professor of Medicine, Bone Marrow Transplant Program, Division of Hematology/Oncology, University of Florida College of Medicine, Gainesville, Florida

HANS H. HIRSCH, MD, MS
Department of Biomedicine, Transplantation Virology, Institute for Medical Microbiology, University of Basel; Department of Internal Medicine, Infectious diseases and Hospital Epidemiology, University Hospital Basel, Basel, Switzerland

JACK HSU, MD
Assistant Professor of Medicine, Bone Marrow Transplant Program, Division of Hematology/Oncology, University of Florida College of Medicine, Gainesville, Florida

ATUL HUMAR, MD, MSc, FRCPC
Department of Medicine, Transplant Infectious Diseases, University of Alberta, Edmonton, Alberta, Canada

MICHAEL G. ISON, MD, MS
Assistant Professor, Divisions of Infectious Diseases and Organ Transplantation, Northwestern University Feinberg School of Medicine, Chicago, Illinois

NICOLAS C. ISSA, MD
Instructor in Medicine, Division of Infectious Disease, Massachusetts General Hospital, Harvard Medical School, Boston, Massachusetts

DIMITRIOS P. KONTOYIANNIS, MD, ScD
Department of Infectious Diseases, Infection Control and Employee Health, The University of Texas MD Anderson Cancer Center, Houston, Texas

SOPHIA KOO, MD
Clinical and Research Fellow, Division of Infectious Diseases, Brigham and Women's Hospital; Division of Infectious Diseases, Dana-Farber Cancer Institute; Harvard Medical School, Boston, Massachusetts

PETRI KOSKINEN, MD, PhD
Department of Medicine, Division of Nephrology; Helsinki University Hospital, and University of Helsinki, Helsinki, Finland

DEEPALI KUMAR, MD, MSc, FRCPC
Department of Medicine, Transplant Infectious Diseases, University of Alberta, Edmonton, Alberta, Canada

IRMELI LAUTENSCHLAGER, MD, PhD
Transplant Unit Research Laboratory, Transplantation and Liver Surgery Clinic; Department of Virology, Helsinki University Hospital, and University of Helsinki, Helsinki, Finland

PER LJUNGMAN, MD, PhD
Department of Hematology, Karolinska University Hospital; Division of Hematology, Department of Medicine Huddinge, Karolinska Institutet, Stockholm, Sweden

FRANCISCO M. MARTY, MD
Assistant Professor of Medicine, Division of Infectious Diseases, Brigham and Women's Hospital; Division of Infectious Diseases, Dana-Farber Cancer Institute; Harvard Medical School, Boston, Massachusetts

MARIAN G. MICHAELS, MD, MPH
Professor, Department of Pediatrics and Surgery, Children's Hospital of Pittsburgh, Pittsburgh, Pennsylvania

MICHELE I. MORRIS, MD
Assistant Professor, Division of Infectious Diseases, University of Miami Miller School of Medicine, Miami, Florida

PATRICIA MUÑOZ, MD, PhD
Professor of Clinical Microbiology and Infectious Diseases, Department of Clinical Microbiology and Infectious Diseases, Hospital General Universitario Gregorio Marañón; Facultad de Medicina, Universidad Complutense de Madrid, Madrid, Spain

ANNA K. PERSON, MD
Division of Infectious Diseases, Department of Medicine, Duke University Health System, Duke University School of Medicine, Durham, North Carolina

DANIEL PUGA, MD
Infectious Diseases Fellow, Department of Clinical Microbiology and Infectious Diseases, Hospital General Universitario Gregorio Marañón, Madrid, Spain

KEVIN SHILEY, MD
Division of Infectious Diseases, Hospital of the University of Pennsylvania, Philadelphia, Pennsylvania

LYNNE STRASFELD, MD
Assistant Professor, Division of Infectious Diseases, Oregon Health and Science University, Portland, Oregon

MARICELA VALERIO, MD
Infectious Diseases Specialist, Department of Clinical Microbiology and Infectious Diseases, Hospital General Universitario Gregorio Marañón, Madrid, Spain

JOHN R. WINGARD, MD
Professor of Medicine, Bone Marrow Transplant Program, Division of Hematology/ Oncology, University of Florida College of Medicine, Gainesville, Florida

Contents

Preface xiii

Kieren A. Marr and Aruna K. Subramanian

Hematopoietic Stem Cell Transplantation: An Overview of Infection Risks and Epidemiology 257

John R. Wingard, Jack Hsu, and John W. Hiemenz

Hematopoietic stem cell transplantation (HSCT) is a treatment for multiple medical conditions that result in bone marrow failure and as an antineoplastic adoptive immunotherapy for hematologic malignancies. HSCT is associated with profound compromises in host barriers and all arms of innate and acquired immunity. The degree of immune compromise varies by type of transplant and over time. Immune reconstitution occurs within several months after autologous HSCT but takes up to a year or longer after allogeneic HSCT. In those patients who develop chronic graft-versus-host disease, immune reconstitution may take years or may never completely develop. Over time, with strengthening immune reconstitution and control of graft-versus-host disease, the risk for infection dissipates.

Infection in Organ Transplantation: Risk Factors and Evolving Patterns of Infection 273

Jay A. Fishman and Nicolas C. Issa

The nature of infections after solid-organ transplantation has changed with increasingly potent immunosuppressive regimens, routine use of antimicrobial prophylaxis, and improved microbiologic diagnostic tools. New pathogens have been identified in this population including many with significant antimicrobial resistance. Intensification of immunosuppressive regimens, including the use of T- and B-lymphocyte depleting agents, presents an increased risk for infection and requires linkage to microbiologic monitoring and prophylaxis against opportunistic infections. The effect of these regimens is reflected in the increased recognition of viral and fungal infections beyond 1 year after transplantation. Donor-derived infections represent a challenge to organ transplantation in terms of microbiologic screening of donors and the need for communication among clinical centers, organ procurement organizations, and public health authorities. New approaches to microbiologic assessment of organ donors and recipients are needed. In the future, improved assays for microbiologic and immunologic monitoring will allow individualization of prophylactic strategies to reduce the risk of infection in this highly susceptible population.

Infectious Complications Associated with Immunomodulating Biologic Agents 285

Sophia Koo, Francisco M. Marty, and Lindsey R. Baden

The armamentarium of biologic therapies targeting specific elements of the immune system is rapidly expanding. This review describes the spectrum of infectious complications associated to date with each of the immunomodulating biologic therapies approved by the US Food and Drug Administration.

Infections Transmitted by Transplantation **497**

Michele I. Morris, Staci A. Fischer, and Michael G. Ison

Infections are frequently transmitted through solid-organ and, to a lesser extent, stem cell transplantation. There are 2 major types of donor-derived infections that are transmitted: those that would be expected secondary to donor and recipient screening (ie, transmission of cytomegalovirus, Epstein-Barr virus, or toxoplasmosis from a seropositive donor to a seronegative recipient) and those that are unexpected despite routine donor screening (ie, human immunodeficiency virus and hepatitis C virus transmitted from a seronegative donor). Expected transmissions occur frequently and screening and prophylaxis strategies are applied to at-risk individuals in nearly all transplant centers globally. Several high profile donor-derived infectious disease transmissions have been recognized; these reports have raised awareness of this rare complication of transplantation. Issues related to the epidemiology of, screening for, and management of proven or probable donor-derived infections are reviewed in this article.

Immunotherapy and Vaccination After Transplant: The Present, the Future **515**

Vincent C. Emery, Hermann Einsele, Sowsan Atabani, and Tanzina Haque

Vaccination and adoptive immunotherapy for herpes virus infections has become an attractive option for the control of a virus family that negatively affects transplantation. In the future, enhanced ability to select antigen-specific T cells without significant in vitro manipulation should provide new opportunities for refining and enhancing adoptive immunotherapeutic approaches. This article focuses on advances in the area of vaccinology for some of these infections and in the use of adoptive immunotherapy. At present, many of these approaches in transplant recipients have focused on infections such as human cytomegalovirus, but the opportunity to use these examples as proof of concept for other infections is discussed.

Index **531**

FORTHCOMING ISSUES

September 2010

Emerging Respiratory Infections in the 21st Century
Alimuddin Zumla, FRCP, PhD(Lond), FRCPath, Wing-Wai Yew, MBBS, FRCP (Edinb), FCCP, and David SC Hui, MD(UNSW), FRACP, FRCP, *Guest Editors*

December 2010

Diseases of the Gastrointestinal Tract and Associated Infections
Guy D. Eslick, PhD, *Guest Editor*

March 2011

Infection Prevention and Control in the Hospital
Keith S. Kaye, MD, MPH, *Guest Editor*

RECENT ISSUES

March 2010

The Atypical Pneumonias
Burke A. Cunha, MD, MACP, *Guest Editor*

December 2009

Antibacterial Therapy and Newer Agents
Keith S. Kaye, MD, MPH, and
Donald Kaye, MD,*Guest Editors*

September 2009

Infections in the Intensive Care Unit
Marin H. Kollef, MD, and
Scott T. Micek, PharmD,*Guest Editors*

ISSUES OF RELATED INTEREST

Critical Care Clinics April 2010 (Vol. 26, No. 2)
Optimizing Hemodynamic Support in Septic Shock
Dane Nichols, MD, *Guest Editor*
Available at: http://www.criticalcare.theclinics.com/

Clinics in Laboratory Medicine December 2009 (Vol. 29, No. 4)
Respiratory Viruses in Pediatric and Adult Populations
Alexander J. McAdam, MD, PhD, *Guest Editor*
Available at: http://www.labmed.theclinics.com/

VISIT THE CLINICS ONLINE!

Access your subscription at:
www.theclinics.com

Preface

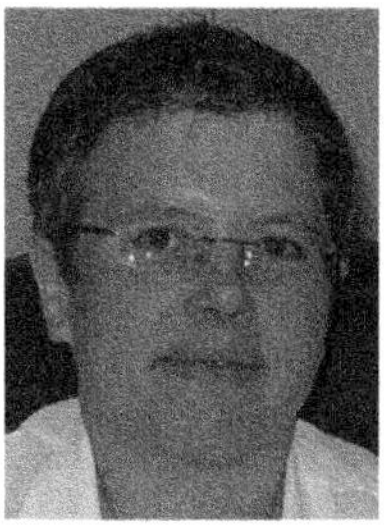 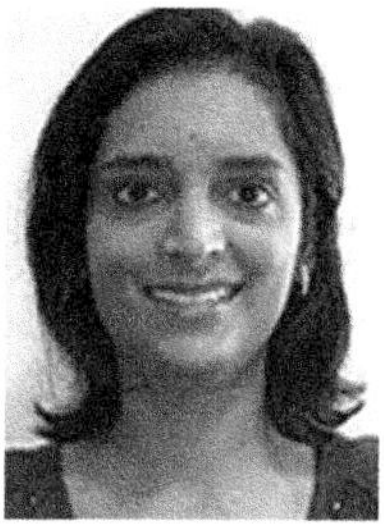

Kieren A. Marr, MD   Aruna K. Subramanian, MD
Guest Editors

The 50-year anniversaries of solid organ transplantation (SOT) and hematopoietic stem cell transplantation (HSCT) have recently been celebrated. Transplantation represents one of the true modern advances in medicine, presenting new and effective treatments for organ and bone marrow failure and neoplastic disorders. For discoveries of transplantation, the two pioneers—Dr Joseph Murray and Dr E. Donnall Thomas—won the Nobel Prize in Medicine in 1990. In the 2 decades since then, treatment of oncologic disorders has evolved, with therapies ranging from cytotoxic drugs to more targeted therapies; the importance of new contributions was underscored in October 2009, with modern pioneers (Brian Druker, Nicholas Lydon, and Charles Sawyers) winning the Lasker Awards for discovery of novel targeted therapies for chronic myeloid leukemia. The approach to treating organ failure and oncologic disorders has evolved rapidly and continues to change.

Changes in transplantation and oncology have driven changes in immunity in the general population and the hospitalized population, leading ultimately to changes in infectious diseases (IDs). Not only have groups of organisms, such as herpesviruses and opportunistic fungi, gained prominence largely as a result of transplant-related immunosuppression but also transplant and oncology patients now serve as the sentinel for recognition of new pathogens, such as arenaviruses. These changes have led to the development of a new field within infectious diseases, focused specifically on the care of transplant and oncology patients. This field is distinguished within the subspecialty not only by the broad differential of infectious and noninfectious syndromes specific to these populations but also by an increased attention to preventive practices in guiding the approach to anti-infective therapies. Transplant and oncology, similar to HIV medicine, require a detailed understanding of the host, with a multidisciplinary background; thus, specialized programs within ID divisions, societies, and new journals have resulted, fostering a focused academic and clinical development.

This volume of *Infectious Disease Clinics of North America* is focused on this specialized population. Its mission is to provide a comprehensive, updated review

Infect Dis Clin N Am 24 (2010) xiii–xv
doi:10.1016/j.idc.2010.02.004

0891-5520/10/$ – see front matter © 2010 Elsevier Inc. All rights reserved.

of important areas in this dynamically evolving field. The volume starts with reviews of the host and basic transplant practices, covered by Wingard and colleagues (HSCT) and by Fishman and Issa (SOT). Knowledge of the hosts and immunologic risks is requisite in the approach to transplant IDs, and these 2 articles cover these broad topics expertly. Immunologic agents and infectious complications associated with these increasingly used biologic therapies are covered in the article by Koo and coworkers, who not only cover the appreciated (reported) infectious risks to date but also provide an exhaustive listing of the current repertoire of monoclonal antibodies and other biologics. Children represent a special population when considering transplant ID, as their underlying diseases and infectious exposures are different than in adults, dictating variance in epidemiology and outcomes. This subject is discussed in depth in the article by Michaels and Green.

The issue transitions from host-directed articles to those that are focused on some of the most important infectious pathogens, syndromes, and problems. As many of the current complications are caused by the several herpesviruses, various aspects of these infections—and those caused by other viruses—are discussed. Ljungman and colleagues review the prominent issues surrounding cytomegalovirus (CMV) in HSCT recipients, and Helanterä and coworkers provide a comprehensive discussion of the impact of different viruses on graft function, focused in particular on kidney grafts, where a great amount of data has been generated. Shiley and Blumberg provide an up-to-date and comprehensive discussion of the direct and indirect effects of other herpesviruses, herpes simplex virus (HSV), varicella-zoster virus (VZV), Epstein-Barr virus, and human herpesvirus, on SOT and HSCT recipients. Finally, the major issues that have developed with antiviral drug resistance—specifically with CMV, HSV, VZV, and hepatitis B—are eloquently discussed by Strasfeld and Chou.

Respiratory viruses and fungi cause a large amount of current morbidity and mortality. These issues are discussed as overviews by Kumar and Humar (respiratory viruses) and Person and colleagues (fungal infections). Parasites and protozoa present unique issues in transplant and oncology patients and, although infection is less common, establishing diagnosis and using appropriate screening tests is imperative; this subject is exhaustively reviewed in the article by Munoz and coworkers.

Finally, this issue ends with a discussion of the up-to-date issues appreciated with infections transmitted by grafts, provided by Morris and colleagues, and an intriguing contemporary and futuristic review of immunotherapy and vaccination by Emery and coworkers. The discussion by Emery and colleagues presents significant advances that have been made in preventing infections by vaccination and sets the stage for issues of prominence in the future, namely, use of immunotherapies, which are being developed in many sophisticated laboratories worldwide.

The authors of this issue are exceptional clinicians and investigators, true experts in this field. We thank them for their contributions. We also thank the editors, especially Barbara Cohen-Kligerman and Dr Bob Moellering, for the invitation to compile an issue on transplant and oncology ID. We would like to dedicate this issue to the memory of Dr Pamela Tucker, a mentor and teacher in transplant and oncology ID at Johns Hopkins. Her determination, energy, and commitment to excellence enriched our institution and the field.

We hope that this issue is informative and triggers new questions and avenues of investigation.

Kieren A. Marr, MD
Division of Infectious Diseases
Johns Hopkins University School of Medicine
720 Rutland Avenue Ross 1064
Baltimore, MD 21212, USA

Aruna K. Subramanian, MD
Division of Infectious Diseases
Johns Hopkins University School of Medicine
1830 East Monument Street Room 450D
Baltimore, MD 21287, USA

E-mail addresses:
kmarr4@jhmi.edu (K.A. Marr)
asubra@jhmi.edu (A.K. Subramanian)

Hematopoietic Stem Cell Transplantation: An Overview of Infection Risks and Epidemiology

John R. Wingard, MD*, Jack Hsu, MD, John W. Hiemenz, MD

KEYWORDS

- Hematopoietic stem cell transplantation
- Opportunistic infections • GVHD

Hematopoietic stem cell transplantation (HSCT) (also known as "bone marrow transplantation") is associated with a variety of infectious complications that pose serious threats to transplant recipients. The risk of infectious complications, type of pathogens, and timing of infectious threats varies substantially according to type of HSCT and the manner in which it is performed. In recent years there have been a number of changes in transplant practices that have altered the epidemiology of infectious complications.

HSCT is used to treat two categories of medical conditions. The first category consists of nonmalignant diseases that result in failure of bone marrow function or bone marrow–derived cells including aplastic anemia; myelodysplastic syndromes; immunodeficiency syndromes, such as severe combined immunodeficiency or chronic granulomatous disease; genetic diseases, such as the mucopolysaccharidoses or glycogen storage diseases; or the hemoglobinopathies of thalassemia and sickle cell anemia. The second category is far more prevalent and consists of neoplastic diseases, particularly hematopoietic malignancies, such as acute or chronic leukemia, lymphomas, multiple myeloma, and myeloproliferative diseases. In the first category of diseases, the transplant serves to replace a defective tissue, much in the same way kidney transplantation is performed for kidney failure. In the second category of diseases, the transplant serves two functions. The first function is to facilitate the safe use of cytotoxic therapies (intensive chemotherapy with or without total body irradiation) by reversing the myelosuppressive or myeloablative

Bone Marrow Transplant Program, Division of Hematology/Oncology, University of Florida College of Medicine, PO Box 100278, 1600 SW Archer Road, Gainesville, FL 32610-0278, USA
* Corresponding author.
E-mail address: wingajr@ufl.edu

Infect Dis Clin N Am 24 (2010) 257–272
doi:10.1016/j.idc.2010.01.010
id.theclinics.com
0891-5520/10/$ – see front matter © 2010 Elsevier Inc. All rights reserved.

effects of the cytotoxic therapy; the second function is to provide immune cells to directly attack neoplastic cells that express tumor-specific or tumor-associated antigens.

There are two major types of HSCT: autologous and allogeneic. Autologous refers to the patient serving as his or her own donor. Allogeneic refers to someone else serving as the donor. The hematopoietic stem cells are collected from the autologous patient before the transplant procedure and cryopreserved. The allogeneic hematopoietic stem cells are collected from the donor (a family member, a volunteer donor, or banked cord blood cells) either before or synchronously with the transplant procedure and are infused into the recipient after receiving a pretransplant conditioning regimen. For allogeneic transplantation, stringent HLA matching between donor and recipient is required to minimize the risk for graft rejection; reduce the risk for graft-versus-host disease (GVHD), which can be viewed as the donor immunity attempting to "reject" the recipient; and to facilitate the development of robust donor protective immunity. When cord blood is used as the source of hematopoietic stem cells, less stringent HLA matching is required because of the naive state of the newborn's immunity, in which case greater donor and recipient HLA disparity is tolerated. Rarely, individuals may have an identical twin, allowing for "syngeneic" HSCT. Although this may be the most optimal source of stem cells for many patients with nonmalignant marrow disorders, the lack of an allogeneic graft versus tumor effect makes this less desirable for patients with malignant disorders, particularly the leukemias and some lymphoproliferative disorders. Autologous transplantation is most commonly used in the treatment of malignant diseases to facilitate intensive antineoplastic cytotoxic therapy.

The hematopoietic stem cell graft may be obtained either from harvesting of bone marrow or by apheresis of the peripheral blood. Bone marrow is the traditional source of stem cells used in HSCT, and is collected by needle aspirations of 1 to 1.5 L of bone marrow obtained from the posterior iliac crests. Ordinarily, hematopoietic stem cells rarely traffic in the circulation, but after chemotherapy, or after administration of granulocyte colony–stimulating factor or plerixafor, large numbers of stem cells are "mobilized" from the bone marrow into the circulation and can be collected from peripheral or central veins by apheresis. Peripheral blood grafts contain more lymphocytes and a greater risk for GVHD when this donor source is used. Bone marrow and peripheral blood grafts consist of a mixture of immature hematopoietic cells, mature hematopoietic cells, and immune cells. Hematopoietic potency of the graft is generally measured by enumeration of the cells expressing the CD34 antigen, an antigen expressed on the cell surface of primitive hematopoietic progenitors. The larger the CD34 count, the faster the neutrophil recovery. Immune potency is measured by enumeration of the lymphocytes (the CD3 count). The larger numbers of $CD3^+$ cells, natural killer cells, and dendritic cells, the more rapid is posttransplant immune reconstitution and greater adoptive immunotherapeutic potency. In some cases the graft may be manipulated ex vivo before administration to the recipient. The most common manipulation of allogeneic grafts is T-cell depletion, which is done to reduce the risk of GVHD. An unintended consequence of T-cell depletion is a greater risk of graft rejection, a higher risk for relapse of the cancer being treated, and slower T-cell reconstitution after transplant.

A conditioning regimen is given before intravenous infusion of the hematopoietic stem cell graft. For patients with cancer, the conditioning regimen consists of intensive chemotherapy with or without total body irradiation, with agents chosen to destroy as much residual cancer as possible. For patients undergoing allogeneic HSCT, suppression of the recipient immunity is also a goal of the conditioning regimen. Agents are chosen to optimize therapeutic goals and minimize toxicities. For autologous transplants, the regimens consist of drugs found to be active against the type of cancer being treated, whose toxicities spare as much as possible nonhematopoietic tissues, and where an antitumor dose-response association is demonstrable. There is a wide array of effective regimens used that vary from cancer to cancer and center to center. For allogeneic HSCT, similar antitumor considerations are also important, but even more important is the immunosuppressive properties of the agents selected. The most widely used agents in allogeneic HSCT are cyclophosphamide, total body irradiation, and antithymocyte globulin. In recent years purine analogs with potent immunosuppressive properties, such as fludarabine, pentostatin, and cladrabine, are increasingly used because they have been found to have less severe nonhematopoietic tissue toxicity. Many elderly individuals and patients with comorbid conditions unrelated to cancer are unable to tolerate intensive conditioning regimens because of high transplant-related morbidity and mortality. With the increasing recognition that much of the anticancer potency of allogeneic HSCT resides in the adoptive immunotherapeutic effects of the graft and the advent of less toxic immunosuppressive agents, a growing body of experience with reduced-intensity (nonablative) conditioning regimens has developed. Increasingly, reduced-intensity regimens are being used in allogeneic HSCT. To facilitate the development of robust anticancer effects, many such nonablative regimens are coupled with acceleration of the tapering of the posttransplant immunosuppressive regimen. Nonablative regimens are associated with shorter times of neutropenia and less injury to the mucosa because the regimens have less cytotoxicity to nonlymphohematopoietic tissues. This has allowed many such transplants to be performed in an outpatient setting with a less intense need for multiple transfusions of blood products, antibiotic support, parenteral analgesics, and fluid and electrolyte supplementation.

After transplantation, a variety of supportive care measures are provided. A tunneled central venous catheter is usually placed for administration of the chemotherapy, stem cell infusion, intravenous medications, electrolyte supplements, nutritional support, and blood products. An immunosuppressive regimen consisting most commonly of a calcineurin inhibitor (cyclosporine or tacrolimus) plus a short course of intravenous methotrexate is given after transplantation both to prevent graft rejection and to prevent GVHD. Other immunosuppressive regimens are sometimes used. After transplantation the immunosuppressive regimen is usually tapered over 4 to 6 months and eventually discontinued, unless GVHD develops and a more prolonged course of immunosuppressive therapy is required. Because no immunosuppressive therapy is given after autologous transplant, immune reconstitution occurs much faster, with humoral and T-cell responses recovering in 3 to 9 months. In contrast, immune reconstitution after allogeneic HSCT is much slower and may take a year or longer. Immune reconstitution may be even slower if GVHD occurs. Even in the absence of GVHD, immune reconstitution is slower if a cord blood, T-cell depleted graft, or graft from a mismatched donor is used as the source of hematopoietic stem cells.

THE DYNAMIC NATURE OF DAMAGE TO HOST DEFENSES AND RESTORATION OF HOST DEFENSES AND IMMUNITY AFTER HSCT

The risk for infection and the spectrum of infectious syndromes differs by type of transplant, type of conditioning regimen, type of stem cell graft, and type of posttransplant therapies and whether or not certain posttransplant complications occur, such as GVHD. **Table 1** illustrates some of these considerations. The risk of infection can be divided into three time intervals. The time periods and infectious risks are illustrated in **Table 2**.

Table 1
Effect of transplant characteristics on infectious risk

Transplant Parameter	Effect on Host Barriers and Immunity	Infectious Consequences
Type of transplant	Allogeneic: slower B- and T-cell immune reconstitution	Greater risk for infections of all types, but especially invasive fungal and herpesvirus infections; longer interval of risk
Type of allogeneic donor	Unrelated or mismatched donor: slower B- and T-cell immune reconstitution	Greater risk for infections of all types, but especially invasive fungal and herpesvirus infections; longer interval of risk
Type of stem cell graft	Peripheral blood: faster neutrophil engraftment, more chronic GVHD Cord blood: slower neutrophil engraftment, less GVHD, slower B- and T-cell immune reconstitution	Different risks for infections associated with neutropenia and GVHD
Stem cell graft manipulation	T-cell depletion: greater risk for graft rejection, slower B- and T-cell immune reconstitution	Greater risk for neutropenic infections, lower risk for infections associated with chronic GVHD, greater and longer risk for herpesvirus and invasive fungal infections
Conditioning regimen	Intensive regimens: more mucosal injury, shorter time to neutropenia and longer neutropenia	Greater risk for neutropenic infections, especially typhlitis
Immunosuppressive regimen (allogeneic)	ATG: more profound deficiency of T-cell immunity Methotrexate: more mucosal injury, longer time to neutrophil recovery	Greater risk for invasive fungal and herpesvirus infections
Central venous catheter	Breach in skin barrier	Greater risk for bacterial and (less frequently) fungal infections

Abbreviations: ATG, antithymocyte globulin; GVHD, graft-versus-host disease.

Early, before engraftment, the major compromises in host defenses are neutropenia and mucosal injury. The duration of neutropenia is 10 to 14 days after autologous HSCT, 15 to 30 days after allogeneic HSCT using an ablative conditioning regimen, and only 5 to 7 days using a nonablative conditioning regimen. The infectious threats are principally the same bacterial and (less commonly) fungal pathogens (eg, *Candida* species and molds) as seen in neutropenic cancer patients who are not transplant recipients. The evaluation and management strategies of these infectious complications are similar to the ones that have been developed for chemotherapy-induced

Table 2
Types of infections encountered at various times after HSCT

Type of Infectious Pathogen	Early Preengraftment (First 2–4 wk)	Early Postengraftment (Second and Third Month)	Late Postengraftment (After Second or Third Month)	Time Independent
Bacteria	Gram-negative bacteria (related to mucosal injury and neutropenia) Gram-positive bacteria (related to venous catheters) *Clostridium difficile* (related to neutropenia, antibiotics, antiacid medications)	Gram-positive bacteria (related to venous catheters) Gram-negative bacteria (related to enteric involvement of GVHD, venous catheters)	Encapsulated bacteria (related to poor opsonization with chronic GVHD) *Nocardia* (related to chronic GVHD)	
Fungi	*Candida* (related to mucosal injury and neutropenia)	*Aspergillus*, other molds and *Pneumocystis jirovecii* (related to GVHD)	*Aspergillus*, other molds and *P jirovecii* (related to GVHD)	
Herpesviruses	HSV	CMV (related to GVHD and impaired cellular immunity) EBV (in patients who have T-cell depleted grafts, receive ATG, or whose donor is mismatched)	CMV and VZV (related to GVHD and impaired cellular immunity and viral latency before transplant) EBV (in patients who have T-cell depleted grafts, receive ATG, or whose donor is mismatched)	
Other viruses		BK virus (related to GVHD and cyclophosphamide in conditioning regimen)		Respiratory viruses (temporally tracks with community outbreaks) Adenoviruses

Abbreviations: ATG, antithymocyte globulin; CMV, cytomegalovirus; EBV, Epstein-Barr virus; GVHD, graft-versus-host disease; HSV, herpes simplex virus; VZV, varicella-zoster virus.

neutropenic fever. Herpes simplex virus (HSV) reactivates in most HSV-seropositive patients during this time period between 1 and 2 weeks after transplantation. Engraftment demarcates the transition to the second time interval.

The early postengraftment period is categorized by progressive recovery in cell-mediated immunity. This occurs much more rapidly after autologous than allogeneic transplant. The infectious threat then recedes dramatically. After autologous HSCT, many early posttransplant infections are associated with the presence of the central venous catheter. Although the venous catheter is generally removed as early as possible, this may be technically challenging in this group of patients and the catheter may need to remain in place if the patient continues to require transfusion support, supplemental medications, nutrition, intravenous fluid, or electrolyte supplements. Gram-positive bacteria are frequent causes of central venous catheter–associated infections, with gram-negative and mixed bacterial infections less common but occasionally seen. After allogeneic HSCT, there is a similar risk for catheter-associated infections, but GVHD also poses an additional risk for bacterial infections. Bacteremias from enteric organisms are especially problematic in patients with GVHD of the intestinal tract. Infections caused by *Candida* species occasionally occur in patients with GVHD, and are often associated with indwelling venous catheters especially in the presence of intravenous administration of nutritional supplementation. *Aspergillus* species and other mold infections and *Pneumocystis jirovecii* pneumonia (PCP) occur in patients with GVHD and in those on high doses of steroids for GVHD treatment. Cytomegalovirus (CMV) viremia occurs chiefly in patients who were seropositive before transplantation and who develop GVHD. Untreated, CMV viremia often is followed by pneumonia or enterocolitis after allogeneic HSCT, which can be associated with substantial morbidity and mortality.

Beyond 3 months, the risk for opportunistic infection in autologous HSCT patients is small. After allogeneic HSCT, there is gradual reconstitution of humoral and cellular immunity, which approaches normality by 1 year if GVHD does not occur. Immunization of the recipient with the childhood vaccines is recommended at that time.[1,2] The development of chronic GVHD leads to delays in immune reconstitution and necessitates prolonged courses of immunosuppressive therapy that compounds the immunodeficiency caused by the GVHD. Late infections in patients are caused by similar pathogens as those in the early posttransplant period (*Candida* species, *Aspergillus* species and other molds, PCP, and CMV) but also include encapsulated bacteria because of poor opsonization and varicella zoster virus (VZV) infections.

COMMON INFECTIOUS SYNDROMES AFTER HSCT AND THEIR ETIOLOGIES

Neutropenic Fever

Fever occurring in the neutropenic transplant recipient is frequent during the pre-engraftment period. Neutropenic fever is less frequent in patients receiving reduced-intensity conditioning regimens. Fever typically occurs 3 to 5 days after the onset of neutropenia and may be the sole manifestation of infection. Bacterial infections are by far the most common infectious causes of the first fever during neutropenia, but in most cases no microbiologic etiology is documented with the prompt initiation of broad-spectrum empiric antibiotic therapy. Likely sites of infection are lungs; skin (especially catheter insertion sites and the perianal area); and genitourinary tract. In addition, the oral cavity and intestinal tract are also possible sites of infection. Gram-positive bacteria are the most frequently isolated bacterial pathogens, with *Staphylococcus epidermidis* making up approximately half, viridians streptococci making up approximately one third, and *Staphylococcus aureus* and several other species making up the remainder of episodes. Gram-negative bacteria make up about 30% to 45% of bacterial infections and include *Enterobacter* spp, *Escherichia coli*, *Klebsiella* spp, *Pseudomonas aeruginosa*, and *Stenotrophomonas maltophilia*. Cultures of blood and from suspected sites of infection should be obtained and empiric antibiotics instituted promptly.

Persistent fever is more problematic. Possible explanations included a delayed response to the initial antibiotic regimen, presence of a gram-positive organism not adequately treated with the initial antibiotic regimen, or antibiotic-resistant gram-negative bacteria. In addition, other types of pathogens are also possible explanations, especially invasive fungal infections by *Candida* spp, *Aspergillus* spp, or other molds. A detailed discussion of the evaluation and approaches to management of neutropenic fever is beyond the scope of this article but is discussed in detail in several authoritative guidelines.[3,4]

Nonneutropenic Fever

Most fevers in the neutropenic transplant recipient resolve at the time of neutrophil recovery. Fever may sometimes occur, however, at the time of engraftment. Although an infectious etiology is possible and should be vigorously pursued, fever often is caused by what has been referred to as the "engraftment syndrome," a noninfectious syndrome of uncertain etiology that consists of fever alone or with rash, pneumonitis, hyperbilirubinemia, or diarrhea. Cultures should be obtained and CT scans of the chest and abdomen should be performed as part of the investigation to assess for a possible infectious focus. If the investigation does not reveal an infectious source, a short course of high-dose corticosteroids may be considered and is often very effective.

Later after engraftment, fever sometimes occurs in the absence of other symptoms. CMV infection, occult sinusitis, central venous catheter–associated infection, or occult fungal infection are frequent causes. Evaluation should include elicitation of infectious symptoms and physical signs; blood cultures for bacteria, fungi, and mycobacteria; urine analysis; and blood samples for CMV polymerase chain reaction (PCR) or antigen. Imaging studies with CT scans of the chest, sinuses, and abdomen should also be considered. Medications can cause fever, so discontinuation of discretionary medications is advisable. If fever persists and no etiology can be discerned, one should consider removal of the venous catheter.

Pneumonia and Pulmonary Infiltrates

Pneumonia is a common complication after HSCT.[5] There are both infectious and noninfectious causes of pneumonia and pulmonary infiltrates in the HSCT recipient, and the likely etiologies vary over time (**Table 3**).

The types of pneumonias can be categorized according to their radiologic appearance into diffuse and localized infiltrates. High-resolution CT scans are the most sensitive radiologic procedure[6,7] because standard radiographs are less sensitive. Diffuse infiltrates can be alveolar, interstitial, mixed alveolar interstitial, or diffuse micronodular. Localized infiltrates may present as lobar consolidation; macronodules (>1 cm); cavities; or wedge-shaped infiltrates.

Before engraftment, most episodes of pneumonia and pulmonary infiltrates are not related to infection. Volume overload may occur during this time period. Congestive heart failure from cardiotoxic drugs or the acute respiratory distress syndrome caused by pulmonary toxicity from the pretransplant conditioning regimen, other antecedent therapy, or prior medical conditions are frequent. Hemorrhagic alveolitis may also occur because of toxicity from the conditioning regimen or inflammatory cytokines

Table 3
Infectious and noninfectious causes of pneumonia after HSCT

Type of Pulmonary Infiltrate		Preengraftment	Early Postengraftment	Late
Diffuse	Noninfectious	Adult respiratory distress syndrome	Idiopathic interstitial pneumonitis	Bronchiolitis obliterans or bronchiolitis obliterans with organizing pneumonia
		Congestive heart failure Fluid overload Hemorrhagic alveolitis	Hemorrhagic alveolitis	
	Infectious	Respiratory virus	CMV Respiratory virus PCP Adenovirus	CMV Respiratory virus PCP Adenovirus
Localized	Noninfectious	Aspiration Pulmonary thromboembolism Micronodules caused by chemotherapy		
	Infectious	Bacterial pneumonia *Aspergillus* or other mold pneumonia	Bacterial pneumonia *Aspergillus* or other mold pneumonia *Nocardia*	Bacterial pneumonia *Aspergillus* or other mold pneumonia *Nocardia*

Abbreviations: CMV, cytomegalovirus; PCP, *Pneumocystis jirovecii* pneumonia.

released as a consequence of the transplant procedure. These noninfectious pulmonary syndromes typically produce diffuse infiltrates. Aspiration pneumonia or bacterial or mold pneumonia also occur but are less frequent and typically produce localized infiltrates. Mold pneumonias are characterized by macronodules, some with halo signs, which later become cavitary. *Aspergillus* spp are by far the most common mold pathogens, with Zygomycetes accounting for 10% to 20% of mold pneumonias, and *Scedosporium* spp, *Fusarium* spp, and other genera accounting for a small percent of mold pneumonias.

Early after engraftment, diffuse pneumonias are evenly divided between infectious and noninfectious causes. Idiopathic pneumonia accounts for half of diffuse pneumonias.[8] The risk for idiopathic pneumonia is associated with higher-intensity conditioning regimens. CMV accounts for approximately 40% of diffuse pneumonias and is most commonly seen in patients with acute GVHD.[9] PCP (if the patient is not taking PCP prophylaxis), legionella, adenovirus, or various respiratory viruses are other possible causes of diffuse pneumonia. Increasingly, respiratory virus infections are being recognized as important causes of diffuse pneumonias.[10–17] Bacterial or mold pneumonias are the most common causes of localized pulmonary infiltrates. The most important risk factor for pulmonary aspergillosis and other mold pneumonias is GVHD.[18,19] Pulmonary aspergillosis most frequently presents as macronodules on CT imaging of the chest. In a large series, 94% of patients had at least one nodule and 79% had multiple nodules.[20] Halo signs, which occur early in infection, were present in 61% of patients with pulmonary aspergillosis. In another single-center series, pulmonary infection with Zygomycetes was observed to have more nodules on CT imaging than commonly occurs in pulmonary aspergillosis.[21]

During the late postengraftment period, there is a more heterogeneous spectrum of infectious causes of pneumonia.[22] Patients with chronic GVHD are particularly susceptible to sinopulmonary infections caused by encapsulated bacteria and increasingly susceptible to mold pneumonias.[23,24] *Nocardia* is an occasional pathogen that can cause pneumonia with similar clinical and radiographic features as infection with *Aspergillus* spp.[25] Bronchiolitis obliterans with organizing pneumonia (cryptogenic organizing pneumonia) is a manifestation of chronic GVHD. PCP may also occur (if the patient is not taking PCP prophylaxis). In the past, CMV pneumonia rarely occurred late, but increasingly, late CMV pneumonia is becoming more common.[26] GVHD and early CMV viremia are risk factors for late CMV pneumonia.

In some cases pneumonias may be caused by multiple pathogens. For example, CMV may be accompanied by superinfection with bacterial pathogens or *Aspergillus* spp. Infection with *Aspergillus* species may similarly be accompanied by bacterial, CMV, or Zygomycetes coinfections. Accordingly, assessment should be thorough and one should not ignore cultures or other tests indicating more than one pathogen.

Although radiology is essential in the assessment of pneumonia, some clinical features suggest certain etiologies. Hemoptysis is suggestive of hemorrhagic alveolitis or thromboembolism. Hemoptysis with pleuritic pain or pleural friction rub is suggestive of infection with *Aspergillus* spp or another mold. Cough is usually nonproductive of sputum with CMV, respiratory virus, PCP, and most noninfectious pneumonias. Although useful, these findings are not sufficiently specific to be diagnostic.

Assessment of diffuse infiltrates should include nasal and throat swabs for viral diagnostic assays with culture or direct fluorescence assay, enzyme-linked immunosorbent assay, or PCR assays for the respiratory viruses. After engraftment, blood should be collected for CMV PCR or antigen assay. Bronchoscopy with bronchoalveolar lavage (BAL) can be quite useful in further assessment.[27,28] The sensitivity and specificity of testing of BAL fluid for infectious etiologies causing diffuse infiltrates (eg, PCP, CMV, or respiratory viruses) are quite good.

Assessment of localized infiltrates should include blood cultures for bacteria and fungi. Sputum, if available, should be cultured. When infection with *Aspergillus* species is suspected, serum for galactomannan[29–31] can be helpful. One should consider bronchoscopic evaluation with cultures and stains in this setting, although the yield in the investigation of nodular infiltrates is lower. Bronchoscopy with BAL can still be useful because it may detect or exclude certain coinfecting pathogens and allow a more focused antimicrobial therapy. For peripheral nodules or infiltrates, CT-guided needle, video-assisted thoracoscopy guided, or even open lung biopsies may be useful if the patient is not significantly thrombocytopenic.

While evaluation of pneumonia proceeds, one should presumptively initiate therapy for the most likely etiologies because delay in initiating therapy may compromise the prospects for a successful outcome. Presumptive therapy should not be used in lieu of a proper assessment, because the spectrum of possible pathogens is large and toxicities of multiple therapies can lead to harm. Once the etiology is established it is important to discontinue the unneeded therapies. If the etiology has not been definitively established, evaluation should be continued.

Diarrhea

Diarrhea may have multiple etiologies (**Table 4**). Shortly after the conditioning regimen, cytotoxic mucosal injury may result in noninfectious diarrhea. During the pre-engraftment period, typhlitis and *Clostridium difficile* enterocolitis are potentially serious complications. Both infections are typically accompanied by fever, abdominal discomfort, and distention. Guarding and ileus may also be present. CT scan shows bowel wall thickening and may also demonstrate bowel distention. With typhlitis, the ascending colon is often involved but other portions of the large and small intestine may also be involved.[32–34] The microbiologic etiology of typhlitis is rarely determined, but is presumed to be caused mostly by gram-negative and anaerobic bacteria. Invasion of the compromised bowel wall by *Candida* species has been noted.[35,36] Toxic megacolon, perforation, and septic shock may result from severe typhlitis and can result in death.

Enteritis caused by *C difficile* is one of the most common nosocomial infections. Strains that produce highly potent toxins have been noted to cause outbreaks and such infections may result in perforation, shock, and death.[37–41] The use of fluoroquinolones and the use of gastric acid suppressants are risk factors for overgrowth in the bowel and infection with *C difficile*.

Table 4
Infectious and noninfectious causes of diarrhea after HSCT

Preengraftment	Early Postengraftment	Late
Mucosal injury from conditioning regimen	GVHD	GVHD
Neutropenic enterocolitis (typhlitis)	*C difficile* enterocolitis	*C difficile* enterocolitis
Clostridium difficile enterocolitis	CMV	CMV
Enteric viruses	Adenovirus	Adenovirus
	Enteric viruses	Enteric viruses

Abbreviations: CMV, cytomegalovirus; GVHD, graft-versus-host disease.

Enteric viruses, including enteroviruses, caliciviruses, and astroviruses, are potential causes of diarrhea[42–45] in the patient undergoing HSCT. Generally, HSCT patients become vulnerable to such pathogens as viral outbreaks occur in the community. Adenoviruses and CMV also can cause diarrhea.[46–48] Infrequently, enteropathic bacteria, such as *Shigella* spp and *Salmonella* spp, protozoa, and helminthic infections can cause enterocolitis.

After engraftment, GVHD is a major noninfectious cause of diarrhea in addition to the previously noted infectious causes. GVHD of the gastrointestinal tract is most commonly associated with the presence of cutaneous GVHD, but occasionally it may occur in the absence of other manifestations of GVHD. GVHD of the gut typically occurs in the early postengraftment period as part of acute GVHD (rather than chronic GVHD). With changing transplant practices, however, which have included the increasing use of peripheral blood as a source of stem cells, donor lymphocyte infusions, and reduced intensity transplant regimens, the spectrum of clinical manifestations of acute and chronic GVHD are blending over time.

Evaluation should include stool samples for assays for *C difficile* antigen or toxin, viral cultures or enzyme-linked immunosorbent assays, CMV antigen or PCR testing, and examination of stool for presence of ova and parasites. For more severe episodes of diarrhea, abdominal CT provides assessment of bowel wall thickening or the development of intra-abdominal abscesses. In patients with typhlitis or severe *C difficile* enterocolitis, serial kidneys-ureter-bladder radiographs can be useful to monitor for evidence of toxic megacolon. For cases where the etiology remains uncertain, colonoscopy should be considered for visual inspection to determine if there are pseudomembranes and to obtain biopsy for histologic examination to assess for GVHD and presence of CMV or other infections by immunostaining, culture, or PCR.

CMV

Decades ago, CMV pneumonia was the predominant infectious life-threatening complication after HSCT. Although pneumonia is the most common CMV syndrome, esophagitis, gastritis, or enterocolitis are other infections that may be caused by CMV. Unlike the patient with severe immunodeficiency caused by infection with HIV, CMV chorioretinitis rarely occurs in patients undergoing HSCT. Although CMV infection occurs after both autologous and allogeneic HSCT, CMV disease is uncommon after autologous HSCT. In allogeneic HSCT patients, seropositivity and GVHD are the major risk factors for CMV reactivation and disease.[49,50] CMV viremia generally precedes pneumonia by 1 to 2 weeks. Because of the adoption of close monitoring for reactivation of CMV and antiviral management strategies routinely used after allogeneic HSCT, CMV disease has receded as a serious threat early after HSCT. In the past, CMV disease most commonly occurred during the early postengraftment period. Recently, however, late-onset CMV disease has been increasing in occurrence.[26] Risk factors for late CMV disease include early viremia posttransplantation and the development of GVHD.

Clinical presentation of CMV pneumonia is low-grade fever, nonproductive cough, and dyspnea. Progressive hypoxia ensues over several days. Examination of the chest may be unrevealing or demonstrate scattered rales. Chest radiographic examination demonstrates alveolar, interstitial, or mixed alveolar-interstitial diffuse infiltrates. Bronchoscopy with BAL specimens for immunostaining or PCR assays is diagnostic with sensitivity and specificity of 90% or higher. Bronchoscopy may also reveal coinfection by bacteria, PCP, or *Aspergillus* spp. For gastrointestinal CMV syndromes, endoscopic examination of the gastrointestinal tract with biopsy should be performed.

Hepatitis

Hepatocellular injury is common after HSCT. Two patterns are seen: cholestasis (elevations of bilirubin and alkaline phosphatase) and hepatitis (elevations of hepatic transaminases). Abnormalities of liver function tests after HSCT are most commonly of noninfectious causes that can give rise to either pattern. These abnormalities can be in the form of cholestasis from hepatic veno-occlusive disease (VOD) (sinusoidal obstruction syndrome) caused by the conditioning regimen, either cholestasis or hepatitis caused by various medications, or cholestasis caused by acute or chronic GVHD. VOD almost always occurs before day 30, GVHD almost always occurs after engraftment. Iron overload from red cell transfusions before the transplant often leads to a hepatocellular injury pattern that can occur at any time after HSCT. Exacerbation of viral hepatitis present before the transplant can produce a hepatitis pattern that may wax and wane periodically after HSCT. This can lead to serious and progressive hepatic injury with tapering of immunosuppressive therapy as immune reconstitution strengthens. In the late postengraftment period, fulminent hepatitis may occur from severe infection with VZV, which may occur even in the absence of vesicular skin lesions. In some cases of hepatic syndromes, the cause may be multifactorial because of multiple etiologies, both infectious and noninfectious. Biliary obstruction caused by a stone may give rise to a cholestatic pattern. Cholecystitis has also been reported to occasionally occur, with an association with busulfan in the conditioning regimen.

Evaluation of liver function abnormalities occurring in the HSCT recipient depends on the type of pattern and time posttransplant. A patient with a cholestatic picture should undergo ultrasonongraphy of the abdomen first to exclude biliary obstruction. A review of medications should be performed and discontinuation of any implicated medications should be considered. Before engraftment cholestasis is frequently caused by VOD. Biopsy is often not possible at this time because of significant thrombocytopenia. After engraftment, GVHD is a strong consideration and biopsy should be performed if possible to confirm the diagnosis. HSCT recipients with the hepatitis pattern should be evaluated with viral hepatitis PCR assays and serum iron studies. Although the latter may be difficult to interpret in the presence of ongoing inflammation, HSCT recipients with a history of multiple red cell transfusions and a serum ferritin in excess of 1000 ng/mL should be considered at risk for iron overload syndrome. Any medications that might be suspected should be discontinued if possible and if the etiology remains uncertain, liver biopsy should be considered.

Rash

Rashes frequently occur after HSCT from a variety of causes. The rash of acute GVHD typically presents as an erythematous maculopapular rash, especially of the palms, soles, and earlobes, but the entire body may be affected along with the mucosal surfaces. In the setting of chronic GVHD, lichenoid or sclerodermatoid changes of skin and mucosal surfaces predominate. Skin involvement by infections usually produces localized lesions. Common manifestations of disseminated infections may include subcutaneous nodules of the skin. These lesions may be macronodular erythematous lesions, sometimes with a necrotic center. Vesicular lesions are characteristic of VZV either in a dermatomal or widely disseminated distribution. Paronychia may be caused by bacteria or yeasts; however, they can commonly be caused by *Fusarium* spp or other molds in the severely immunocompromised HSCT recipient and can lead to life-threatening systemic fungal infection.

Punch biopsy of skin lesions can be diagnostic. If a fungal infection is suspected, special stains for fungal organisms, such as the Gomori methenamine silver stain, are necessary because routine histologic stains, such as hematoxylin and eosin, may not be sufficient to visualize the presence of fungi in the tissues. Where disseminated infection is suspected bacterial and fungal blood cultures should also be part of the evaluation. Vesicles found on the skin should be unroofed with a tuberculin-sized syringe and needle to collect fluid for viral cultures, immunostains, or PCR for VZV and HSV.

PREVENTION AND TREATMENT APPROACHES

Management strategies are beyond the scope of this article. Consensus guidelines for infection prevention for HSCT patients were first published in 2000[51] and recently have been updated.[1] Evaluation and management guidelines for neutropenic fever have been published.[3,4] Prevention and treatment guidelines for *Candida* and *Aspergillus* have been published.[52,53] Discussions of CMV treatment have been published.[49,54]

SUMMARY

HSCT has become a common treatment of bone marrow failure and certain malignancies. Types of transplant, including types of stem cells and conditioning regimens vary, impacting the magnitude and duration of primary risk periods. Risks for infections caused by numerous bacterial, viral, and fungal pathogens can extend over a long period of time, dictating preventative strategies and differential diagnoses.

REFERENCES

1. Tomblyn M, Chiller T, Einsele H, et al. Guidelines for preventing infectious complications among hematopoietic cell transplant recipients: a global perspective. Bone Marrow Transplant 2009;15(10):1143–238.
2. Ljungman P, Engelhard D, Da La Camara R, et al. Vaccination of stem cell transplant recipients: recommendations of the Infectious Diseases Working Party of the EBMT. Bone Marrow Transplant 2005;35:737–46.
3. Hughes WT, Armstrong D, Bodey GP, et al. 2002 guidelines for the use of antimicrobial agents in neutropenic patients with cancer. Clin Infect Dis 2002;34(6):730–51.
4. Friefeld AG, Baden LR, Brown AE, et al. The NCCN fever and neutropenia clinical practice guidelines in oncology. Version 1. 2005.
5. Gosselin MV, Adams RH. Pulmonary complications in bone marrow transplantation. J Thorac Imaging 2002;17(2):132–44.
6. Heussel CP, Kauczor HU, Heussel G, et al. Early detection of pneumonia in febrile neutropenic patients: use of thin-section CT. AJR Am J Roentgenol 1997;169(5):1347–53.
7. Conces DJ Jr. Noninfectious lung disease in immunocompromised patients. J Thorac Imaging 1999;14(1):9–24.
8. Wingard JR, Mellits ED, Sostrin MB, et al. Interstitial pneumonitis after allogeneic bone marrow transplantation: nine-year experience at a single institution. Medicine (Baltimore) 1988;67(3):175–86.
9. Wingard JR, Piantadosi S, Burns WH, et al. Cytomegalovirus infections in bone marrow transplant recipients given intensive cytoreductive therapy. Rev Infect Dis 1990;12(Suppl 7):S793–804.

10. Harrington RD, Hooton TM, Hackman RC, et al. An outbreak of respiratory syncytial virus in a bone marrow transplant center. J Infect Dis 1992;165(6):987–93.
11. Ljungman P. Respiratory virus infections in bone marrow transplant recipients: the European perspective. Am J Med 1997;102(3A):44–7.
12. Whimbey E, Champlin RE, Couch RB, et al. Community respiratory virus infections among hospitalized adult bone marrow transplant recipients. Clin Infect Dis 1996;22(5):778–82.
13. Whimbey E, Englund JA, Couch RB. Community respiratory virus infections in immunocompromised patients with cancer. Am J Med 1997;102(3A):10–8.
14. Bowden RA. Respiratory virus infections after marrow transplant: the Fred Hutchinson Cancer Research Center experience. Am J Med 1997;102(3A): 27–30.
15. Nichols WG, Gooley T, Boeckh M. Community-acquired respiratory syncytial virus and parainfluenza virus infections after hematopoietic stem cell transplantation: the Fred Hutchinson Cancer Research Center experience. Biol Blood Marrow Transplant 2001;7(Suppl):11S–5S.
16. Whimbey E, Vartivarian SE, Champlin RE, et al. Parainfluenza virus infection in adult bone marrow transplant recipients. Eur J Clin Microbiol Infect Dis 1993; 12(9):699–701.
17. Ljungman P. Respiratory virus infections in stem cell transplant patients: the European experience. Biol Blood Marrow Transplant 2001;7(Suppl):5S–7S.
18. De La Rosa GR, Champlin RE, Kontoyiannis DP. Risk factors for the development of invasive fungal infections in allogeneic blood and marrow transplant recipients. Transpl Infect Dis 2002;4(1):3–9.
19. Fukuda T, Boeckh M, Carter RA, et al. Risks and outcomes of invasive fungal infections in recipients of allogeneic hematopoietic stem cell transplants after nonmyeloablative conditioning. Blood 2003;102(3):827–33.
20. Greene RE, Schlamm HT, Oestmann JW, et al. Imaging findings in acute invasive pulmonary aspergillosis: clinical significance of the halo sign. Clin Infect Dis 2007;44(3):373–9.
21. Chamilos G, Marom EM, Lewis RE, et al. Predictors of pulmonary zygomycosis versus invasive pulmonary aspergillosis in patients with cancer. Clin Infect Dis 2005;41(1):60–6.
22. Wingard JR, Santos GW, Saral R. Late-onset interstitial pneumonia following allergenic bone marrow transplantation. Transplantation 1985;39(1):21–3.
23. Marr KA, Carter RA, Boeckh M, et al. Invasive aspergillosis in allogeneic stem cell transplant recipients: changes in epidemiology and risk factors. Blood 2002; 100(13):4358–66.
24. Yamasaki S, Heike Y, Mori S, et al. Infectious complications in chronic graft-versus-host disease: a retrospective study of 145 recipients of allogeneic hematopoietic stem cell transplantation with reduced- and conventional-intensity conditioning regimens. Transpl Infect Dis 2008;10:252–9.
25. Daly AS, McGeer A, Lipton JH. Systemic nocardiosis following allogeneic bone marrow transplantation. Transpl Infect Dis 2003;5:16–20.
26. Boeckh M, Leisenring W, Riddell SR, et al. Late cytomegalovirus disease and mortality in recipients of allogeneic hematopoietic stem cell transplants: importance of viral load and T-cell immunity. Blood 2003;101(2):407–14.
27. Dunagan DP, Baker AM, Hurd DD, et al. Bronchoscopic evaluation of pulmonary infiltrates following bone marrow transplantation. Chest 1997;111(1):135–41.
28. Feller-Kopman D, Ernst A. The role of bronchoalveolar lavage in the immunocompromised host. Semin Respir Infect 2003;18(2):87–94.

29. Maertens J, Theunissen K, Verhoef G, et al. Galactomannan and computed tomography-based preemptive antifungal therapy in neutropenic patients at high risk for invasive fungal infection: a prospective feasibility study. Clin Infect Dis 2005;41(9):1242–50.
30. Maertens J, Van Eldere J, Verhaegen J, et al. Use of circulating galactomannan screening for early diagnosis of invasive aspergillosis in allogeneic stem cell transplant recipients. J Infect Dis 2002;186(9):1297–306.
31. Pfeiffer CD, Fine JP, Safdar N. Diagnosis of invasive aspergillosis using a galactomannan assay: a meta-analysis. Clin Infect Dis 2006;42:1417–27.
32. Gorschluter M, Mey U, Strehl J, et al. Neutropenic enterocolitis in adults: systematic analysis of evidence quality. Eur J Haematol 2005;75(1):1–13.
33. Cardona AF, Ramos PL, Casasbuenas A. From case reports to systematic reviews in neutropenic enterocolitis. Eur J Haematol 2005;75(5):445–6.
34. Aksoy DY, Tanriover MD, Uzun O, et al. Diarrhea in neutropenic patients: a prospective cohort study with emphasis on neutropenic enterocolitis. Ann Oncol 2007;18(1):183–9.
35. Cardona Zorrilla AF, Reveiz HL, Casasbuenas A, et al. Systematic review of case reports concerning adults suffering from neutropenic enterocolitis. Clin Transl Oncol 2006;8(1):31–8.
36. Gorschluter M, Mey U, Strehl J, et al. Invasive fungal infections in neutropenic enterocolitis: a systematic analysis of pathogens, incidence, treatment and mortality in adult patients. BMC Infect Dis 2006;6:35.
37. Weiss K. Poor infection control, not fluoroquinolones, likely to be primary cause of *Clostridium difficile*-associated diarrhea outbreaks in Quebec. Clin Infect Dis 2006;42(5):725–7.
38. McDonald LC, Killgore GE, Thompson A, et al. An epidemic, toxin gene-variant strain of *Clostridium difficile*. N Engl J Med 2005;353(23):2433–41.
39. Pepin J, Saheb N, Coulombe MA, et al. Emergence of fluoroquinolones as the predominant risk factor for *Clostridium difficile*-associated diarrhea: a cohort study during an epidemic in Quebec. Clin Infect Dis 2005;41(9):1254–60.
40. Kuijper EJ, van den Berg RJ, Debast S, et al. *Clostridium difficile* ribotype 027, toxinotype III, the Netherlands. Emerg Infect Dis 2006;12(5):827–30.
41. Loo VG, Poirier L, Miller MA, et al. A predominantly clonal multi-institutional outbreak of *Clostridium difficile*-associated diarrhea with high morbidity and mortality. N Engl J Med 2005;353(23):2442–9.
42. Yolken RH, Bishop CA, Townsend TR, et al. Infectious gastroenteritis in bone-marrow-transplant recipients. N Engl J Med 1982;306(17):1010–2.
43. Townsend TR, Bolyard EA, Yolken RH, et al. Outbreak of coxsackie A1 gastroenteritis: a complication of bone-marrow transplantation. Lancet 1982;1(8276):820–3.
44. Cox GJ, Matsui SM, Lo RS, et al. Etiology and outcome of diarrhea after marrow transplantation: a prospective study. Gastroenterology 1994;107(5): 1398–407.
45. van Kraaij MG, Dekker AW, Verdonck LF, et al. Infectious gastro-enteritis: an uncommon cause of diarrhoea in adult allogeneic and autologous stem cell transplant recipients. Bone Marrow Transplant 2000;26(3):299–303.
46. La Rosa AM, Champlin RE, Mirza N, et al. Adenovirus infections in adult recipients of blood and marrow transplants. Clin Infect Dis 2001;32(6):871–6.
47. Shields AF, Hackman RC, Fife KH, et al. Adenovirus infections in patients undergoing bone-marrow transplantation. N Engl J Med 1985;312(9):529–33.
48. Hale GA, Heslop HE, Krance RA, et al. Adenovirus infection after pediatric bone marrow transplantation. Bone Marrow Transplant 1999;23(3):277–82.

49. Boeckh M, Nichols WG, Papanicolaou G, et al. Cytomegalovirus in hematopoietic stem cell transplant recipients: current status, known challenges, and future strategies. Biol Blood Marrow Transplant 2003;9(9):543–58.
50. Boeckh M, Nichols WG. The impact of cytomegalovirus serostatus of donor and recipient before hematopoietic stem cell transplantation in the era of antiviral prophylaxis and preemptive therapy. Blood 2004;103(6):2003–8.
51. Dykewicz CA, Jaffe HW, Spira TJ, et al. Guidelines for preventing opportunistic infections among hematopoietic stem cell transplant recipients. MMWR Recomm Rep 2000;49(RR-10):1–125.
52. Walsh TJ, Anaissie EJ, Denning DW, et al. Treatment of aspergillosis: clinical practice guidelines of the Infectious Diseases Society of America. Clin Infect Dis 2008;46(3):327–60.
53. Pappas PG, Rex JH, Sobel JD, et al. Infectious Diseases Society of America. Guidelines for treatment of candidiasis. Clin Infect Dis 2004;38(2):161–89.
54. Boeckh M, Ljungman P. How we treat cytomegalovirus in hematopoietic cell transplant recipients. Blood 2009;113(23):5711–9.

Infection in Organ Transplantation: Risk Factors and Evolving Patterns of Infection

Jay A. Fishman, MD[a,b,c,*], Nicolas C. Issa, MD[c]

KEYWORDS

- Solid-organ transplantation • Infection • Viral infection
- Epidemiology

GENERAL CONCEPTS

The evolution of immunosuppression for organ transplantation has reduced the incidence of acute graft rejection but has increased the risk for infection and virally mediated malignancie[1–6] The clinical diagnosis of infection is complicated by the relative absence of signs and symptoms of inflammation, alterations in anatomy caused by transplantation surgery, denervation of grafts, and underlying diseases such as diabetes or cirrhosis. Several noninfectious causes of fever (graft rejection, drug reactions, autoimmune disorders) may mimic infection. Established infection is poorly tolerated in transplant recipients with a high level of associated morbidity. Equally important, the toxicities and interactions of antimicrobial agents with the standard immunosuppressive agents used to prevent graft rejection are often amplified because of underlying organ dysfunction. As a result, early and specific microbiologic diagnoses and rapid treatment of infections are essential. Advanced radiologic techniques and invasive diagnostic procedures may be required to establish firm microbiologic diagnoses. The relatively recent availability of quantitative molecular and antibody-based diagnostic assays has facilitated such early diagnoses and these are now used routinely in transplant infectious disease management.

[a] Transplant Infectious Disease & Compromised Host Program, Massachusetts General Hospital, Harvard Medical School, 55 Fruit Street, GRJ 504, Boston, MA 02114, USA
[b] Transplant Center, Massachusetts General Hospital, Harvard Medical School, 55 Fruit Street, GRJ 504, Boston, MA, USA
[c] Division of Infectious Disease, Massachusetts General Hospital, Harvard Medical School, 55 Fruit Street, GRJ 504, Boston, MA 02114, USA
* Corresponding author. Division of Infectious Disease, Massachusetts General Hospital, Harvard Medical School, 55 Fruit Street, GRJ 504, Boston, MA 02114.
E-mail address: jfishman@partners.org

Infect Dis Clin N Am 24 (2010) 273–283
doi:10.1016/j.idc.2010.01.005
id.theclinics.com
0891-5520/10/$ – see front matter © 2010 Elsevier Inc. All rights reserved.

The epidemiology of transplant-associated infections has changed. The incidence of previously common infections caused by cytomegalovirus (CMV) or *Pneumocystis jiroveci* (PCP) have been reduced by the routine use of antimicrobial prophylaxis. Prophylactic antimicrobials and nosocomial exposures have also contributed to the emergence of bacteria (eg, *Stentotrophomonas* species) or viruses (ganciclovir-resistant CMV) carrying antimicrobial resistance. At the same time, a variety of factors have contributed to the emergence of new infections and changes in epidemiology in transplant recipients (**Box 1**).

Each type of allograft presents some unique infectious risks (eg, renal grafts and urinary tract infections after catheter placement or ureteric stenting; biliary, pancreatic, and gastrointestinal anastamotic leaks; drive line infections from cardiac assist devices; tracheal anastamotic infections), but the general patterns of infection are similar. Healing at vascular or other anastamoses and at cut surfaces (livers, lungs) is impaired as a result of tissue ischemia, local infection, and immunosuppression, with the associated risk for wound dehiscence and leakage. The result is a fluid collection (blood, bile, urine, lymph) prone to infection. Catheters and drains (surgical, T-tubes, and so forth) become conduits for infection from the outside world. The patient is bathed in a sea of antimicrobial-resistant, nosocomial flora including methicillin-resistant *Staphylococcus aureus* (MRSA), vancomycin-resistant enterococci (VRE), extended-spectrum β-lactamase (ESBL)-producing gram-negative bacilli, and fluconazole-resistant *Candida* species.[7–11] Improved microbiological diagnostic techniques have allowed recognition of previously undiagnosed infections; notably nucleic acid detection assays have increasingly led to recognition of viral infections (eg, BK polyomavirus, human herpes virus (HHV)-6, -7, and -8).

RISK FOR INFECTION IN SOLID-ORGAN TRANSPLANT RECIPIENTS

The risk for infection is determined by 2 factors: the epidemiologic exposures and a complex function that encompasses all factors contributing to an individual's infectious risk: "the net state of immunosuppression." This equation of risk may be further altered by 2 factors: deployment of antimicrobial prophylaxis and adjustment of immunosuppression based on measures of either global or pathogen-specific immunity. These 4 factors must be considered in the development of a differential diagnosis for infectious syndrome in the transplant recipient. Clinically useful assays that measure

Box 1
Factors contributing to the emergence of novel infections in organ transplant recipients

- Prolonged patient survival (exposures via travel, employment, hobbies)
- Shifts in nosocomial flora (antimicrobial resistance) with antimicrobial exposures (prophylaxis and therapy) and prolonged pretransplant hospitalization
- Intensified immunosuppression (based on exposures and colonization of individual)
- Improved diagnostic assays (molecular), detection of previously unrecognized pathogens
- New technologies (contamination of ventricular assist devices, stem cell transplantation)
- Organ shortage with greater organ dysfunction (sicker patients)
- Donor-derived infections, use of marginal donors?
- Broader epidemiologic exposures, transplantation in developing regions of the world with endemic pathogens

immune function relevant to the graft (ie, risk for rejection) or for specific pathogens remain largely experimental and are an important area for future development. However, the lack of such assays predicts that most patients will suffer excessive or inadequate immunosuppression at some point during their posttransplant course.

EPIDEMIOLOGIC EXPOSURES

Epidemiologic exposures can be divided into multiple categories: donor- and recipient-derived infections, community-acquired infections including those related to travel, and nosocomial infections.

Donor-derived Infections

Medical histories coupled with serologic and culture-based screening of organ donors and recipients have successfully prevented the transmission of most infections with transplanted organs. However, with the emergence of antimicrobial resistance in hospitals and, now, in the community, routine surgical prophylaxis for transplantation surgery may fail to prevent transmission of common organisms including MRSA, VRE, and azole-resistant yeasts.[12–16] This observation has been compounded by the observation of the transmission, although rare, of unusual viral infections (lymphocytic choriomeningitis virus [LCMV], West Nile virus, rabies virus, human immunodeficiency virus [HIV], human herpes virus 8 [HHV-8], human T-cell lymphotropic virus [HTLV]) with allografts.[2,17–26] These infections may be amplified in the setting of immunosuppression. The degree of amplification is illustrated by the increased neurovirulence of West Nile virus in transplant recipients and by the inability to identify LCMV in the deceased donors of organs in clusters of LCMV transmission.[19] Thus, donor-derived infections must be considered in posttransplant recipients with unexplained infectious syndromes. Improved deployment of molecular assays and antigen-detection–based diagnostics may help to prevent such transmissions in the future.[2,23,27] Such diagnostic assays are not available for all potential pathogens, are not universally available, are generally expensive, and require validation and standardization. Controversy exists regarding the optimal testing strategy for microbiologic screening of deceased organ donors given differences in the populations tested in terms of risk for various infections, the characteristics of the assays, and the potential risk for false-negative (risking transmission) and false-positive (risking loss of good organs) assays. To facilitate communication of clinical data between transplant centers, the United Network for Organ Sharing in the United States (UNOS) mandates reporting of suspected donor-derived infections and, with the Centers for Disease Control and Prevention (CDC), is developing a web-based system to provide real-time tracking for organs and tissues for all donors and recipients (Transplantation Transmission Sentinel Network or TTSN) in the United States.[28]

Recipient-derived Infections

Transplant candidates should be free of infection, to the degree possible, before transplantation. The medical history and microbiologic screening should detect common and endemic pathogens and prophylactic strategies developed according to microbiologic data and organ-specific considerations. Thus, a history should reveal prior infections and unique exposures (eg, to mycobacteria or hepatitis), residence in regions with endemic fungi (*Histoplasma capsulatum*, *Coccidioides immitis*, *Blastomyces dermatitidis*), and travel (*Strongyloides stercoralis*, *Trypanosoma cruzi*, *Leishmania*). Increasingly, patients with chronic infections (biliary, pulmonary, ventricular assist devices) are treated with an array of antimicrobial agents before transplantation.

Thus, like organ donors, recipients may carry nosocomial, antimicrobial-resistant flora through complex transplant surgery. Technical mishaps are, again, amplified in the setting of immunosuppression and tissue ischemia. Thus, new or resistant pathogens (CMV, Epstein-Barr virus [EBV], herpes simplex virus [HSV], varicella zoster [VZV], HIV, hepatitis B virus [HBV], hepatitis C virus [HCV], syphilis; HTLV I and II, *Toxoplasma gondii*, HHV-8) may emerge despite antimicrobial prophylaxis or microbiologic monitoring applied to common pathogens detected by pretransplant screening. Adequate courses of antimicrobial agents with documentation of clinical responses should be used for documented infections before transplantation.

Community-acquired Infections

Compared with the general population, community-acquired infections in organ recipients are of greater severity (eg, disseminated adenovirus) and, in the case of respiratory viral processes, may be complicated by superinfection. Newer pathogens, including human metapneumovirus, have been identified in transplant recipients. Certain daily activities (gardening, pigeon rearing, farming, well water, travel) may expose transplant recipients to pathogens including *Aspergillus* or *Nocardia* species, *Cryptococcus neoformans* and *gattii* species, *Paracoccidioides* species, *Leishmania* species that may emerge following transplantation. Thus, counseling regarding the risk of infection associated with daily activities, food preparation and consumption, travel, and other activities are integral to the pretransplantation evaluation.

Nosocomial Infections

Patients awaiting transplantation, and many organ donors, are at risk for colonization with nosocomial organisms (discussed earlier). These pathogens are resistant to routine surgical prophylaxis and may be transmitted to other organ transplant recipients.[9,14,29–31] Colonization with such pathogens may preclude transplantation and is an area of controversy.

THE NET STATE OF IMMUNOSUPPRESSION

The net state of immunosuppression is a concept used to describe all factors that may contribute to the individual's risk for infection.[2] This risk is largely determined by the dose, duration, and sequence of immunosuppressive therapies (**Table 1**). However, postoperative fluid collections, vascular catheters and surgical drains, tissue ischemia, drug-induced neutropenia, underlying immune deficits (eg, diabetes), organ dysfunction, metabolic derangements, antimicrobial exposures, and other factors may contribute to the infectious risk.

Indirect Effects of Viral Infection

One factor that is often overlooked in the equation of immunosuppression is the effect of viral infection on immune function. These effects are best described for CMV and include proliferative graft injury (bronchiolitis obliterans syndrome in lungs, accelerated atherogenesis in hearts), enhanced viral replication (of other herpes viruses, HCV), and increased susceptibility to PTLD and other opportunistic infections (*Aspergillus* species, bacteria, PCP).[2,32–37] Similar effects have been observed for other viruses. These immune alterations and syndromes have generally been termed indirect effects, a misnomer as these seem to be linked directly to latent infection, low level viral replication, or to diminished function by infected immunocytes. The term microinfection has also been applied to these syndromes. Much of the effect of these infections on opportunistic infection is at the interface of the innate immune system

Table 1
Immunosuppressive therapies and infectious risk

Agent	Common Pathogens/Problems
Corticosteroids, chronic	Pneumocystis, bacteria, molds, poor wound healing, hepatitis B virus
Corticosteroids, bolus (graft rejection)	CMV, BK polyomavirus nephropathy (PVAN)
Azathioprine	Neutropenia, papillomavirus?
Mycophenylate mofetil	Early bacteria, late CMV?, neutropenia, esophagitis
Calcineurin inhibitors (CNI)	Viruses, gingival infections, posttransplant lymphoproliferative disorder (PTLD), skin cancers
Rapamycin	Pneumonitis (excess infections in combinations with CNIs)
T-lymphocyte depletion (agent specific)[a]	Herpes virus activation, PVAN, late fungal and viral infections, PTLD, hepatitis C
B-lymphocyte depletion, plasmapheresis	Encapsulated bacteria, sepsis
IL2R antagonists (induction)	Limited data, no evident effect
Abatacept, belatacept	Possibly increased PTLD

Individual risks vary based on total immunosuppressive dose, duration and temporal sequence, viral coinfection, graft dysfunction, or metabolic disorders and other factors. Limited experience with newer agents (eg, JAK/STAT inhibitors, sphingosine 1-phosphate receptor-1 agonist) precludes comment.

[a] Effects greater after use in graft rejection than with use in induction therapy.

(monocytes, macrophages, dendritic cells, and natural killer [NK] cells) and the adaptive immune system (lymphocytes, antibodies). Although many facets of immunity are altered, antigen presentation, dendritic cell maturation, and leukocyte mobilization are among the major deficits. Other virally mediated effects are the result of alterations in the milieu of cytokines, toll-like receptors, and other inflammatory mediators, locally and systemically. The net effect of viral infection is that subsequent infection should be anticipated, often as a result of colonizing organisms or previous infections that have been incompletely treated.

Antilymphocyte Therapies and the Risk of Infection

Current antilymphocyte therapies can be divided into 3 groups: T-lymphocyte depleting agents (antithymocyte globulins [ATGs], OKT3, alemtuzumab), nondepleting costimulatory blockade therapies (interleukin-2 receptor [IL2-R] antagonists (basiliximab and daclizumab), CTLA-4 antagonists [belatacept, abatacept], and B-cell depleting agents [rituximab, anti-CD20 antibody]). Rituximab has been used as an induction therapy agent in ABO-incompatible and positive cross-match kidney transplant recipients, and in the treatment of humoral graft rejection. A variety of newer agents targeting antibody-mediated graft rejection are also under development.

UNOS data for the past decade shows an increased rate of infections in renal allograft recipients. This has been attributed, in part, to use of potent induction therapies and maintenance regimens.[4] Antithymocyte therapies provide a dose-dependent depletion of T cells.[38,39] Effects of various ATGs on the risk for infection depend on other immunosuppressive therapies, the individual's immune function, the type of ATG used, and the total dose and duration of therapy. ATG used in induction therapy or in treatment of graft rejection, if not coupled with adequate CMV prophylaxis, is associated with increased incidence of CMV and an increased severity of symptoms.[40–45] ATG used in induction therapy and in graft rejection is also associated with an increased risk for BK viremia and BKV-associated nephropathy.[46–52] Most studies suggest an association between ATG therapy and risk for development of PTLD.[53–57] OKT3 has been associated with an increased rate of severe infection (CMV, fungal infections)[58,59] and an increased risk of PTLD.[60,61] Alemtuzumab is a humanized monoclonal antibody directed against the membrane glycoprotein CD52 found on lymphoid cells (T cells and B cells), cells of monocyte lineage (monocytes and macrophages) and NK cells. Pan-T cell depletion is profound and persists at least 9 months after treatment.[62] Data regarding infectious complications associated with alemtuzumab are limited, but greater risk for late invasive viral and fungal infections has been observed.[63] Interleukin-2α-receptor (IL-2R) antagonists seem to have a lower rate of infectious complications (including CMV) compared with other induction therapies.[64–66] However, clinical experience remains limited.

Rituximab is a humanized chimeric monoclonal antibody directed against CD20, a transmembrane protein located on pre-B and mature cells but not on plasma cells. There are few data regarding the infectious complications associated with its use in solid-organ transplant recipients, but skin and soft tissue infections and blood stream infections may be increased.[67]

TIME LINE OF INFECTION AFTER ORGAN TRANSPLANTATION

The time line of infection after transplantation is determined by the nature and intensity of an individual's epidemiologic exposures and the net state of immunosuppression. The time line has been reviewed in detail elsewhere.[2] The risk for infection is reset by intensified immunosuppression (ie, for graft rejection). Risk is delayed, but only temporarily, by antimicrobial prophylaxis and reductions in immunosuppression. In the early posttransplantation period (1–2 months), donor- and recipient-derived infections predominate, with nosocomial infections (eg, *Clostridium difficile* colitis, MRSA or VRE bacteremias, *Aspergillus* pneumonia) occurring on a center-specific basis.

After the first month, viral infections predominate, notably in patients receiving antimicrobial prophylaxis with trimethoprim-sulfamethoxazole (TMP-SMZ). TMP-SMZ prophylaxis prevents most infections caused by PCP, *Listeria monocytogenes*, *Toxoplasma gondii* and *Nocardia* species. Reactivation of latent infections may be observed in this time period including *Mycobacterium tuberculosis*, *Trypanosoma cruzi*, *Leishmania* species, *Strongyloides stercoralis*, *Cryptococcus neoformans*, *Histoplasma capsulatum*, *Coccidioides*. and *Paracoccidioides* species.

Newer viruses have emerged as a function of intensified immunosuppression and improved (molecular) diagnostic assays. A reduction in herpes virus infections has been observed as a result of antiviral prophylaxis (CMV, HSV, VZV, HHV-6, -7, and -8). HBV has also been controlled by successful antiviral strategies. BK polyomavirus nephropathy (PVAN) has also emerged, primarily in renal graft recipients. HCV remains a major pathogen in transplant recipients in the relative absence of effective antiviral therapies. Parvovirus B19 is associated with persistent anemia unresponsive to erythropoietin, carditis, and leukopenia. Community-acquired respiratory viruses remain a common hazard. In these immunocompromised hosts these common pathogens may present with pneumonitis, viremia, or tissue-invasive disease (hepatitis, carditis).

In the period 1 to 6 months after transplantation, development of opportunistic infections seems to be driven largely by viral coinfection (discussed earlier see in the section on indirect effects). Further, histologic patterns previously attributed to chronic rejection seem to be attributable at least in part to immunologically mediated processes and cellular proliferation driven by various viruses, notably CMV. These include bronchiolitis obliterans syndrome in lung recipients and accelerated anthropogenesis in cardiac recipients. These immunomodulating viruses (CMV, EBV, HHV-6, HBV, HCV) may predispose to other opportunistic infections, accelerated HCV infection, EBV-mediated PTLD, and an increased risk for acute and chronic graft injury or rejection.

The risk for infection more than 6 months after transplantation is largely a function of residual immunosuppression, exposure to T-cell depleting therapies, graft function, and individual epidemiology. Thus, common community-acquired respiratory infections tend to be more severe or prolonged than in normal hosts. PTLD and skin cancers may occur. The greatest shifts in the epidemiology of infection fall into 2 categories: new exposures and residual immune deficits. New infections often reflect aging (herpes zoster), travel (Lyme disease, malaria), or dietary indiscretions (*Listeria monocytogenes*). Residual defects may reflect treatment of graft rejection in the absence of appropriate prophylaxis (PCP or CMV infections). Increasingly, late viral and fungal infections are observed as a result of T-cell depletion used in initial induction therapy or in graft rejection. Thus, the linkage of immune suppression and prevention (vaccines, prophylaxis, monitoring) must be reemphasized.

FUTURE DIRECTIONS AND SUMMARY

The absence of assays that measure general infectious risk maintains transplant infectious disease as a clinical art form as much as a science. The gradual development of pathogen-specific assays for immune function T-cell subsets, HLA-restricted lymphocyte sorting using tetramers, antigen-specific interferon-γ release assays may allow determination of individual risk for specific infections.[68–71] In the meantime, vaccine development for immunocompromised hosts remains an important area of clinical investigation.

The epidemiology of infections after solid-organ transplantation has shifted as a result of changes in immunosuppressive strategies and improved survival. Immunosuppression must be linked with appropriate vaccinations, donor and recipient screening, patient education regarding infectious risks and lifestyle, monitoring, and antimicrobial prophylaxis. The risk for infections has increased with the use of lymphocyte depleting agents. Some drugs that alter the mobilization of lymphocytes (eg, FTY 720, a high-affinity agonist for the sphingosine 1-phosphate receptor-1) or other components of the inflammatory response may alter the histology of infection and further confound diagnosis. Thus, it should be anticipated that with the introduction of each new immunosuppressive agent, there will be unique effects on the presentation and epidemiology of infection in the organ transplant recipient.

REFERENCES

1. Ciancio G, Burke GW, Miller J. Induction therapy in renal transplantation: an overview of current developments. Drugs 2007;67:2667.
2. Fishman JA. Infection in solid-organ transplant recipients. N Engl J Med 2007; 357:2601.
3. Meier-Kriesche HU, Li S, Gruessner RW, et al. Immunosuppression: evolution in practice and trends, 1994–2004. Am J Transplant 2006;6:1111.
4. Parasuraman R, Nizaar A, Karthikeyan V, et al. Significant increase in infection-associated renal allograft failure over the past decade: UNOS data analysis. In American Transplant Congress. Toronto, Ontario, Canada, 2008.

5. Pascual M, Theruvath T, Kawai T, et al. Strategies to improve long-term outcomes after renal transplantation. N Engl J Med 2002;346:580.
6. Smith JM, McDonald RA. Emerging viral infections in transplantation. Pediatr Transplant 2006;10:838.
7. Husain S, Tollemar J, Dominguez EA, et al. Changes in the spectrum and risk factors for invasive candidiasis in liver transplant recipients: prospective, multicenter, case-controlled study. Transplantation 2003;75:2023.
8. Paterson DL, Singh N, Rihs JD, et al. Control of an outbreak of infection due to extended-spectrum beta-lactamase–producing *Escherichia coli* in a liver transplantation unit. Clin Infect Dis 2001;33:126.
9. Rebuck JA, Olsen KM, Fey PD, et al. Characterization of an outbreak due to extended-spectrum beta-lactamase-producing *Klebsiella pneumoniae* in a pediatric intensive care unit transplant population. Clin Infect Dis 2000;31:1368.
10. Singh N, Gayowski T, Rihs JD, et al. Evolving trends in multiple-antibiotic-resistant bacteria in liver transplant recipients: a longitudinal study of antimicrobial susceptibility patterns. Liver Transpl 2001;7:22.
11. Singh N, Paterson DL, Chang FY, et al. Methicillin-resistant *Staphylococcus aureus*: the other emerging resistant gram-positive coccus among liver transplant recipients. Clin Infect Dis 2000;30:322.
12. Fishman JA. Vancomycin-resistant enterococcus in liver transplantation: what have we left behind? Transpl Infect Dis 2003;5:109.
13. Hashimoto M, Sugawara Y, Tamura S, et al. *Pseudomonas aeruginosa* infection after living-donor liver transplantation in adults. Transpl Infect Dis 2009;11:11.
14. Herrero IA, Issa NC, Patel R. Nosocomial spread of linezolid-resistant, vancomycin-resistant enterococcus faecium. N Engl J Med 2002;346:867.
15. Keven K, Basu A, Re L, et al. *Clostridium difficile* colitis in patients after kidney and pancreas-kidney transplantation. Transpl Infect Dis 2004;6:10.
16. West M, Pirenne J, Chavers B, et al. *Clostridium difficile* colitis after kidney and kidney-pancreas transplantation. Clin Transplant 1999;13:318.
17. Barozzi P, Luppi M, Facchetti F, et al. Post-transplant Kaposi sarcoma originates from the seeding of donor-derived progenitors. Nat Med 2003;9:554.
18. DeSalvo D, Roy-Chaudhury P, Peddi R, et al. West Nile virus encephalitis in organ transplant recipients: another high-risk group for meningoencephalitis and death. Transplantation 2004;77:466.
19. Fischer SA, Graham MB, Kuehnert MJ, et al. Transmission of lymphocytic choriomeningitis virus by organ transplantation. N Engl J Med 2006;354:2235.
20. Iwamoto M, Jernigan DB, Guasch A, et al. Transmission of West Nile virus from an organ donor to four transplant recipients. N Engl J Med 2003;348:2196.
21. Kumar D, Prasad GV, Zaltzman J, et al. Community-acquired West Nile virus infection in solid-organ transplant recipients. Transplantation 2004;77:399.
22. Kusne S, Smilack J. Transmission of rabies virus from an organ donor to four transplant recipients. Liver Transpl 2005;11:1295.
23. Palacios G, Druce J, Du L, et al. A new arenavirus in a cluster of fatal transplant-associated diseases. N Engl J Med 2008;358:991.
24. Toro C, Benito R, Aguilera A, et al. Infection with human T lymphotropic virus type I in organ transplant donors and recipients in Spain. J Med Virol 2005;76:268.
25. Toro C, Rodes B, Poveda E, et al. Rapid development of subacute myelopathy in three organ transplant recipients after transmission of human T-cell lymphotropic virus type I from a single donor. Transplantation 2003;75:102.

26. Wilck M, Fishman JA. The challenges of infection in transplantation: donor-derived infections. Curr Opin Organ Transplant 2005;10:301.
27. Relman DA. New technologies, human-microbe interactions, and the search for previously unrecognized pathogens. J Infect Dis 2002;186(Suppl 2):S254.
28. Fishman JA, Strong DM, Kuehnert MJ. Organ and tissue safety workshop 2007: advances and challenges. Cell Tissue Bank 2009;10:271.
29. Angelis M, Cooper JT, Freeman RB. Impact of donor infections on outcome of orthotopic liver transplantation. Liver Transpl 2003;9:451.
30. Delmonico FL. Cadaver donor screening for infectious agents in solid organ transplantation. Clin Infect Dis 2000;31:781.
31. Freeman RB, Giatras I, Falagas ME, et al. Outcome of transplantation of organs procured from bacteremic donors. Transplantation 1999;68:1107.
32. George MJ, Snydman DR, Werner BG, et al. The independent role of cytomegalovirus as a risk factor for invasive fungal disease in orthotopic liver transplant recipients. Boston Center for Liver Transplantation CMVIG-Study Group. Cytogam, MedImmune, Inc. Gaithersburg, Maryland. Am J Med 1997;103:106.
33. Perez-Sola MJ, Caston JJ, Solana R, et al. Indirect effects of cytomegalovirus infection in solid organ transplant recipients. Enferm Infecc Microbiol Clin 2008; 26:38.
34. Potena L, Holweg CT, Chin C, et al. Acute rejection and cardiac allograft vascular disease is reduced by suppression of subclinical cytomegalovirus infection. Transplantation 2006;82:398.
35. Potena L, Valantine HA. Cytomegalovirus-associated allograft rejection in heart transplant patients. Curr Opin Infect Dis 2007;20:425.
36. Varani S, Frascaroli G, Landini MP, et al. Human cytomegalovirus targets different subsets of antigen-presenting cells with pathological consequences for host immunity: implications for immunosuppression, chronic inflammation and autoimmunity. Rev Med Virol 2009;19:131.
37. Wagner JA, Ross H, Hunt S, et al. Prophylactic ganciclovir treatment reduces fungal as well as cytomegalovirus infections after heart transplantation. Transplantation 1995;60:1473.
38. Mohty M. Mechanisms of action of antithymocyte globulin: T-cell depletion and beyond. Leukemia 2007;21:1387.
39. Simon T, Opelz G, Weimer R, et al. The effect of ATG on cytokine and cytotoxic T-lymphocyte gene expression in renal allograft recipients during the early post-transplant period. Clin Transplant 2003;17:217.
40. Buchler M, Hurault de Ligny B, Madec C, et al. Induction therapy by anti-thymocyte globulin (rabbit) in renal transplantation: a 1-yr follow-up of safety and efficacy. Clin Transplant 2003;17:539.
41. Huurman VA, Kalpoe JS, van de Linde P, et al. Choice of antibody immunotherapy influences cytomegalovirus viremia in simultaneous pancreas-kidney transplant recipients. Diabetes Care 2006;29:842.
42. Lebranchu Y, Bridoux F, Buchler M, et al. Immunoprophylaxis with basiliximab compared with antithymocyte globulin in renal transplant patients receiving MMF-containing triple therapy. Am J Transplant 2002;2:48.
43. Ozaki KS, Pestana JO, Granato CF, et al. Sequential cytomegalovirus antigenemia monitoring in kidney transplant patients treated with antilymphocyte antibodies. Transpl Infect Dis 2004;6:63.
44. von Muller L, Schliep C, Storck M, et al. Severe graft rejection, increased immunosuppression, and active CMV infection in renal transplantation. J Med Virol 2006;78:394.

45. Zamora MR. Controversies in lung transplantation: management of cytomegalovirus infections. J Heart Lung Transplant 2002;21:841.
46. Awadalla Y, Randhawa P, Ruppert K, et al. HLA mismatching increases the risk of BK virus nephropathy in renal transplant recipients. Am J Transplant 2004;4:1691.
47. Dadhania D, Snopkowski C, Ding R, et al. Epidemiology of BK virus in renal allograft recipients: independent risk factors for BK virus replication. Transplantation 2008;86:521.
48. Dharnidharka V, Cherikh W. Analysis of OPTN/UNOS data for rate of treatment for, and risk factors for, BK virus nephropathy (BKVN) in kidney transplant recipients. In American Transplant Congress. Toronto, Ontario, Canada, 2008.
49. Hirsch HH, Brennan DC, Drachenberg CB, et al. Polyomavirus-associated nephropathy in renal transplantation: interdisciplinary analyses and recommendations. Transplantation 2005;79:1277.
50. Hirsch HH, Knowles W, Dickenmann M, et al. Prospective study of polyomavirus type BK replication and nephropathy in renal-transplant recipients. N Engl J Med 2002;347:488.
51. Smith JM, Dharnidharka VR, Talley L, et al. BK virus nephropathy in pediatric renal transplant recipients: an analysis of the North American Pediatric Renal Trials and Collaborative Studies (NAPRTCS) registry. Clin J Am Soc Nephrol 2007;2:1037.
52. Srinivas TR, Schold JD, Eagan GA, et al. Total rabbit ATG dose is a risk factor for onset of BK viremia in kidney transplant recipients. Am J Transplant 2007;7(Suppl 2):234.
53. Bustami RT, Ojo AO, Wolfe RA, et al. Immunosuppression and the risk of post-transplant malignancy among cadaveric first kidney transplant recipients. Am J Transplant 2004;4:87.
54. Caillard S, Dharnidharka V, Agodoa L, et al. Posttransplant lymphoproliferative disorders after renal transplantation in the United States in era of modern immunosuppression. Transplantation 2005;80:1233.
55. Cherikh W, Ring M, Kauffman HM, et al. Updated analysis of dissociation of depletion and PTLD in kidney recipients treated with alemtuzumab induction therapy. Am J Transplant 2007;7(Suppl 2).
56. Cherikh WS, Kauffman HM, McBride MA, et al. Association of the type of induction immunosuppression with posttransplant lymphoproliferative disorder, graft survival, and patient survival after primary kidney transplantation. Transplantation 2003;76:1289.
57. Dharnidharka VR, Stevens G. Risk for post-transplant lymphoproliferative disorder after polyclonal antibody induction in kidney transplantation. Pediatr Transplant 2005;9:622.
58. Hibberd PL, Tolkoff-Rubin NE, Cosimi AB, et al. Symptomatic cytomegalovirus disease in the cytomegalovirus antibody seropositive renal transplant recipient treated with OKT3. Transplantation 1992;53:68.
59. Oh CS, Stratta RJ, Fox BC, et al. Increased infections associated with the use of OKT3 for treatment of steroid-resistant rejection in renal transplantation. Transplantation 1988;45:68.
60. Meier-Kriesche HU, Arndorfer JA, Kaplan B. Association of antibody induction with short- and long-term cause-specific mortality in renal transplant recipients. J Am Soc Nephrol 2002;13:769.
61. Swinnen LJ, Costanzo-Nordin MR, Fisher SG, et al. Increased incidence of lymphoproliferative disorder after immunosuppression with the monoclonal antibody OKT3 in cardiac-transplant recipients. N Engl J Med 1990;323:1723.

62. Morris EC, Rebello P, Thomson KJ, et al. Pharmacokinetics of alemtuzumab used for in vivo and in vitro T-cell depletion in allogeneic transplantations: relevance for early adoptive immunotherapy and infectious complications. Blood 2003;102: 404.
63. Peleg AY, Husain S, Kwak EJ, et al. Opportunistic infections in 547 organ transplant recipients receiving alemtuzumab, a humanized monoclonal CD-52 antibody. Clin Infect Dis 2007;44:204.
64. Issa NC, Fishman JA. Infectious complications of antilymphocyte therapies in solid organ transplantation. Clin Infect Dis 2009;48:772.
65. Vincenti F, Kirkman R, Light S, et al. Interleukin-2-receptor blockade with daclizumab to prevent acute rejection in renal transplantation. Daclizumab Triple Therapy Study Group. N Engl J Med 1998;338:161.
66. Webster AC, Playford EG, Higgins G, et al. Interleukin 2 receptor antagonists for renal transplant recipients: a meta-analysis of randomized trials. Transplantation 2004;77:166.
67. Grim SA, Pham T, Thielke J, et al. Infectious complications associated with the use of rituximab for ABO-incompatible and positive cross-match renal transplant recipients. Clin Transplant 2007;21:628.
68. Cummins NW, Deziel PJ, Abraham RS, et al. Deficiency of cytomegalovirus (CMV)-specific CD8+ T cells in patients presenting with late-onset CMV disease several years after transplantation. Transpl Infect Dis 2009;11:20.
69. Mattes FM, Vargas A, Kopycinski J, et al. Functional impairment of cytomegalovirus specific CD8 T cells predicts high-level replication after renal transplantation. Am J Transplant 2008;8:990.
70. Walker S, Fazou C, Crough T, et al. Ex vivo monitoring of human cytomegalovirus-specific CD8+ T-cell responses using QuantiFERON-CMV. Transpl Infect Dis 2007;9:165.
71. Westall GP, Mifsud NA, Kotsimbos T. Linking CMV serostatus to episodes of CMV reactivation following lung transplantation by measuring CMV-specific CD8+ T-cell immunity. Am J Transplant 2008;8:1749.

Infectious Complications Associated with Immunomodulating Biologic Agents

Sophia Koo, MD[a,b,c,*], Francisco M. Marty, MD[a,b,c], Lindsey R. Baden, MD[a,b,c]

KEYWORDS

- Monoclonal antibodies • Biologic therapies
- Infectious complications

The repertoire of monoclonal antibodies and other biologic therapies targeted at precise components of the immune response continues to expand rapidly. In theory, these therapies should carry fewer infectious risks than traditional immunosuppressive therapies, but with increasing clinical use, it seems that many of these agents have a wide array of unintended, sometimes fatal, infectious consequences. Given the low frequency of these infectious events, an increase in specific infectious risks is often not appreciable in initial randomized controlled trials, and the discernment of these patterns often relies on ongoing surveillance during the postmarketing period, with the accumulation of a larger volume of patient exposures and reporting to national registries or voluntary reporting systems. Because patients who require immunomodulating biologic therapy are usually at higher risk of developing infections at baseline given their underlying disease and prior and concurrent treatment with other immunosuppressive agents, it is often difficult to discern a pattern of infection attributable to the addition of biologic therapies to this background, even when a pattern is present. In addition, biologic therapies may have different target affinities, be used at various dosages, and given with different frequencies, all of which may affect their immunosuppressive consequences. Furthermore, the use of prophylactic antimicrobial agents

Funding support: none.

[a] Division of Infectious Diseases, Brigham and Women's Hospital, 75 Francis Street, PBB-A4, Boston, MA 02115, USA

[b] Division of Infectious Diseases, Dana-Farber Cancer Institute, Boston, MA, USA

[c] Harvard Medical School, Boston, MA, USA

* Corresponding author. Division of Infectious Diseases, Brigham and Women's Hospital, 75 Francis Street, PBB-A4, Boston, MA 02115.

E-mail address: skoo@partners.org

Infect Dis Clin N Am 24 (2010) 285–306
doi:10.1016/j.idc.2010.01.006 id.theclinics.com
0891-5520/10/$ – see front matter © 2010 Elsevier Inc. All rights reserved.

(eg, acyclovir and trimethoprim/sulfamethoxazole) or preemptive monitoring (eg, cytomegalovirus [CMV] viral load surveillance) may alter disease diagnosis and presentation. This review describes the range of infectious complications associated to date with each of the immunomodulating biologic therapies approved by the US Food and Drug Administration (FDA). Monoclonal antibodies used to treat infections and to diagnose disease on radiology studies are beyond the scope of this discussion.

B-LYMPHOCYTE DEPLETION: RITUXIMAB

Rituximab is a chimeric murine-human monoclonal IgG1 that targets CD20 on normal and malignant B lymphocytes, with rapid and durable depletion of these cells for 6 to 9 months. Serum immunoglobulin levels remain largely stable, although prolonged hypogammaglobulinemia has been described in some patients with non-Hodgkin lymphoma (nHL) receiving rituximab concurrently with autologous hematopoietic stem cell transplantation (HSCT).[1] Rituximab does not significantly affect CD3, CD4, CD8 or natural killer (NK) T-cell populations, and in theory has minimal effects on cell-mediated immunity.[2]

Rituximab was initially approved by the FDA in 1997 for the treatment of relapsed or refractory low-grade or follicular nHL, and has subsequently been approved for the treatment of several other CD20+ B-cell lymphomas, either alone or in combination with other chemotherapy, and treatment of moderate to severe rheumatoid arthritis (RA) in combination with methotrexate in patients with an inadequate response to tumor necrosis factor α (TNF-α) antagonists. According to the manufacturer, there have been more than a million patient exposures since its approval, giving rituximab the most extensive clinical use of any biologic therapy to date.

No appreciable increase in infectious complications was observed with rituximab therapy over placebo in several randomized controlled trials for the treatment of nHL or B-cell chronic lymphocytic leukemia (CLL),[3,4] although 2 recent meta-analyses of randomized trials of rituximab maintenance therapy in lymphoma patients have reported a higher relative risk (2.90) of grade 3 to 4 infections with rituximab therapy.[5,6]

In some studies of human immunodeficiency virus (HIV)-associated nHL, addition of rituximab to standard chemotherapy was associated with a higher incidence of serious infections, particularly in patients with profound CD4 lymphopenia. A pooled assessment of 3 phase II randomized trials in which patients with HIV-associated nHL and a median CD4 count of 161 cells/μL receiving rituximab with standard chemotherapy reported a 14% incidence of serious opportunistic infections (OIs) within 3 months of chemotherapy completion despite trimethoprim-sulfamethoxazole and fluconazole prophylaxis, with the development of infections typically associated with impaired cellular immunity, including CMV retinitis, tuberculosis (TB), *Pneumocystis jirovecii* pneumonia (PCP), and salmonellosis.[7] Another phase III trial of patients with HIV-associated nHL treated with rituximab or placebo plus cyclophosphamide, hydroxydaunomycin, oncovin (vincristine), and prednisone (CHOP) reported a significant difference in infectious mortality, 14% with rituximab (R-CHOP) compared with 2% with placebo.[8] Of patients treated with R-CHOP, the incidence of infectious mortality was far higher in patients with baseline CD4 counts less than 50 cells/μL (36%) than patients with CD4 counts 50 cells/μL or greater (6%). Several OIs developed within 6 months of rituximab therapy in patients treated with R-CHOP, including PCP, CMV, invasive candidiasis, and *Mycobacterium avium intercellulare* (MAI), whereas no OIs were observed in the CHOP arm. Using more stringent enrollment criteria (exclusion of patients with CD4 <100 cells/μL, prior OIs, or poor performance status), a phase II study of R-CHOP in HIV-associated patients with nHL reported a lower incidence of infection.[9] The depletion of B lymphocytes in patients with severe deficits in cellular immunity seems to increase the risk of developing OIs.

Hepatitis B virus (HBV) reactivation has been consistently associated with rituximab treatment in postmarketing reports. Humoral immunity to HBV surface antigen is known to play an important role in the containment of HBV infection, and several reports describe a reverse seroconversion phenomenon, with loss of protective HBV surface antibody and sometimes fulminant reactivation of HBV infection in rituximab recipients, particularly in patients with chronic HBV and detectable surface antigen before treatment.[10,11] A recent study of patients with resolved HBV infection (positive HBV core antibody and negative surface antigen) in an HBV-endemic area receiving R-CHOP or CHOP for nHL described a 23.8% reactivation rate at 6 months in patients receiving R-CHOP, including 1 case of progression to hepatic failure, and 0% reactivation in patients receiving CHOP alone.[12] The investigators associated rituximab exposure, male gender, and a lack of HBV surface antibody with HBV reactivation in this setting. Although most HBV reactivation seems to occur within 6 months of starting rituximab-containing therapy, reactivations as late as a year following therapy have been reported.[13] Assessment of HBV status before starting rituximab-containing chemotherapy is essential in patients from endemic areas or with risk factors for prior HBV infection. Lamivudine prophylaxis during rituximab-containing chemotherapy has been reported to prevent HBV reactivation,[11,14] and some groups recommend prophylactic HBV antiviral therapy in HBV surface antigen-positive patients for at least 6 months after completing chemotherapy.[15] Optimal management of patients with resolved HBV infection receiving rituximab chemotherapy is less well defined, but patients should at a minimum have HBV surface antigen, HBV viral load, and liver function test monitoring every few months to assess for HBV reactivation.

From the initial FDA approval of rituximab in 1997 to 2008, 76 cases of progressive multifocal leukoencephalopathy (PML) associated with rituximab use have been reported to the manufacturer's global safety database.[16] PML is traditionally associated with profound deficits in cellular immunity, and the role of rituximab-induced impairments in humoral immunity in the development of PML is far less clear. Most cases have been reported in patients with lymphoproliferative disorders, although cases have also been reported in patients receiving rituximab therapy for systemic lupus erythematosus, RA, and immune thrombocytopenic purpura.[17] Most of these patients were previously or concurrently exposed to other immunosuppressive therapies. Patients received a median of 6 rituximab doses and were exposed to rituximab for a median of 16 months before their PML diagnosis. The case fatality rate was high (90%), and the clinical course of these patients was rapidly progressive, with a 2-month median time to death after PML diagnosis. In 9 of 14 cases with available data, CD4 counts were less than 500 cells/μL. Although the absolute overall incidence of PML cases in patients exposed to rituximab is low, rituximab has carried a black box warning for PML since 2007, and active postmarketing surveillance is ongoing.

A case-control study of patients with persistent, relapsing *Babesia microti* infection and severe morbidity and death despite repeated courses of antiparasitic therapy identified rituximab treatment as an important factor in the inability to clear this infection. Patients required prolonged courses of antiparasitic therapy for cure, for at least 2 weeks after clearance of parasites on blood smear.[18]

A case series reported a higher rate of PCP infection in patients receiving rituximab in combination with CHOP-based chemotherapy for lymphoma (6%–13%) compared with patients receiving comparable CHOP-based regimens alone (4%). PCP has been linked to rituximab therapy in other case series and reports, although patients concurrently received steroids and other immunosuppressive therapy.[19–21] Although PCP infection has been classically associated with CD4 lymphocyte deficits, B-cell deficient mice are exquisitely sensitive to PCP infection and are unable to generate a protective CD4 memory and effector T-cell response to PCP.[22,23]

There have been several reports of TB and nontuberculous mycobacterial (NTM) infections in association with rituximab. A recent survey-based study of mycobacterial infections reported by members of the Emerging Infections Network identified 3 cases of TB and 5 cases of NTM associated with rituximab use.[24] Severe MAI infection and disseminated *M kansasii* and *M wolinskyi* infections have been reported in patients receiving rituximab, although patients in these cases also received other concurrent immunosuppression.[25,26] B lymphocytes seem to be important in the containment of TB in murine infection models, and B-lymphocyte knockout mice are unable to contain TB infections, with an increased pulmonary mycobacterial burden compared with mice with normal B-cell function.[27] B lymphocytes are present in the periphery of tuberculous granulomas in active folliclelike centers associated with antigen-presenting cells and CD4 and CD8 T lymphocytes in human TB infection, and are believed to help orchestrate containment of infection.[28]

Several other severe infections have been linked to rituximab use at a sporadic case report level, including persistent enteroviral meningoencephalitis,[29–31] CMV disease,[32–34] disseminated varicella-zoster virus (VZV),[35,36] pure red cell aplasia from parvovirus B19 infection,[37–39] West Nile virus meningoencephalitis,[40–42] and nocardiosis,[43,44] although all patients received rituximab in combination with other immunosuppressive therapies, and the causal role of rituximab itself is unclear.

ANTI-TNF-α- THERAPIES: INFLIXIMAB, ADALIMUMAB, ETANERCEPT, CERTOLIZUMAB PEGOL, GOLIMUMAB

Infliximab, adalimumab, and golimumab are monoclonal antibodies directed against TNF-α, certolizumab pegol is a pegylated fragment antigen-binding (Fab) fragment of a humanized anti-TNF-α monoclonal antibody, and etanercept is a soluble receptor for TNF-α. All of these therapies abrogate TNF-α activity to varying degrees, and are effective treatment modalities for various inflammatory conditions. The monoclonal antibodies bind soluble and cell-surface TNF-α, with fixation of complement and lysis of T lymphocytes and neutrophils expressing surface TNF-α, whereas etanercept is able to bind only to soluble TNF-α and does not seem to have the same lytic effect on cells expressing membrane-bound TNF-α.[45] TNF-α is essential for macrophage activation, phagosome activation, differentiation of monocytes into macrophages, recruitment of neutrophils and macrophages, granuloma formation, and maintenance of granuloma integrity, and therapy with TNF-α blockers is associated with a particularly increased risk of granulomatous and intracellular infections.[46–48]

Infliximab was approved in 1998 for the treatment of RA, psoriatic arthritis and plaque psoriasis, ankylosing spondylitis, ulcerative colitis, and Crohn disease. Adalimumab was approved in 1999, and has the same treatment indications as infliximab, except for ulcerative colitis. Etanercept was approved in 2001 for the treatment of RA, psoriasis and psoriatic arthritis, and ankylosing spondylitis. In 2009, the FDA approved golimumab for RA, psoriatic arthritis, and ankylosing spondylitis, and certolizumab for RA and Crohn disease refractory to conventional therapy.

The overall incidence of serious infections associated with anti-TNF-α therapy has been estimated from comprehensive national registry data of RA patients from the United Kingdom[49] and Germany[50] at 5.2 to 6.2 per 100 patient-years in patients with infliximab, 6.3 per 100 patient-years with adalimumab, and 5.3 to 6.4 per 100 person-years with etanercept. The German biologics register study adjusted for differences in patient characteristics using propensity scores, and reported an adjusted relative risk for total serious adverse infectious events of 2.2 with etanercept and 3.0 with infliximab use. An observational cohort study of the Swedish biologics register of RA patients assessed the risk of hospitalization with infection with anti-TNF-α therapy, and reported an increased relative risk of 1.43 during the first year, 1.15 during the second year, and no difference in the risk of hospitalization in subsequent years compared with RA patients not receiving anti-TNF-α therapy.[51] A meta-analysis of anti-TNF-α therapy trials in RA reported an odds ratio (OR) of 2.0 for serious infections and 3.3 for malignancy in patients receiving anti-TNF-α therapy, compared with placebo, with only 12 granulomatous infections (10 cases of TB, 1 of histoplasmosis, and 1 of coccidioidomycosis) in 126 serious infections.[52]

An association between anti-TNF-α therapy and TB was noted a few years after the initial approval of infliximab.[53] A query of the FDA MedWatch spontaneous reporting system in 2001 showed 70 TB cases developing a median of 12 weeks after initial infliximab exposure, with a high proportion of extrapulmonary dissemination (57%), and a frequent lack of granuloma formation in patients with biopsy samples. In the United States, the rate of granulomatous and intracellular infection in patients receiving anti-TNF-α therapy has been estimated from the FDA adverse event reporting system, which relies on spontaneous reporting of cases, unlike national registries. These infections were more common in patients receiving infliximab (129 events per 100,000 patients) than etanercept (60 events per 100,000 patients).[54,55] The rate of TB was 54 per 100,000 patients in infliximab patients, with a rate ratio of 1.9 compared with etanercept patients, and the median time to TB was substantially shorter in infliximab patients (17 weeks) than etanercept patients (48 weeks). A case-control study of RA patients in an American pharmaceutical claims database also identified a higher rate ratio in patients treated with biologic therapy (1.5) compared with patients receiving nonbiologic RA therapy, and also reported an earlier median time to TB in patients receiving infliximab (17 weeks) than in patients receiving etanercept (79 weeks).[56] A Monte Carlo simulation of time to reactivation of latent TB calculated a median monthly rate of TB reactivation of 20.8% in patients receiving infliximab, 12.1-fold higher than patients receiving etanercept.[57] There was a clustering of infliximab-associated TB reactivation cases in the first year; the risk of progression of new TB infection to active disease was comparable in infliximab and etanercept patients, suggesting that much of the excess risk of TB with infliximab therapy over etanercept is a consequence of more efficient latent TB reactivation shortly after starting anti-TNF-α therapy, whereas both infliximab and etanercept fairly equally increase the risk of active incident disease. In TB patients receiving anti-TNF-α therapy, an immune reconstitution inflammatory syndrome-like reaction has been described after withdrawal of these agents, sometimes requiring the reinitiation of these agents to control an overly exuberant and deleterious host immune response.[58,59]

NTM infections have also been associated with anti-TNF-α therapy. The rate of NTM in the United States has been estimated at 9 cases per 100,000 patients with infliximab and 6 cases per 100,000 patients with etanercept.[54] A recent survey asking members of the Emerging Infections Network to identify all cases of TB and NTM in patients receiving anti-TNF-α therapy in their clinical practice during the prior 6 months found that reports of NTM (65%) exceeded reports of TB.[24] Most cases were MAI infections, but cases of *M chelonae*, *M abscessus*, *M marinum*, *M fortuitum*, *M haemophilum*, *M kansasii*, and *M scrofulaceum* were also reported. Cases of lepromatous leprosy have been reported in patients from Louisiana, Texas, and the Brazilian Amazon receiving anti-TNF-α therapy for various indications, with high numbers of bacilli on biopsy.[60–62] The progression of disease has been observed to be faster than usual in these patients. A type 1 reversal reaction was described in the 2 North American patients a month after discontinuing anti-TNF-α therapy and starting antibiotic therapy, with exacerbation of skin lesions, malaise, and greater organization of the inflammatory infiltrate on skin biopsy.[61] Severe infections with other rare mycobacterial pathogens, such as *M peregrinum*,[63] *M aurum*,[64] *M bovis*,[65] and *M szulgai*[66] have been described on a case report level in patients receiving anti-TNF-α therapy.

Histoplasmosis has been associated with anti-TNF-α therapy, with a significantly higher rate in infliximab (19 cases per 100,000 patients) than etanercept recipients (3 cases per 100,000 patients) in the United States.[54] Most cases have been reported within 6 months of initiation of anti-TNF-α therapy,[67] and many of the reported cases have been associated with disseminated disease.[68,69]

Coccidioidomycosis has been reported in association with anti-TNF-α therapy, also with significantly higher rates with infliximab (11 cases per 100,000 patients) than etanercept (1 case per 100,000 patients) exposure in the United States.[54,70] An assessment of patients with inflammatory arthritis living in *Coccidioides immitis*–endemic areas reported a relative risk of approximately 5 for coccidioidomycosis with infliximab compared with other antirheumatic drugs.[71]

The rate of cryptococcosis in the United States is estimated at 9 cases per 100,000 patients exposed to anti-TNF-α therapy, and there is no notable difference in patients treated with infliximab or etanercept.[54]

TNF-α is essential for normal activation of macrophage phagosomes and clearance of intracellular pathogens, and several intracellular infections have been associated with anti-TNF-α therapy, including *Listeria* bacteremia and meningitis,[54,72,73] which has been reported at higher rates in infliximab (9 cases per 100,000 patients) than etanercept (1 case per 100,000 patients) recipients, *Legionella* pneumonia,[54,74,75] and salmonellosis.[54,76,77] Several intracellular protozoal pathogens have been reported in association with anti-TNF-α therapy, including relapsing cutaneous and visceral leishmaniasis in endemic areas,[78–80] overwhelming *Plasmodium falciparum* parasitemia,[81] and a report of an eventually fatal progressive myositis caused by *Brachiola algerae*.[82]

TNF-α enhances conidial phagocytosis by alveolar macrophages, augments the effectiveness of polymorphonuclear cells against *Aspergillus hyphae*, and contributes to the recruitment and activation of neutrophils and mononuclear cells in the lung; anti-TNF-α therapy has been associated with an increased risk of invasive fungal infections, with overall invasive aspergillosis (IA) and invasive candidasis rates of approximately 7 to 8 cases per 100,000 exposed patients.[54,83] A review of invasive fungal infections associated with TNF-α inhibition identified 281 cases, most associated with infliximab therapy, and many associated with concurrent corticosteroid therapy.[70] IA was associated with TNF-α therapy in 64 reports, invasive candidiasis in 64 cases, and zygomycosis in 4 cases. Other fungi that generally cause localized disease, such as *Trichophyton rubrum* and *Sporothrix schenckii* infection, have been associated with disseminated disease in recipients of anti-TNF-α therapy.[84,85]

Other infections associated with anti-TNF-α therapy include PCP,[86–88] nocardiosis (~4 cases per 100,000 infliximab recipients),[54] toxoplasmosis (~2 cases per 100,000 infliximab recipients),[54,89] bartonellosis,[54] and brucellosis.[54]

The relationship between TNF-α inhibition and reactivation of latent and chronic viral infections is less well defined. A recent assessment of herpes zoster in the large German biologics registry reported 86 episodes, with a crude incidence rate of 11.1 per 1000 patient-years with monoclonal antibodies (adalimumab, infliximab), 8.9 for etanercept, and 5.6 with conventional disease-modifying antirheumatic therapy. Adjusting for other factors, the hazard ratio of herpes zoster with monoclonal antibody therapy compared with conventional therapy was 1.8, and there was no discernible increase in risk with etanercept.[90] An assessment of large patient databases from the United States and the United Kingdom identified an increased risk of zoster with conventional disease-modifying RA therapy and a higher risk (OR 1.5) in patients receiving biologic therapy.[91] Reactivation of other herpesviruses has not clearly been associated with anti-TNF-α therapy, although 3 cases of herpes simplex virus encephalitis were recently reported in patients receiving infliximab or adalimumab.[92] Several cases of severe HBV reactivation in patients with positive surface antigen at the start of anti-TNF-α therapy have been reported,[93–95] although concurrent lamivudine treatment may decrease the risk of reactivation in these patients.[96]

Allogeneic HSCT recipients with severe steroid-refractory acute graft-versus-host disease (GVHD) have a high risk of invasive fungal disease (IFD) and CMV reactivation, likely because of the loss of normal mucosal barrier integrity and heavy concurrent immune suppression; the addition of anti-TNF-α therapy further increases the risk of these infections. A retrospective evaluation of 21 patients receiving infliximab for steroid-refractory GVHD reported the development of bacterial infections in 81%, viral reactivations in 67% (predominantly CMV), and invasive fungal infections in 48% of patients.[97] Patients receiving infliximab for severe steroid-refractory GVHD at the authors' institution had a high incidence rate of IFD (6.8 cases per 1000 GVHD patient-days) compared with 0.53 cases per 1000 GVHD patient-days in patients not exposed to infliximab.[98] The adjusted hazard ratio for IFD in patients exposed to infliximab was 13.6 compared with patients who were not exposed.

Clinical experience with certolizumab pegol and golimumab is limited. Some studies of certolizumab for Crohn disease and RA have reported an increased incidence of serious infections compared with placebo, including several cases of TB.[99–101] Although many randomized trials of golimumab have shown no increase in the overall incidence of serious infections compared with placebo, a trial in RA patients also treated with methotrexate[102] and a trial in patients with severe asthma refractory to high-dose inhaled steroids and β2 agonists[103] reported a higher incidence of serious infections with golimumab therapy, with 1 case of TB and 1 case of *Legionella* pneumonia. As golimumab is similar in structure to infliximab, it is likely that a comparable pattern of OIs will emerge with further clinical use.

A consensus group statement on the use of biologic agents in patients with RA recommends measures to reduce infectious complications in patients receiving anti-TNF-α therapy, including screening for latent TB infection and assessment for latent or chronic HBV and hepatitis C virus infection before starting therapy.[104]

ANTI-INTERLEUKIN 1 THERAPIES: ANAKINRA, RILONACEPT

The cytokine interleukin 1 (IL-1) is secreted by numerous cell types in response to inflammatory antigens, and has a wide range of biologic activity, including mediation of the febrile response to infection and inflammation, B-cell activation, induction of IL-2 with subsequent stimulation of T-cell maturation, and induction of IL-6, TNF-γ, and IL-8.

Anakinra, a recombinant IL-1 receptor antagonist, was approved for the treatment of moderate to severe RA in 2001. It competitively inhibits binding of IL-1 to IL-1 type I receptor, with a decrease in the response to inflammatory stimuli. The German biologics registry reported a rate of 3.2 serious infections per 100 patient-years in patients exposed to anakinra, although the total number of patients receiving anakinra was small.[50] A meta-analysis of all randomized placebo-controlled trials evaluating anakinra in RA reported a 1.4% incidence of serious infections with anakinra, compared with 0.5% with placebo, and the OR of serious infection was 3.40 in patients treated with high-dose anakinra versus placebo, although this difference was not significant when results were adjusted for underlying comorbidities.[105] Pneumonia and other bacterial infections accounted for most events; no OIs were reported. One case of TB was reported in a patient enrolled in an RA study who had underlying pneumoconiosis from mining,[106] and 1 case of visceral leishmaniasis was reported in a child living in an endemic area of France receiving anakinra for systemic onset juvenile idiopathic arthritis 6 months after starting treatment.[107]

Rilonacept is a dimeric fusion protein of the ligand-binding domain of the extracellular portion of the human IL-1 receptor and IL-1 receptor accessory protein linked to the Fc portion of human IgG1. It acts as a soluble decoy receptor and binds IL-1β, preventing its normal binding to IL-1 receptors. Rilonacept was approved in 2008 for the treatment of cryopyrin-associated periodic syndromes (CAPS), characterized by excessive IL-1β production. In a study of 47 patients with CAPS, rilonacept was associated with upper respiratory infections in 26% of patients, compared with 4% in patients receiving placebo.[108] One case of *Streptococcus pneumoniae* meningitis developed during the open-label extension period, but was believed not to be related to the study drug. The rilonacept package insert reported a case of MAI olecranon bursitis in a patient receiving rilonacept for an unapproved indication and intra-articular glucocorticoid injections.

ALEMTUZUMAB

Alemtuzumab is a humanized monoclonal IgG1 that targets CD52 on normal and neoplastic B and T lymphocytes, monocytes, macrophages, and NK cells, with lysis of these cell populations and substantial sustained deficits in cell-mediated and humoral immunity. CD4 and CD8 T-lymphocyte counts reach their nadir approximately 4 weeks after administration, and median counts remain at less than 25% of baseline values for approximately 9 months.[109]

Alemtuzumab received accelerated approval by the FDA in 2001 for the treatment of B-cell CLL refractory to alkylating agents and fludarabine, and regular approval for single-agent therapy for B-cell CLL in 2007.

A wide spectrum of infections has been associated with alemtuzumab therapy, particularly herpesvirus reactivations, incident viral infections, and invasive fungal infections. Before the routine use of PCP and herpesvirus prophylaxis in these patients, a phase II study of alemtuzumab for the treatment of fludarabine-refractory CLL reported a 41.7% incidence of OIs, including reactivation of latent herpesviruses (CMV, disseminated VZV) and invasive fungal infections (PCP, IA, candidiasis). Severe infections were reported in 8% of patients in the first, 6% in the second, and 7% in the third month of therapy.[110] Another phase II study of alemtuzumab in this patient population used PCP prophylaxis and valacyclovir herpesvirus prophylaxis but still reported a 20% incidence of CMV reactivation, and cases of disseminated VZV, probable IA, sinus zygomycosis, and disseminated NTM infection.[111] A larger multicenter study in this population mandated PCP and herpesvirus prophylaxis in all patients, and reported a lower incidence of overall grade 3 to 4 infection (26.9%) and CMV reactivation (8%). Several OIs developed after alemtuzumab treatment despite prophylaxis, including PCP, IA, rhinocerebral zygomycosis, cryptococcal pneumonia, invasive candidiasis, herpes zoster, and *Listeria* meningitis.[112]

A retrospective evaluation of 27 patients receiving alemtuzumab for lymphoproliferative disorders, primarily CLL, at the authors' institution showed a high rate of OIs (33%) and non-OIs (82%) despite PCP and herpesvirus prophylaxis.[113] Patients developed a diverse array of OIs (IA, disseminated histoplasmosis, adenovirus pneumonia, PML, cerebral toxoplasmosis, CMV disease, and disseminated acathamebiasis) a median of 169 days after starting alemtuzumab. Many patients (44%) developed asymptomatic CMV viremia on hybrid-capture assay. Infections contributed to mortality in 7 of 10 patients who died.

A lower incidence of infection has been reported in studies of alemtuzumab as first-line therapy for CLL, compared with studies in patients heavily exposed to prior chemotherapy regimens for refractory CLL. In a phase II study of first-line treatment of patients with symptomatic CLL, only 10% of patients developed CMV reactivation and no patients developed CMV disease.[114] In a large study of treatment-naive CLL patients randomized to either alemtuzumab or chlorambucil single-agent therapy, 15.6% of patients in the alemtuzumab arm developed symptomatic CMV infection without CMV disease, although 52.4% of patients receiving alemtuzumab had asymptomatic CMV viremia, compared with only 7.5% in patients receiving chlorambucil.[115] No other OIs were reported in this study.

Several cases of severe mycobacterial infections have been reported in patients with CLL treated with alemtuzumab, including disseminated MAI,[116] disseminated *M bovis* in a patient concurrently receiving intravesical bacille Calmette-Guérin therapy for localized bladder cancer,[117] cutaneous *M haemophilum* infection,[118] and cutaneous *M chelonae* infection.[119]

The use of alemtuzumab for T-cell depletion in nonmyeloablative allogeneic HSCT is associated with a particularly high incidence of CMV reactivation (50%–85%),[113,120–123] severe adenovirus infection and disease (40%), particularly in patients with low absolute lymphocyte counts,[122] respiratory virus infections, including influenza, parainfluenza, and respiratory syncytial virus (30%), with frequent progression to lower respiratory tract infection,[124] and symptomatic *Human herpesvirus 6* encephalitis (11.6%).[125] A recent large retrospective evaluation of posttransplant lymphoproliferative disorder (PTLD) cases in allogeneic HSCT recipients identified alemtuzumab T-cell depletion as a significant risk factor for the development of PTLD, with a relative risk of 3.1, although the risk of PTLD with alemtuzumab was substantially lower than with other T-cell depleting modalities.[126]

A retrospective assessment of a large number of solid-organ transplant patients receiving alemtuzumab for prevention or treatment of allograft rejection described a 10% incidence of OIs, including CMV disease in 3% of patients, and several cases of BK virus infection, PTLD, esophageal candidiasis, cryptococcosis, other IFDs, nocardiosis, mycobacterial infections, and isolated cases of *Parvovirus B19* infection, *Balamuthia mandrillaris*, and toxoplasmosis. The incidence of OI was higher in patients receiving alemtuzumab for treatment of rejection (21%) compared with patients treated with alemtuzumab for induction (4.5%). The OR for the development of an OI after alemtuzumab exposure was particularly high in lung (3.7) and intestinal transplant (8.3) recipients.[127]

All patients receiving alemtuzumab should receive PCP and herpesvirus prophylaxis. Given the high incidence of CMV infection with alemtuzumab treatment, CMV prophylaxis or close monitoring with preemptive therapy may be warranted. One study reported the effectiveness of prompt initiation of preemptive CMV therapy in preventing CMV disease despite a high rate of CMV reactivation.[128] A recent study randomized patients receiving alemtuzumab for various hematologic malignancies to prophylactic valacyclovir 500 mg daily or valganciclovir 450 mg twice daily, and reported no CMV reactivation in the valganciclovir arm, versus 35% in the acyclovir arm.[129]

BLOCKING ACTIVATED T-LYMPHOCYTE PROLIFERATION: DACLIZUMAB, BASLIXIMAB

Daclizumab and basiliximab are monoclonal antibodies that target CD25, the α chain of the IL-2 receptor complex expressed on activated alloantigen-reactive T lymphocytes, with competitive inhibition of IL-2 binding and abatement of IL-2-mediated lymphocyte proliferation, differentiation, and cytokine release. Antigen-specific alloreactive T cells are depleted, with a blunted response to antigenic challenge. The FDA approved daclizumab in 1997 and basiliximab in 1998 for the prophylaxis of acute allograft rejection in renal transplant recipients in combination with other immunosuppressive therapy.

Daclizumab does not seem to be associated with an increased risk of infectious complications in solid-organ transplantation. In randomized controlled trials of daclizumab in renal transplantation, a decreased incidence of acute rejection has been reported with daclizumab compared with placebo, with a lower requirement for antirejection therapy, and possibly a lower incidence of CMV reactivation.[130,131] Daclizumab for prophylaxis of acute rejection in cardiac transplantation has also been reported to reduce the risk of rejection, with a comparable incidence of serious OI at 6 months (6.9%) compared with placebo.[132] One retrospective study of lung transplant patients at a single national center reported daclizumab use in induction as a risk factor for the development of IA, with an OR of 2.05 compared with polyclonal induction regimens, but this has not been corroborated by other reports.[133]

A high rate of infectious mortality has been reported in allogeneic HSCT recipients receiving daclizumab for steroid-refractory acute GVHD, although a causal role for daclizumab is unclear, given the high baseline risk of OI in this population. In 1 series, 10 of 43 patients died of GVHD and infection and 7 patients died of infection. Three patients, all of whom were T-cell-depleted unrelated-donor HSCT recipients, developed EBV-associated PTLD during or after daclizumab exposure.[134] In a retrospective assessment of patients receiving daclizumab for steroid-refractory GVHD, 95% of patients developed OIs by 6 months, and infection contributed to mortality in 79% of patients who died.[135] Bacterial infections were reported in 88% of all patients, viral infections in 53%, with CMV infection in 35% and EBV-associated PTLD in 7%, and IFD in 51%, with IA in 12% of patients, 1 *Scedosporium apiospermum* infection, and 1 *Cunninghamella* infection. Other OIs reported in this study included 3 MAI infections, and 1 case each of TB, toxoplasmosis, nocardiosis, and *Legionella* infection.

Similar to daclizumab, basiliximab does not seem to be generally associated with an increased risk of serious infection in renal,[136–138] cardiac,[139,140] or liver transplantation.[141,142] A large randomized study comparing basiliximab with antithymocyte globulin identified a higher incidence of acute rejection episodes in patients randomized to basiliximab and a higher incidence of CMV disease in the basiliximab arm (17.5 vs 7.8%) in this context.[143]

Data on basiliximab use for treatment of steroid-refractory acute GVHD are limited; a single prospective phase II study reported infections in 65% of patients, with CMV reactivation in 22% of patients, 2 cases of IFD, and 1 case of cerebral toxoplasmosis.

SELECTIVE T-CELL COSTIMULATION BLOCKADE: ABATACEPT, BELATACEPT

Abatacept and belatacept are soluble fusion proteins comprised of the extracellular domain of anticytotoxic T-lymphocyte-associated antigen 4 and the Fc portion of IgG1. These proteins block the costimulatory engagement of CD80 or CD86 on antigen-presenting cells with CD28 on T lymphocytes, preventing full T-lymphocyte activation. Abatacept was approved by the FDA in 2005 for the treatment of RA, and belatacept is currently being reviewed for approval. Some randomized controlled trials of abatacept in RA have reported a higher incidence of serious infections than placebo, particularly in patients receiving other concurrent biologic therapy,[144–146] with approximately 5 cases of serious infection per 100 patient-years in patients treated with prolonged courses of therapy,[147,148] although a recent meta-analysis of trials in RA patients did not show a statistically significant increase in infections overall.[105] Most of these serious infections are pneumonias and pyogenic bacterial infections, although a single case of IA and a possible case of TB have been reported. Exposure to abatacept confers a lesser risk of TB reactivation than exposure to murine anti-TNF-α therapy in a mouse TB infection model; mice treated with abatacept for 16 weeks were able to control their *M tuberculosis* infection and all animals survived to the end of the experiment, whereas 100% of mice treated with anti-TNF-α therapy died with disseminated TB infection.[149] Mice treated with abatacept had similar activated T-lymphocyte, macrophage, B-lymphocyte, and neutrophil counts compared with mice treated only with the carrier vehicle and produced a comparable IFN-γ response to infection. The clinical experience with belatacept is limited; in a randomized controlled trial of belatacept versus cyclosporine in combination with basiliximab, mycophenolate mofetil, and corticosteroids for induction therapy in patients receiving renal transplantation, 1 patient developed PTLD while receiving intensive belatacept, and 2 additional patients in the belatacept arm developed PTLD after belatacept was replaced with conventional agents.[150]

THERAPIES INTERFERING WITH T-LYMPHOCYTE MIGRATION: NATALIZUMAB, EFALIZUMAB

Natalizumab is a humanized IgG4 that targets the α_4 subunit of $\alpha_4\beta_1$ and $\alpha_4\beta_7$ integrins on the surface of activated T lymphocytes, inhibiting binding to cellular adhesion molecules in the central nervous system and the gastrointestinal tract and blocking migration of T lymphocytes into these tissues. Treatment is associated with a profound decrease in CD4, CD8, and CD19 lymphocytes in the cerebrospinal fluid.[151] Natalizumab was initially approved for the treatment of relapsing multiple sclerosis (MS) in 2004, then withdrawn from the market a few months later after 3 cases of PML were reported in clinical trials in patients with prolonged exposure to natalizumab and interferon β-1a combination therapy,[152–154] with an overall risk of 1 case per 1000 exposed patients treated for an average of 17.9 months.[155] Natalizumab was reintroduced as MS monotherapy in 2006 with a black box warning about the risk of PML. Additional cases of PML in patients receiving prolonged natalizumab monotherapy (12–31 months) have been reported since that time, with an associated mortality of 23%.[16] In addition to PML, other sporadic OIs were reported in natalizumab recipients during the FDA hearing for market reapproval, including viral meningitis and encephalitis, CMV infection, pulmonary IA, PCP pneumonia, VZV pneumonia, and MAI, although many patients were receiving concurrent immunosuppression.[151] Natalizumab was recently approved for the treatment of refractory Crohn disease.

Efalizumab is a monoclonal IgG1 that binds to CD11a, the α-subunit of leukocyte functional antigen 1 (LFA-1) on activated T lymphocytes, inhibiting lymphocyte binding to endothelial cellular adhesion molecules and blocking migration of these cells through the endothelium during inflammation. It was initially approved for the treatment of plaque psoriasis in 2003, and received a black box warning in 2008, when 3 confirmed PML cases and 1 possible case were reported in patients exposed to efalizumab monotherapy for more than 3 years, with a risk of 1 case per 400 exposed patients. None of these patients had other underlying chronic conditions, and patients were not receiving concurrent immunosuppression with other agents.[16] Other sporadic OIs typically associated with impairment in cell-mediated immunity were reported in association with efalizumab therapy, including visceral leishmaniasis in a patient living in an endemic area,[156] disseminated cryptococcosis,[157] and CMV reactivation.[158] Given its unfavorable risk-benefit profile, efalizumab was voluntarily withdrawn from the market in 2009.

ALEFACEPT

Alefacept is a recombinant fusion protein of human lymphocyte function-associated antigen-3 (LFA-3) and a portion of human IgG1. It binds to CD2 receptors on T lymphocytes to block their activation and to FcγRIII on NK cells, with apoptosis of CD2 memory-effector T-lymphocytes and dose-dependent reductions in CD4 and CD8 T-lymphocyte counts for approximately 28 weeks. Despite the depletion of CD4+CD45RO+ and CD8+CD45RO+ cell populations, naive T-cell populations are relatively preserved, and the T-cell-dependent humoral immune response to extrinsic antigens seems to be preserved in patients receiving alefacept challenged with neoantigen (ϕX174) vaccination.[159] Responses to a recall antigen (tetanus toxoid) were also preserved despite a quantitative loss of memory-effector cells. Alefacept was approved in 2003 for the treatment of moderate to severe plaque psoriasis. A meta-analysis of randomized controlled trials of alefacept for plaque psoriasis reported no discernible increase in serious infections in alefacept recipients compared with placebo.[160] Despite a depletion of CD4 counts, OIs have only rarely been reported in patients receiving alefacept to date: 1 patient receiving alefacept and infliximab concurrently developed disseminated *Nocardia farcinica* infection,[161] and a patient receiving alefacept for psoriasis with a CD4 count of 298 cells/μL developed MAI olecranon bursitis.[162]

PROLONGED NEUTROPENIA: GEMTUZUMAB OZOGAMICIN

Gemtuzumab ozogamicin (GO) is a humanized monoclonal antibody directed at CD33 conjugated to calicheamicin, an antibiotic with potent antitumor activity that cleaves double-stranded DNA at specific sequences. Most myeloid blast cells in acute myelogenous leukemia (AML) express CD33, as do normal hematopoietic progenitor cells. GO was approved in 2000 for the treatment of CD33+ AML in first relapse in patients 60 years of age or older who are not candidates for other cytotoxic chemotherapy. Because it targets normal hematopoietic progenitor cells along with malignant myeloid cells, GO is associated with prolonged myelosuppression, with neutropenia lasting approximately 40 days in patients with a clinical response to GO, accompanied by risk of bacteremia and pneumonia.[163] Despite prolonged neutropenia, an increased risk of IFD has not been described in GO recipients.

SUMMARY

Our understanding of the infectious risks associated with the use of these targeted therapies is nascent. Each biologic target (eg, CD20, CD33) may predispose a different infectious susceptibility. Altering the disease targeted, using the biologic therapy at a different point in the disease process (eg, initial vs salvage therapy) or for off-label indications, and altering the dose or the frequency of administration may all substantively affect the infectious risk engendered with these immunotherapies. Optimal minimization of infectious complications associated with the use of these agents requires vigilance. Patients receiving certain targeted biologic immunomodulators are at higher risk for the reactivation of latent or chronic infections and the acquisition of incident infection than patients not exposed to these therapies. Patients should be screened for latent and chronic infections associated with these biologic agents before starting therapy, and receive prophylactic or preemptive therapy for these infections if screening is positive. Careful assessment for emergent illness is required, as usual presenting symptoms of infection may be altered or absent.

REFERENCES

1. Shortt J, Spencer A. Adjuvant rituximab causes prolonged hypogammaglobulinaemia following autologous stem cell transplant for non-Hodgkin's lymphoma. Bone Marrow Transplant 2006;38:433.
2. McLaughlin P, Grillo-Lopez AJ, Link BK, et al. Rituximab chimeric anti-CD20 monoclonal antibody therapy for relapsed indolent lymphoma: half of patients respond to a four-dose treatment program. J Clin Oncol 1998;16:2825.
3. Byrd JC, Rai K, Peterson BL, et al. Addition of rituximab to fludarabine may prolong progression-free survival and overall survival in patients with previously untreated chronic lymphocytic leukemia: an updated retrospective comparative analysis of CALGB 9712 and CALGB 9011. Blood 2005;105:49.
4. Rafailidis PI, Kakisi OK, Vardakas K, et al. Infectious complications of monoclonal antibodies used in cancer therapy: a systematic review of the evidence from randomized controlled trials. Cancer 2007;109:2182.
5. Aksoy S, Dizdar O, Hayran M, et al. Infectious complications of rituximab in patients with lymphoma during maintenance therapy: a systematic review and meta-analysis. Leuk Lymphoma 2009;50:357.
6. Vidal L, Gafter-Gvili A, Leibovici L, et al. Rituximab maintenance for the treatment of patients with follicular lymphoma: systematic review and meta-analysis of randomized trials. J Natl Cancer Inst 2009;101:248.
7. Spina M, Jaeger U, Sparano JA, et al. Rituximab plus infusional cyclophosphamide, doxorubicin, and etoposide in HIV-associated non-Hodgkin lymphoma: pooled results from 3 phase 2 trials. Blood 2005;105:1891.
8. Kaplan LD, Lee JY, Ambinder RF, et al. Rituximab does not improve clinical outcome in a randomized phase 3 trial of CHOP with or without rituximab in patients with HIV-associated non-Hodgkin lymphoma: AIDS-Malignancies Consortium Trial 010. Blood 2005;106:1538.
9. Boue F, Gabarre J, Gisselbrecht C, et al. Phase II trial of CHOP plus rituximab in patients with HIV-associated non-Hodgkin's lymphoma. J Clin Oncol 2006;24:4123.
10. Dervite I, Hober D, Morel P. Acute hepatitis B in a patient with antibodies to hepatitis B surface antigen who was receiving rituximab. N Engl J Med 2001;344:68.
11. Tsutsumi Y, Tanaka J, Kawamura T, et al. Possible efficacy of lamivudine treatment to prevent hepatitis B virus reactivation due to rituximab therapy in a patient with non-Hodgkin's lymphoma. Ann Hematol 2004;83:58.
12. Yeo W, Chan TC, Leung NW, et al. Hepatitis B virus reactivation in lymphoma patients with prior resolved hepatitis B undergoing anticancer therapy with or without rituximab. J Clin Oncol 2009;27:605.
13. Garcia-Rodriguez MJ, Canales MA, Hernandez-Maraver D, et al. Late reactivation of resolved hepatitis B virus infection: an increasing complication post rituximab-based regimens treatment? Am J Hematol 2008;83:673.
14. Hamaki T, Kami M, Kusumi E, et al. Prophylaxis of hepatitis B reactivation using lamivudine in a patient receiving rituximab. Am J Hematol 2001;68:292.

15. Yeo W, Johnson PJ. Diagnosis, prevention and management of hepatitis B virus reactivation during anticancer therapy. Hepatology 2006;43:209.
16. Carson KR, Focosi D, Major EO, et al. Monoclonal antibody-associated progressive multifocal leucoencephalopathy in patients treated with rituximab, natalizumab, and efalizumab: a review from the Research on Adverse Drug Events and Reports (RADAR) Project. Lancet Oncol 2009;10:816.
17. Carson KR, Evens AM, Richey EA, et al. Progressive multifocal leukoencephalopathy after rituximab therapy in HIV-negative patients: a report of 57 cases from the Research on Adverse Drug Events and Reports project. Blood 2009;113:4834.
18. Krause PJ, Gewurz BE, Hill D, et al. Persistent and relapsing babesiosis in immunocompromised patients. Clin Infect Dis 2008;46:370.
19. Kumar D, Gourishankar S, Mueller T, et al. *Pneumocystis jirovecii* pneumonia after rituximab therapy for antibody-mediated rejection in a renal transplant recipient. Transpl Infect Dis 2009;11:167.
20. Teichmann LL, Woenckhaus M, Vogel C, et al. Fatal *Pneumocystis pneumonia* following rituximab administration for rheumatoid arthritis. Rheumatology (Oxford) 2008;47:1256.
21. Venhuizen AC, Hustinx WN, van Houte AJ, et al. Three cases of *Pneumocystis jirovecii* pneumonia (PCP) during first-line treatment with rituximab in combination with CHOP-14 for aggressive B-cell non-Hodgkin's lymphoma. Eur J Haematol 2008;80:275.
22. Lund FE, Hollifield M, Schuer K, et al. B cells are required for generation of protective effector and memory CD4 cells in response to pneumocystis lung infection. J Immunol 2006;176:6147.
23. Marcotte H, Levesque D, Delanay K, et al. *Pneumocystis carinii* infection in transgenic B cell-deficient mice. J Infect Dis 1996;173:1034.
24. Winthrop KL, Yamashita S, Beekmann SE, et al. Mycobacterial and other serious infections in patients receiving anti-tumor necrosis factor and other newly approved biologic therapies: case finding through the Emerging Infections Network. Clin Infect Dis 2008;46:1738.
25. Chen YC, Jou R, Huang WL, et al. Bacteremia caused by *Mycobacterium wolinskyi.* Emerg Infect Dis 2008;14:1818.
26. Lutt JR, Pisculli ML, Weinblatt ME, et al. Severe nontuberculous mycobacterial infection in 2 patients receiving rituximab for refractory myositis. J Rheumatol 2008;35:1683.
27. Maglione PJ, Xu J, Chan J. B cells moderate inflammatory progression and enhance bacterial containment upon pulmonary challenge with *Mycobacterium tuberculosis.* J Immunol 2007;178:7222.
28. Ulrichs T, Kosmiadi GA, Trusov V, et al. Human tuberculous granulomas induce peripheral lymphoid follicle-like structures to orchestrate local host defence in the lung. J Pathol 2004;204:217.
29. Archimbaud C, Bailly JL, Chambon M, et al. Molecular evidence of persistent echovirus 13 meningoencephalitis in a patient with relapsed lymphoma after an outbreak of meningitis in 2000. J Clin Microbiol 2003;41:4605.
30. Padate BP, Keidan J. Enteroviral meningoencephalitis in a patient with non-Hodgkin's lymphoma treated previously with rituximab. Clin Lab Haematol 2006;28:69.
31. Quartier P, Tournilhac O, Archimbaud C, et al. Enteroviral meningoencephalitis after anti-CD20 (rituximab) treatment. Clin Infect Dis 2003;36:e47.
32. Goldberg SL, Pecora AL, Alter RS, et al. Unusual viral infections (progressive multifocal leukoencephalopathy and cytomegalovirus disease) after high-dose

chemotherapy with autologous blood stem cell rescue and peritransplantation rituximab. Blood 2002;99:1486.
33. Lee MY, Chiou TJ, Hsiao LT, et al. Rituximab therapy increased post-transplant cytomegalovirus complications in non-Hodgkin's lymphoma patients receiving autologous hematopoietic stem cell transplantation. Ann Hematol 2008;87:285.
34. Suzan F, Ammor M, Ribrag V. Fatal reactivation of cytomegalovirus infection after use of rituximab for a post-transplantation lymphoproliferative disorder. N Engl J Med 2001;345:1000.
35. Bermudez A, Marco F, Conde E, et al. Fatal visceral varicella-zoster infection following rituximab and chemotherapy treatment in a patient with follicular lymphoma. Haematologica 2000;85:894.
36. McIlwaine LM, Fitzsimons EJ, Soutar RL. Inappropriate antidiuretic hormone secretion, abdominal pain and disseminated varicella-zoster virus infection: an unusual and fatal triad in a patient 13 months post rituximab and autologous stem cell transplantation. Clin Lab Haematol 2001;23:253.
37. Crowley B, Woodcock B. Red cell aplasia due to parvovirus b19 in a patient treated with alemtuzumab. Br J Haematol 2002;119:279.
38. Isobe Y, Sugimoto K, Shiraki Y, et al. Successful high-titer immunoglobulin therapy for persistent parvovirus B19 infection in a lymphoma patient treated with rituximab-combined chemotherapy. Am J Hematol 2004;77:370.
39. Sharma VR, Fleming DR, Slone SP. Pure red cell aplasia due to parvovirus B19 in a patient treated with rituximab. Blood 2000;96:1184.
40. Huang C, Slater B, Rudd R, et al. First isolation of West Nile virus from a patient with encephalitis in the United States. Emerg Infect Dis 2002;8:1367.
41. Levi ME, Quan D, Ho JT, et al. Impact of rituximab-associated B-cell defects on West Nile virus meningoencephalitis in solid organ transplant recipients. Clin Transplant 2009. [Epub ahead of print].
42. Mawhorter SD, Sierk A, Staugaitis SM, et al. Fatal West Nile Virus infection after rituximab/fludarabine–induced remission for non-Hodgkin's lymphoma. Clin Lymphoma Myeloma 2005;6:248.
43. Flohr TR, Sifri CD, Brayman KL, et al. Nocardiosis in a renal transplant recipient following rituximab preconditioning. Ups J Med Sci 2009;114:62.
44. Kundranda MN, Spiro TP, Muslimani A, et al. Cerebral nocardiosis in a patient with NHL treated with rituximab. Am J Hematol 2007;82:1033.
45. Scallon B, Cai A, Solowski N, et al. Binding and functional comparisons of two types of tumor necrosis factor antagonists. J Pharmacol Exp Ther 2002;301:418.
46. Algood HM, Lin PL, Flynn JL. Tumor necrosis factor and chemokine interactions in the formation and maintenance of granulomas in tuberculosis. Clin Infect Dis 2005;41(Suppl 3):S189.
47. Harris J, Hope JC, Keane J. Tumor necrosis factor blockers influence macrophage responses to *Mycobacterium tuberculosis*. J Infect Dis 2008;198:1842.
48. Roach DR, Bean AG, Demangel C, et al. TNF regulates chemokine induction essential for cell recruitment, granuloma formation, and clearance of mycobacterial infection. J Immunol 2002;168:4620.
49. Dixon WG, Symmons DP, Lunt M, et al. Serious infection following anti-tumor necrosis factor alpha therapy in patients with rheumatoid arthritis: lessons from interpreting data from observational studies. Arthritis Rheum 2007;56:2896.
50. Listing J, Strangfeld A, Kary S, et al. Infections in patients with rheumatoid arthritis treated with biologic agents. Arthritis Rheum 2005;52:3403.

51. Askling J, Fored CM, Brandt L, et al. Time-dependent increase in risk of hospitalisation with infection among Swedish RA patients treated with TNF antagonists. Ann Rheum Dis 2007;66:1339.
52. Bongartz T, Sutton AJ, Sweeting MJ, et al. Anti-TNF antibody therapy in rheumatoid arthritis and the risk of serious infections and malignancies: systematic review and meta-analysis of rare harmful effects in randomized controlled trials. JAMA 2006;295:2275.
53. Keane J, Gershon S, Wise RP, et al. Tuberculosis associated with infliximab, a tumor necrosis factor alpha-neutralizing agent. N Engl J Med 2001;345:1098.
54. Wallis RS, Broder M, Wong J, et al. Granulomatous infections due to tumor necrosis factor blockade: correction. Clin Infect Dis 2004;39:1254.
55. Wallis RS, Broder MS, Wong JY, et al. Granulomatous infectious diseases associated with tumor necrosis factor antagonists. Clin Infect Dis 2004;38:1261.
56. Brassard P, Kezouh A, Suissa S. Antirheumatic drugs and the risk of tuberculosis. Clin Infect Dis 2006;43:717.
57. Wallis RS. Mathematical modeling of the cause of tuberculosis during tumor necrosis factor blockade. Arthritis Rheum 2008;58:947.
58. Arend SM, Leyten EM, Franken WP, et al. A patient with de novo tuberculosis during anti-tumor necrosis factor-alpha therapy illustrating diagnostic pitfalls and paradoxical response to treatment. Clin Infect Dis 2007;45:1470.
59. Wallis RS, van Vuuren C, Potgieter S. Adalimumab treatment of life-threatening tuberculosis. Clin Infect Dis 2009;48:1429.
60. Oberstein EM, Kromo O, Tozman EC. Type I reaction of Hansen's disease with exposure to adalimumab: a case report. Arthritis Rheum 2008;59:1040.
61. Scollard DM, Joyce MP, Gillis TP. Development of leprosy and type 1 leprosy reactions after treatment with infliximab: a report of 2 cases. Clin Infect Dis 2006;43:e19.
62. Vilela Lopes R, Barros Ohashi C, Helena Cavaleiro L, et al. Development of leprosy in a patient with ankylosing spondylitis during the infliximab treatment: reactivation of a latent infection? Clin Rheumatol 2009;28:615.
63. Marie I, Heliot P, Roussel F, et al. Fatal *Mycobacterium peregrinum* pneumonia in refractory polymyositis treated with infliximab. Rheumatology (Oxford) 2005;44:1201.
64. Martin-Aspas A, Guerrero-Sanchez F, Garcia-Martos P, et al. Bilateral pneumonia by *Mycobacterium aurum* in a patient receiving infliximab therapy. J Infect 2008;57:167.
65. Larsen MV, Sorensen IJ, Thomsen VO, et al. Re-activation of bovine tuberculosis in a patient treated with infliximab. Eur Respir J 2008;32:229.
66. van Ingen J, Boeree M, Janssen M, et al. Pulmonary *Mycobacterium szulgai* infection and treatment in a patient receiving anti-tumor necrosis factor therapy. Nat Clin Pract Rheumatol 2007;3:414.
67. Lee JH, Slifman NR, Gershon SK, et al. Life-threatening histoplasmosis complicating immunotherapy with tumor necrosis factor alpha antagonists infliximab and etanercept. Arthritis Rheum 2002;46:2565.
68. Asrani NS. Disseminated histoplasmosis associated with the treatment of rheumatoid arthritis with anticytokine therapy. Ann Intern Med 2008;149:594.
69. Wood KL, Hage CA, Knox KS, et al. Histoplasmosis after treatment with anti-tumor necrosis factor-alpha therapy. Am J Respir Crit Care Med 2003;167:1279.
70. Tsiodras S, Samonis G, Boumpas DT, et al. Fungal infections complicating tumor necrosis factor alpha blockade therapy. Mayo Clin Proc 2008;83:181.

71. Bergstrom L, Yocum DE, Ampel NM, et al. Increased risk of coccidioidomycosis in patients treated with tumor necrosis factor alpha antagonists. Arthritis Rheum 2004;50:1959.
72. Pena-Sagredo JL, Hernandez MV, Fernandez-Llanio N, et al. *Listeria monocytogenes* infection in patients with rheumatic diseases on TNF-alpha antagonist therapy: the Spanish Study Group experience. Clin Exp Rheumatol 2008;26: 854.
73. Slifman NR, Gershon SK, Lee JH, et al. *Listeria monocytogenes* infection as a complication of treatment with tumor necrosis factor alpha-neutralizing agents. Arthritis Rheum 2003;48:319.
74. Li Gobbi F, Benucci M, Del Rosso A. Pneumonitis caused by *Legionella pneumoniae* in a patient with rheumatoid arthritis treated with anti-TNF-alpha therapy (infliximab). J Clin Rheumatol 2005;11:119.
75. Wondergem MJ, Voskuyl AE, van Agtmael MA. A case of legionellosis during treatment with a TNFalpha antagonist. Scand J Infect Dis 2004;36:310.
76. Fu A, Bertouch JV, McNeil HP. Disseminated *Salmonella typhimurium* infection secondary to infliximab treatment. Arthritis Rheum 2004;50:3049.
77. Netea MG, Radstake T, Joosten LA, et al. Salmonella septicemia in rheumatoid arthritis patients receiving anti-tumor necrosis factor therapy: association with decreased interferon-gamma production and toll-like receptor 4 expression. Arthritis Rheum 2003;48:1853.
78. Bagalas V, Kioumis I, Argyropoulou P, et al. Visceral leishmaniasis infection in a patient with rheumatoid arthritis treated with etanercept. Clin Rheumatol 2007;26:1344.
79. Fabre S, Gibert C, Lechiche C, et al. Visceral leishmaniasis infection in a rheumatoid arthritis patient treated with infliximab. Clin Exp Rheumatol 2005;23:891.
80. Mueller MC, Fleischmann E, Grunke M, et al. Relapsing cutaneous leishmaniasis in a patient with ankylosing spondylitis treated with infliximab. Am J Trop Med Hyg 2009;81:52.
81. Geraghty EM, Ristow B, Gordon SM, et al. Overwhelming parasitemia with *Plasmodium falciparum* infection in a patient receiving infliximab therapy for rheumatoid arthritis. Clin Infect Dis 2007;44:e82.
82. Coyle CM, Weiss LM, Rhodes LV 3rd, et al. Fatal myositis due to the microsporidian *Brachiola algerae*, a mosquito pathogen. N Engl J Med 2004; 351:42.
83. Roilides E, Dimitriadou-Georgiadou A, Sein T, et al. Tumor necrosis factor alpha enhances antifungal activities of polymorphonuclear and mononuclear phagocytes against *Aspergillus fumigatus*. Infect Immun 1998;66:5999.
84. Gottlieb GS, Lesser CF, Holmes KK, et al. Disseminated sporotrichosis associated with treatment with immunosuppressants and tumor necrosis factor-alpha antagonists. Clin Infect Dis 2003;37:838.
85. Lowther AL, Somani AK, Camouse M, et al. Invasive *Trichophyton rubrum* infection occurring with infliximab and long-term prednisone treatment. J Cutan Med Surg 2007;11:84.
86. Harigai M, Koike R, Miyasaka N. *Pneumocystis pneumonia* associated with infliximab in Japan. N Engl J Med 2007;357:1874.
87. Kaur N, Mahl TC. *Pneumocystis jiroveci* (*carinii*) pneumonia after infliximab therapy: a review of 84 cases. Dig Dis Sci 2007;52:1481.
88. Takeuchi T, Tatsuki Y, Nogami Y, et al. Postmarketing surveillance of the safety profile of infliximab in 5000 Japanese patients with rheumatoid arthritis. Ann Rheum Dis 2008;67:189.

89. Garcia-Vidal C, Rodriguez-Fernandez S, Teijon S, et al. Risk factors for opportunistic infections in infliximab-treated patients: the importance of screening in prevention. Eur J Clin Microbiol Infect Dis 2009;28:331.
90. Strangfeld A, Listing J, Herzer P, et al. Risk of herpes zoster in patients with rheumatoid arthritis treated with anti-TNF-alpha agents. JAMA 2009;301:737.
91. Smitten AL, Choi HK, Hochberg MC, et al. The risk of herpes zoster in patients with rheumatoid arthritis in the United States and the United Kingdom. Arthritis Rheum 2007;57:1431.
92. Bradford RD, Pettit AC, Wright PW, et al. Herpes simplex encephalitis during treatment with tumor necrosis factor-alpha inhibitors. Clin Infect Dis 2009;49:924.
93. Esteve M, Saro C, Gonzalez-Huix F, et al. Chronic hepatitis B reactivation following infliximab therapy in Crohn's disease patients: need for primary prophylaxis. Gut 2004;53:1363.
94. Michel M, Duvoux C, Hezode C, et al. Fulminant hepatitis after infliximab in a patient with hepatitis B virus treated for an adult onset still's disease. J Rheumatol 2003;30:1624.
95. Zingarelli S, Frassi M, Bazzani C, et al. Use of tumor necrosis factor-alpha-blocking agents in hepatitis B virus-positive patients: reports of 3 cases and review of the literature. J Rheumatol 2009;36:1188.
96. Roux CH, Brocq O, Breuil V, et al. Safety of anti-TNF-alpha therapy in rheumatoid arthritis and spondylarthropathies with concurrent B or C chronic hepatitis. Rheumatology (Oxford) 2006;45:1294.
97. Couriel D, Saliba R, Hicks K, et al. Tumor necrosis factor-alpha blockade for the treatment of acute GVHD. Blood 2004;104:649.
98. Marty FM, Lee SJ, Fahey MM, et al. Infliximab use in patients with severe graft-versus-host disease and other emerging risk factors of non-*Candida* invasive fungal infections in allogeneic hematopoietic stem cell transplant recipients: a cohort study. Blood 2003;102:2768.
99. Keystone E, Heijde D, Mason D Jr, et al. Certolizumab pegol plus methotrexate is significantly more effective than placebo plus methotrexate in active rheumatoid arthritis: findings of a fifty-two-week, phase III, multicenter, randomized, double-blind, placebo-controlled, parallel-group study. Arthritis Rheum 2008; 58:3319.
100. Schreiber S, Khaliq-Kareemi M, Lawrance IC, et al. Maintenance therapy with certolizumab pegol for Crohn's disease. N Engl J Med 2007;357:239.
101. Smolen J, Landewe RB, Mease P, et al. Efficacy and safety of certolizumab pegol plus methotrexate in active rheumatoid arthritis: the RAPID 2 study. A randomised controlled trial. Ann Rheum Dis 2009;68:797.
102. Keystone EC, Genovese MC, Klareskog L, et al. Golimumab, a human antibody to tumour necrosis factor {alpha} given by monthly subcutaneous injections, in active rheumatoid arthritis despite methotrexate therapy: the GO-FORWARD Study. Ann Rheum Dis 2009;68:789.
103. Wenzel SE, Barnes PJ, Bleecker ER, et al. A randomized, double-blind, placebo-controlled study of tumor necrosis factor-alpha blockade in severe persistent asthma. Am J Respir Crit Care Med 2009;179:549.
104. Furst DE, Keystone EC, Kirkham B, et al. Updated consensus statement on biological agents for the treatment of rheumatic diseases. Ann Rheum Dis 2008; 67(Suppl 3):iii2.
105. Salliot C, Dougados M, Gossec L. Risk of serious infections during rituximab, abatacept and anakinra treatments for rheumatoid arthritis: meta-analyses of randomised placebo-controlled trials. Ann Rheum Dis 2009;68:25.

106. Le Loet X, Nordstrom D, Rodriguez M, et al. Effect of anakinra on functional status in patients with active rheumatoid arthritis receiving concomitant therapy with traditional disease modifying antirheumatic drugs: evidence from the OMEGA Trial. J Rheumatol 2008;35:1538.
107. Lequerre T, Quartier P, Rosellini D, et al. Interleukin-1 receptor antagonist (anakinra) treatment in patients with systemic-onset juvenile idiopathic arthritis or adult onset still disease: preliminary experience in France. Ann Rheum Dis 2008;67:302.
108. Hoffman HM, Throne ML, Amar NJ, et al. Efficacy and safety of rilonacept (interleukin-1 Trap) in patients with cryopyrin-associated periodic syndromes: results from two sequential placebo-controlled studies. Arthritis Rheum 2008;58:2443.
109. Morris EC, Rebello P, Thomson KJ, et al. Pharmacokinetics of alemtuzumab used for in vivo and in vitro T-cell depletion in allogeneic transplantations: relevance for early adoptive immunotherapy and infectious complications. Blood 2003;102:404.
110. Rai KR, Freter CE, Mercier RJ, et al. Alemtuzumab in previously treated chronic lymphocytic leukemia patients who also had received fludarabine. J Clin Oncol 2002;20:3891.
111. Ferrajoli A, O'Brien SM, Cortes JE, et al. Phase II study of alemtuzumab in chronic lymphoproliferative disorders. Cancer 2003;98:773.
112. Keating MJ, Flinn I, Jain V, et al. Therapeutic role of alemtuzumab (Campath-1H) in patients who have failed fludarabine: results of a large international study. Blood 2002;99:3554.
113. Martin SI, Marty FM, Fiumara K, et al. Infectious complications associated with alemtuzumab use for lymphoproliferative disorders. Clin Infect Dis 2006;43:16.
114. Lundin J, Kimby E, Bjorkholm M, et al. Phase II trial of subcutaneous anti-CD52 monoclonal antibody alemtuzumab (Campath-1H) as first-line treatment for patients with B-cell chronic lymphocytic leukemia (B-CLL). Blood 2002;100:768.
115. Hillmen P, Skotnicki AB, Robak T, et al. Alemtuzumab compared with chlorambucil as first-line therapy for chronic lymphocytic leukemia. J Clin Oncol 2007; 25:5616.
116. Saadeh CE, Srkalovic G. *Mycobacterium avium* complex infection after alemtuzumab therapy for chronic lymphocytic leukemia. Pharmacotherapy 2008;28: 281.
117. Abad S, Gyan E, Moachon L, et al. Tuberculosis due to *Mycobacterium bovis* after alemtuzumab administration. Clin Infect Dis 2003;37:e27.
118. Kamboj M, Louie E, Kiehn T, et al. *Mycobacterium haemophilum* infection after alemtuzumab treatment. Emerg Infect Dis 2008;14:1821.
119. Dungarwalla M, Field-Smith A, Jameson C, et al. Cutaneous *Mycobacterium chelonae* infection in chronic lymphocytic leukaemia. Haematologica 2007; 92:e5.
120. Chae YS, Sohn SK, Kim JG, et al. Impact of alemtuzumab as conditioning regimen component on transplantation outcomes in case of CMV-seropositive recipients and donors. Am J Hematol 2008;83:649.
121. Chakrabarti S, Mackinnon S, Chopra R, et al. High incidence of cytomegalovirus infection after nonmyeloablative stem cell transplantation: potential role of Campath-1H in delaying immune reconstitution. Blood 2002;99:4357.
122. Ho AY, Pagliuca A, Kenyon M, et al. Reduced-intensity allogeneic hematopoietic stem cell transplantation for myelodysplastic syndrome and acute myeloid leukemia with multilineage dysplasia using fludarabine, busulphan, and alemtuzumab (FBC) conditioning. Blood 2004;104:1616.

123. Perez-Simon JA, Kottaridis PD, Martino R, et al. Nonmyeloablative transplantation with or without alemtuzumab: comparison between 2 prospective studies in patients with lymphoproliferative disorders. Blood 2002;100:3121.
124. Chakrabarti S, Avivi I, Mackinnon S, et al. Respiratory virus infections in transplant recipients after reduced-intensity conditioning with Campath-1H: high incidence but low mortality. Br J Haematol 2002;119:1125.
125. Vu T, Carrum G, Hutton G, et al. Human herpesvirus-6 encephalitis following allogeneic hematopoietic stem cell transplantation. Bone Marrow Transplant 2007;39:705.
126. Landgren O, Gilbert ES, Rizzo JD, et al. Risk factors for lymphoproliferative disorders after allogeneic hematopoietic cell transplantation. Blood 2009;113:4992.
127. Peleg AY, Husain S, Kwak EJ, et al. Opportunistic infections in 547 organ transplant recipients receiving alemtuzumab, a humanized monoclonal CD-52 antibody. Clin Infect Dis 2007;44:204.
128. Laurenti L, Piccioni P, Cattani P, et al. Cytomegalovirus reactivation during alemtuzumab therapy for chronic lymphocytic leukemia: incidence and treatment with oral ganciclovir. Haematologica 2004;89:1248.
129. O'Brien S, Ravandi F, Riehl T, et al. Valganciclovir prevents cytomegalovirus reactivation in patients receiving alemtuzumab-based therapy. Blood 2008;111:1816.
130. Hengster P, Pescovitz MD, Hyatt D, et al. Cytomegalovirus infections after treatment with daclizumab, an anti IL-2 receptor antibody, for prevention of renal allograft rejection. Roche Study Group. Transplantation 1999;68:310.
131. Vincenti F, Kirkman R, Light S, et al. Interleukin-2-receptor blockade with daclizumab to prevent acute rejection in renal transplantation. Daclizumab Triple Therapy Study Group. N Engl J Med 1998;338:161.
132. Hershberger RE, Starling RC, Eisen HJ, et al. Daclizumab to prevent rejection after cardiac transplantation. N Engl J Med 2005;352:2705.
133. Iversen M, Burton CM, Vand S, et al. Aspergillus infection in lung transplant patients: incidence and prognosis. Eur J Clin Microbiol Infect Dis 2007;26:879.
134. Przepiorka D, Kernan NA, Ippoliti C, et al. Daclizumab, a humanized anti-interleukin-2 receptor alpha chain antibody, for treatment of acute graft-versus-host disease. Blood 2000;95:83.
135. Perales MA, Ishill N, Lomazow WA, et al. Long-term follow-up of patients treated with daclizumab for steroid-refractory acute graft-vs-host disease. Bone Marrow Transplant 2007;40:481.
136. Keown P, Balshaw R, Khorasheh S, et al. Meta-analysis of basiliximab for immunoprophylaxis in renal transplantation. BioDrugs 2003;17:271.
137. Lawen JG, Davies EA, Mourad G, et al. Randomized double-blind study of immunoprophylaxis with basiliximab, a chimeric anti-interleukin-2 receptor monoclonal antibody, in combination with mycophenolate mofetil-containing triple therapy in renal transplantation. Transplantation 2003;75:37.
138. Sheashaa HA, Bakr MA, Ismail AM, et al. Basiliximab induction therapy for live donor kidney transplantation: a long-term follow-up of prospective randomized controlled study. Clin Exp Nephrol 2008;12:376.
139. Mattei MF, Redonnet M, Gandjbakhch I, et al. Lower risk of infectious deaths in cardiac transplant patients receiving basiliximab versus anti-thymocyte globulin as induction therapy. J Heart Lung Transplant 2007;26:693.
140. Mehra MR, Zucker MJ, Wagoner L, et al. A multicenter, prospective, randomized, double-blind trial of basiliximab in heart transplantation. J Heart Lung Transplant 2005;24:1297.

141. Lupo L, Panzera P, Tandoi F, et al. Basiliximab versus steroids in double therapy immunosuppression in liver transplantation: a prospective randomized clinical trial. Transplantation 2008;86:925.
142. Neuhaus P, Clavien PA, Kittur D, et al. Improved treatment response with basiliximab immunoprophylaxis after liver transplantation: results from a double-blind randomized placebo-controlled trial. Liver Transpl 2002;8:132.
143. Brennan DC, Daller JA, Lake KD, et al. Rabbit antithymocyte globulin versus basiliximab in renal transplantation. N Engl J Med 2006;355:1967.
144. Kremer JM, Genant HK, Moreland LW, et al. Effects of abatacept in patients with methotrexate-resistant active rheumatoid arthritis: a randomized trial. Ann Intern Med 2006;144:865.
145. Weinblatt M, Combe B, Covucci A, et al. Safety of the selective costimulation modulator abatacept in rheumatoid arthritis patients receiving background biologic and nonbiologic disease-modifying antirheumatic drugs: a one-year randomized, placebo-controlled study. Arthritis Rheum 2006;54:2807.
146. Weinblatt M, Schiff M, Goldman A, et al. Selective costimulation modulation using abatacept in patients with active rheumatoid arthritis while receiving etanercept: a randomised clinical trial. Ann Rheum Dis 2007;66:228.
147. Genovese MC, Becker JC, Schiff M, et al. Abatacept for rheumatoid arthritis refractory to tumor necrosis factor alpha inhibition. N Engl J Med 2005;353:1114.
148. Genovese MC, Schiff M, Luggen M, et al. Efficacy and safety of the selective co-stimulation modulator abatacept following 2 years of treatment in patients with rheumatoid arthritis and an inadequate response to anti-tumour necrosis factor therapy. Ann Rheum Dis 2008;67:547.
149. Bigbee CL, Gonchoroff DG, Vratsanos G, et al. Abatacept treatment does not exacerbate chronic *Mycobacterium tuberculosis* infection in mice. Arthritis Rheum 2007;56:2557.
150. Vincenti F, Larsen C, Durrbach A, et al. Costimulation blockade with belatacept in renal transplantation. N Engl J Med 2005;353:770.
151. Goodin DS, Cohen BA, O'Connor P, et al. Assessment: the use of natalizumab (Tysabri) for the treatment of multiple sclerosis (an evidence-based review): report of the Therapeutics and Technology Assessment Subcommittee of the American Academy of Neurology. Neurology 2008;71:766.
152. Kleinschmidt-DeMasters BK, Tyler KL. Progressive multifocal leukoencephalopathy complicating treatment with natalizumab and interferon beta-1a for multiple sclerosis. N Engl J Med 2005;353:369.
153. Langer-Gould A, Atlas SW, Green AJ, et al. Progressive multifocal leukoencephalopathy in a patient treated with natalizumab. N Engl J Med 2005;353:375.
154. Van Assche G, Van Ranst M, Sciot R, et al. Progressive multifocal leukoencephalopathy after natalizumab therapy for Crohn's disease. N Engl J Med 2005;353:362.
155. Yousry TA, Major EO, Ryschkewitsch C, et al. Evaluation of patients treated with natalizumab for progressive multifocal leukoencephalopathy. N Engl J Med 2006;354:924.
156. Balato A, Balato N, Patruno C, et al. Visceral leishmaniasis infection in a patient with psoriasis treated with efalizumab. Dermatology 2008;217:360.
157. Tuxen AJ, Yong MK, Street AC, et al. Disseminated cryptococcal infection in a patient with severe psoriasis treated with efalizumab, methotrexate and ciclosporin. Br J Dermatol 2007;157:1067.

158. Miquel FJ, Colomina J, Marii JI, et al. Cytomegalovirus infection in a patient treated with efalizumab for psoriasis. Arch Dermatol 2009;145:961.
159. Gottlieb AB, Casale TB, Frankel E, et al. CD4+ T-cell-directed antibody responses are maintained in patients with psoriasis receiving alefacept: results of a randomized study. J Am Acad Dermatol 2003;49:816.
160. Brimhall AK, King LN, Licciardone JC, et al. Safety and efficacy of alefacept, efalizumab, etanercept and infliximab in treating moderate to severe plaque psoriasis: a meta-analysis of randomized controlled trials. Br J Dermatol 2008; 159:274.
161. Al-Tawfiq JA, Al-Khatti AA. Disseminated systemic *Nocardia farcinica* infection complicating alefacept and infliximab therapy in a patient with severe psoriasis. Int J Infect Dis 2009;14:e153.
162. Prasertsuntarasai T, Bello EF. *Mycobacterium avium* complex olecranon bursitis in a patient treated with alefacept. Mayo Clin Proc 2005;80:1532.
163. Sievers EL, Larson RA, Stadtmauer EA, et al. Efficacy and safety of gemtuzumab ozogamicin in patients with CD33-positive acute myeloid leukemia in first relapse. J Clin Oncol 2001;19:3244.

Infections in Pediatric Transplant Recipients: Not Just Small Adults

Marian G. Michaels, MD, MPH*, Michael Green, MD, MPH

KEYWORDS

- Immunocompromised children • Pediatric transplantation
- Cytomegalovirus • Epstein-Barr virus • Vaccinations

Transplantation increasingly is being used as treatment for children with end-stage organ diseases, hematopoietic rescue from therapy used to treat malignancies, and as a cure of primary immune deficiencies. The numbers of transplant procedures performed on children is substantially less than those performed on adults, with recipients under the age of 18 years accounting for only 7.7% of all solid organ transplants performed in the United States.[1] Because the numbers are limited, data on specific infections more often are based on retrospective reviews from single institutions and less rigorously defined than data for adults. In addition, data on infections from adult studies often are extrapolated to assist with the management of pediatric patients. Although this approach is reasonable in many cases, it may be less reliable for situations where the underlying disease influences the risk for infection and where age of the recipient has substantial impact upon the risk for infectious complications. This article reviews some of the major concepts of infections that complicate pediatric transplantation, highlighting differences of epidemiology, evaluation, treatment and prevention for children compared with adult recipients.

SOLID ORGAN TRANSPLANTATION

Over the last 20 years, increasing numbers of children have undergone transplantation of kidney, liver, heart, lungs, pancreas, and intestines with survival continuing to improve over time. For example, children who undergo heart transplantation and survive the first year have a median survival well over 15 years.[2] Although both patient and graft survival varies by type of organ and by age of the recipient, observed survival for pediatric solid organ transplantation (SOT) recipients is often as good, if not better

Department of Pediatrics and Surgery, Children's Hospital of Pittsburgh, One Children's Hospital Drive, 4401 Penn Avenue, Pittsburgh, PA 15224, USA
* Corresponding author.
E-mail address: marian.michaels@chp.edu

Infect Dis Clin N Am 24 (2010) 307–318
doi:10.1016/j.idc.2010.02.001
id.theclinics.com
0891-5520/10/$ – see front matter © 2010 Elsevier Inc. All rights reserved.

than that of adults. For example, in the United States, pediatric kidney transplant recipients have a survival over 97% compared with adult 3-year survival of 91%.[3] Infections, however, remain a major cause of morbidity and mortality in these patients. To understand the types of infections that might occur after transplantation, it is useful to consider several sets of key principles related to infectious complications. The first principle is that the type of infection present in an SOT recipient is predicted by the time period after transplantation in which the patient presents. In general, the pattern and timing of infections are similar in both adults and children.[4] Although the actual breakpoints of a time line are indistinct, one can consider the general timing of presentation after SOT to help predict the types of infections that might be occurring in a given child based on stereotypical patterns:

The early period (0 to 4 weeks) is one in which postoperative bacterial surgical infections predominate.

The middle period (generally 1 to 6 months) is the time wherein opportunistic infections and reactivation of latent infections in the recipient or from the donor are prominent.

The late period (usually after 6 months) is a period when community-acquired viruses and infections associated with chronic graft dysfunction predominate.[4–7]

This concept, put forward in the early era of SOT, is generally true today.[7] Not only does it inform the evaluation of fevers in a patient after SOT, but it likewise has led to the tailoring of preventive strategies for specific time periods and patients.[8]

The second major principle informing the understanding of infectious complications of SOT is that there is a defined set of key risk factors that predispose to infection in these children. These risk factors can be categorized as those present before transplantation, those relating to the transplant procedure itself, and postoperative risk factors that are influenced most heavily by the immunosuppression required to prevent rejection. A careful examination of these risk factors identifies the major differences in types and outcome of infection between pediatric and adult recipients.

Pretransplant Risk Factors

The age of the child at the time of undergoing SOT is an important factor that influences the types of infections they may experience after transplantation. Age impacts upon the chance of having had prior exposure to infectious agents. The presence of prior infection can have both negative and positive influences on the transplant recipient. For example, older candidates are more likely to have encountered pathogens that establish lifelong latent infection such as herpes simplex virus (HSV), cytomegalovirus (CMV), tuberculosis, as well as certain endemic fungi. This can be negative, as these microbes can reactivate under the pressure of immune suppression with significant clinical consequences. Accordingly, strategies have been developed to screen for or prevent reactivation of these potential pathogens following transplantation.[4–7] On the positive side, disease associated with reactivation of latent pathogens (or even reinfection with a new strain of a given latent pathogen) tends to be less aggressive than that associated with primary infection occurring after SOT, as the person has some baseline immunity.[4–9] In some cases (eg, Epstein-Barr virus [EBV]), this preexisting immunity provides a high degree of protection against clinical disease after transplantation.[9,10]

The age of a child at the time of SOT impacts on the likelihood that he or she will have acquired immunity against potential pathogens from natural infection. Certain pathogens appear to specifically cause infections in younger SOT recipients. For instance, children who receive a heart transplant before 2 years of age have been noted to be at increased risk for recurrent *Streptococcus pneumoniae* disease including bacteremia, even when they are older and have normal splenic function.[11] It is hypothesized that this may occur because of lack of normal antibody function.[12] Children receiving a transplant before 1 year of age often will not have had exposures to common respiratory pathogens until after transplantation. Respiratory syncytial virus (RSV), influenza, and parainfluenza have been shown to be more severe in the very young transplant recipient who is less than a year of age compared with older individuals.[13–15]

Age also impacts on the likelihood that children undergoing SOT will have had the opportunity to receive their full compliment of immunizations.[16–19] Accordingly, young children who receive a transplant before receiving their routine primary vaccinations will be at higher risk for vaccine-preventable infections. In addition, the authors have found that even with increasing age children who have underlying diseases that require transplantation often miss the opportunity to receive their age-appropriate vaccinations because of time spent in the hospital or primary attention being diverted from routine childhood care (Michaels MG, unpublished observation, 2009).

A second pretransplant factor influencing the risk of infectious complications following SOT is the underlying cause of organ dysfunction. The causes of organ failure in children are typically different than adults. Accordingly, this leads to differences in the risk of infection between pediatric and adult SOT recipients. For example, hepatitis C virus (HCV) is a leading cause of liver disease requiring transplantation in adults, but is rare in the pediatric population. For this reason, recurrent HCV infection following liver transplantation is not typically an issue in pediatric recipients. On the other hand, children are more likely to have congenital anomalies (eg, Biliary atresia) as a cause of end-stage liver disease. These malformations may predispose to recurrent episodes of infection (eg, cholangitis) that might predispose to infection with multidrug-resistant bacteria following the organ transplant. Congenital heart defects that require neonatal transplantation do so at a time when the child is particularly vulnerable to bacterial infections. For example, neonates requiring heart transplantation are at increased risk for mediastinitis caused by gram-negative bacteria compared with older children and adults.[20,21] Small bowel transplantation in childhood is more often associated with neonatal catastrophic events such as necrotizing enterocolitis from prematurity or complicated gastroschisis. These children have been hospitalized for significant periods of their life and have numerous prior intravascular line associated infections and exposures to antibiotics. Accordingly, they often are colonized with bacteria that have resistance to multiple antibiotics.[22]

Intraoperative Factors

In contrast to adult SOT recipients, pediatric patients more often receive organs from adult donors, with a resultant discrepancy in their size because of the relative paucity of pediatric donors. This size discrepancy can lead to an increased risk for anastomotic complications with the potential consequence of leakage, thrombosis, or necrosis, or the potential to leave the body cavity (abdomen or chest) open for a prolonged period of time. In these cases, the child is at an increased risk of bacteria and yeast infections postoperatively.[5,6,22]

Children are also at increased risk for donor-associated transmission of pathogens, as they more frequently lack immunity to this set of organisms. In particular, children are much more likely to be EBV seronegative before transplant, placing them at an increased likelihood of being in a mismatched state and at a marked increased risk of developing post-transplant lymphoproliferative disorders (PTLDs) compared with adult recipients. This in large part explains the much higher frequency of EBV/PTLDs observed in children compared with adults.[9,10,22–24] This is also true for CMV; accordingly primary CMV infections also are seen much more frequently in pediatric recipients compared with adult recipients.[23,25–29]

Post-transplant Risk Factors

As with adult recipients, immunosuppression is the major post-transplant risk factor for infection in children undergoing SOT. Unlike adults, this immunosuppressive therapy can have a substantial impact on growth and development, including the developing immune system. Children requiring higher levels of immune suppression because of rejection are at increased risk for developing more severe infection. This is true not only for common transplant associated pathogens (eg, CMV, EBV), but also for community-acquired viral pathogens such as RSV, parainfluenza, and influenza. Because children are more likely to be immunologically naïve to community pathogens, disease attributable to these agents tends to be more severe in children than adults.[5,6]

The general requirement for immunosuppression also results in decreased immunogenicity of vaccinations that are provided following SOT.[16–19,30–34] Although there are inadequate studies addressing the use of vaccines in pediatric SOT recipients, it is very likely that those children requiring higher levels of immune suppression are less likely to experience the full benefit of these vaccinations. Accordingly, they will be at increased risk of developing vaccine-associated diseases compared with both adults and children requiring lower levels of immunosuppression after transplant. Further, live virus vaccines remain generally contraindicated after transplant.[16–18,35] Although a growing number of transplant centers will administer varicella vaccine and measles-mumps-rubella vaccine after SOT, the numbers of children studied are small, and potential risks of vaccine-associated disease are not inconsequential.[36–39]

Finally, young children, whether immunosuppressed or not, are more likely than adults to share potentially infectious secretions with one another. Children who undergo SOT therefore are more likely to have infectious exposures from their siblings, playmates, and classmates. Their imperfect hygienic practices create an increased risk for exposure to community-acquired pathogens compared with adults.

Prevention

Recommendations for the prevention of infection following SOT are generally similar for both pediatric and adult organ transplant recipients.[4–7] Along with routine serologic screening for human immunodeficiency virus (HIV), hepatitis B virus (HBV), HCV, and syphilis, pediatric transplant centers should evaluate immunity to EBV, CMV, and HSV. In addition, organ candidates who are old enough to have been immunized or have had wild-type infection should have antibody measured against measles and varicella. Results of serologic assays should be interpreted, taking into account the potential of passive antibody presence from the mother (children under 12 to 15 months of age) or from blood products.

One important opportunity to improve post-transplant outcome can be accomplished during the pretransplant evaluation of potential pediatric candidates of SOT. A history of vaccination should be evaluated as early as possible in these candidates, and accelerated schedules should be encouraged to give them as many protective vaccines as possible before transplantation. Primary vaccine series can be started as early as 6 weeks of age and subsequent primary immunizations given every 4 weeks.[18,35] Varicella vaccination and measles-mumps-rubella vaccination should be given at least a month before transplantation.

Following SOT, children with herpes simplex seropositivity should be given acyclovir prophylaxis until the maximal period of immunosuppression has past (generally several months).[5,6] The decision to use prophylaxis against CMV versus virologic monitoring of patients at risk to inform pre-emptive antiviral therapy is similar to decisions used for adult recipients.[28,29,40] In contrast to adults, however, children are more likely to be at risk of developing primary CMV infection. Accordingly, many pediatric transplant centers will use chemoprophylaxis against CMV, as many experts believe this is the preferred strategy for high-risk mismatched patients (seronegative recipients of seropositive donors).[28,41] Finally, because most children are EBV seronegative, many centers have employed strategies of EBV viral load monitoring to inform preemptive reductions in immune suppression in an effort to prevent complications associated with this pathogen.[42,43]

HEMATOPOIETIC STEM CELL TRANSPLANTATION

Replacement of the bone marrow in children can be as a rescue measure after intense chemotherapy or radiation required to eradicate certain malignancies, or for replacement of a deficient bone marrow as seen with primary immune deficiencies, primary bone marrow failure, inborn errors of metabolism, or an assortment of genetic disorders.[44–46] Overall, there are fewer differences in the infections seen between pediatric and adult hematopoietic stem cell transplantation (HSCT) than that for SOT, since both adults and children are rendered immunologically naïve in preparation for the transplant. The source of cells can be autologous (from the individual's own cells) or allogeneic (from another person), and it can be from bone marrow (related or unrelated), peripheral blood that has been stimulated to be enriched for stem cells, or from cord blood. The risk for infection varies with both the underlying reason for HSCT and with the type of donor used, as well as how the cells have been prepared. For example, people undergoing autologous HSCT will have risks for infection before engraftment but fewer risks afterwards. Patients receiving HSCT with a T-cell depleted stem cell product may have less risk of graft-versus-host disease (GVHD) but some increased risk of infection. Cord blood transplants may take longer to engraft, with concomitant increased risks for infection during the pre-engraftment period. In addition to these risk factors, both GVHD and the medications to prevent or treat GVHD put the child at risk for infections. Finally, infections following HSCT can be classified according to specific time periods after transplantation similar to SOT recipients.[44–46] These time periods include the pretransplantation period, pre-engraftment period (0 to 1 month), postengraftment period (1 to 3 months), and the late post-transplantation period (>3 months). Children and adults have specific defects in host defenses that vary during these periods and predispose to infection. The presence of indwelling catheters or mucositis that may occur secondary to radiation or chemotherapy interrupts the normal anatomic barriers creating defects in this important host defense that may be present anytime following transplantation but tend to predominate in the early periods.

Pretransplantation Period

Children come to HSCT with various underlying diseases, differing exposures to chemotherapy, and variable histories of prior infections and amount of immunosuppression. Infections that are present in these children before transplantation, whether because of neutropenia or bone marrow dysfunction from immune or genetic disorders, or the presence of invasive catheters, should be recognized and addressed prior to transplantation. During the pretransplant period, children undergoing autologous HSCT are at similar risk for infection as those undergoing allogeneic transplantation, as the major risks during this period are neutropenia and breaks in the normal barriers of the skin and oropharyngeal and gastrointestinal (GI) mucous membranes.[47] Infection with circulating community viral infections (RSV, influenza, adenovirus) can have an important negative impact.[48–51] Accordingly, having infection control policies to prevent the spread of viruses to these children is imperative.

Pre-engraftment Period

During this period, neutropenia and breeches in the normal anatomic barriers of the body comprise the greatest risk factors for infection. Bacterial infections predominate, with bacteremia being the most commonly documented. Both gram-positive and gram-negative organisms occur. Gram-negative bacilli increase in frequency when the mucosal lining of the GI tract is interrupted.[44–47] Oral mucositis predisposes to the presence of *S viridans,* which can be associated with antibiotic resistance.[44–47,52] Likewise, the presence of extended-spectrum β-lactamase production in the gram-negative bacilli is being noted increasingly.[45,46] Fungal infections occurring during this phase most often are caused by *Candida* species, but *Aspergillus* subspecies are increased in frequency with prolonged neutropenia. More recently, mucormycosis also has been identified in those who have had prolonged neutropenia before HSCT.[53–56]

Viral infections also occur during the pre-engraftment period. Although reactivation of HSV is observed commonly after HSCT in adults,[57] it is less frequent in children, who are less frequently seropositive before transplantation. As noted in the section concerning prevention, children who have had prior infection with HSV should receive prophylaxis to prevent reactivation. Nosocomial or community exposures to circulating viral pathogens represent an important potential source of infection for these children.[48–51] There is growing evidence that community-acquired viruses cause increased morbidity and mortality for HSCT recipients during this time period. Adenovirus is a particularly important viral pathogen that may present earlier in children, although it typically presents after engraftment.[58–60]

Postengraftment Period

The predominant defect in host defenses in the early phase after engraftment is altered cell-mediated immunity.[46] Infectious risks are potentiated by the presence of GVHD. This risk is especially accentuated 50 to 100 days after HSCT, when host immunity is lost and donor immunity is not yet established.[44–46] Opportunistic pathogens predominate during this time period. Without the use of appropriate prophylaxis *Pneumocystis jiroveci* pneumonia presents in this phase early after engraftment.[61] *Aspergillus* is a prominent cause of fungal infection during this period; in addition, other opportunistic mycoses also are being recognized increasingly.[53,55,56] Hepatosplenic candidiasis frequently presents during the postengraftment period, although seeding likely occurred during the neutropenic phase.[62] Reactivation of *Toxoplasma gondii*, a rare cause of disease among pediatric HSCT recipients, also may present after engraftment.[63]

CMV is one of the most important causes of morbidity and mortality among HSCT recipients, and it typically presents during this early postengraftment phase; it is covered in detail in an article on CMV in this journal. Although primary infection from the donor can cause disease, the most prominent problems from CMV after HSCT are caused by reactivation in an HSCT recipient whose donor was naïve to the virus.[64–66] For this reason, the older HSCT patient is at greater risk by virtue of more likely having acquired CMV before transplantation. Disease risk from CMV after HSCT also is increased in recipients of donors who are unrelated, or T-cell depleted and children whose course is complicated by GVHD.[44–46,65] Similar to adults, children with CMV disease present with fevers, with or without associated symptoms including hepatitis, esophagitis, or gastroenteritis, and life-threatening interstitial pneumonitis. Asymptomatic shedding or viremia also can occur. Prophylaxis and monitoring with institution of pre-emptive treatment have helped to decrease the risk of serious fatal disease.[67,68]

Adenovirus is the second most important viral infection during this period in children undergoing HSCT, causing disease in approximately 30% of stem cell recipients.[44] Similar to CMV, children receiving grafts from HLA-matched donors or cord blood cell transplants have an increased risk for disease, along with those who had total body irradiation.[44,45] Polyomaviruses, such as BK virus, are recognized as a cause of hemorrhagic cystitis and renal dysfunction following HSCT.[44,45] Nosocomial acquisition of circulating community-acquired pathogens likewise can occur during this time period.

Late Post-transplantation Period

Late after HSCT, in the absence of GVHD, infections are less of a problem. When present, however, chronic GVHD significantly affects the humoral and cell-mediated immune function and causes a breakdown of some anatomic barriers such as is seen with chronic GVHD of the GI tract or lungs. Encapsulated bacteria such as *S pneumoniae* and *Haemophilus influenzae* have been noted to cause disease during this period.[44–47] Viral infections, in particular reactivation of varicella–zoster virus (VZV), also accounts for infections during this time period.[44–46] Fungal infections are less frequent during the late post-transplantation time period.

Prevention

Similar to preventive strategies for children who are going to undergo SOT, children being evaluated for HSCT should have a thorough history reviewed of their past infections and their risk for infections. Also similar to SOT, many of the decisions on prophylaxis have been derived from studies in adult recipients. Serology should be obtained to determine the prior presence of latent or persistent viruses such as members of the herpesvirus family (HSV, VZV, CMV, EBV), HIV, HBV, HCV, hepatitis A virus (HAV), and syphilis. Many centers also will screen for antibody against *T gondii,* because it can reactivate in seropositive individuals. Similar to adults, the use of prophylaxis is advised to prevent reactivation of specific viruses such as HSV. For those with past disease, acyclovir (either intravenously or orally depending on the patient's clinical status) should be used during the highest periods of immunosuppression. A study in adults suggests a year of prophylaxis is beneficial without adverse side effects.[69] This therapy is also useful for prophylaxis against reactivation of varicella. Although prophylaxis against CMV is efficacious, ganciclovir (the best studied medication) is toxic to the bone marrow. Accordingly, many centers opt to use a stringent monitoring protocol and institute pre-emptive treatment when the viral load is positive.[46,70] Children who are negative for CMV before HSCT also should receive leukocyte-reduced blood products in an effort to avoid exposure to and infection with this pathogen.[46]

Fungal prophylaxis and bacterial prophylaxis usually are instituted during the period of neutropenia with variation on the specific type of drug based on the infectious disease history of the individual child and the type of HSCT he or she is receiving (eg, autologous vs allogeneic).[44–46,71,72] Intravenous immunoglobulin use is somewhat controversial. However, it is used at many centers through the early engraftment phase or when there is significant chronic GVHD.[44–46] Trimethoprim sulfamethoxazole is the mostly widely employed prophylaxis against *P jiroveci* pneumonia (PCP). Because of myelosuppression associated with its use, it usually is given before HSCT and then held until engraftment, at which time it is reinstituted.[44–46]

Vaccination is particularly important among children undergoing HSCT as they may not have even had their full complement of primary vaccines before beginning chemotherapy. The timing to restart vaccination after HCST is based on the risk of disease, the ability for the immune system to respond to the antigen, and the safety of the vaccine. These issues are impacted upon by the type of transplant and donor's immunity, the presence of ongoing GVHD, and the use of passive immunoglobulin. In general, the recipient will acquire the immunity that is found in the donor. Antibody titers to vaccine antigens, however, tend not be long-lasting, and repeat vaccination is warranted.[44–46] Live virus vaccines are the ones that have the potential to cause serious vaccine-associated disease when given to an immunosuppressed host. Recommendations do exist to repeat or reissue non-live vaccines at 12, 14, and 24 months after HSCT.[35,44–46] Studies in children who have undergone HSCT show that vaccinations against measles, mumps, and rubella as a single vaccine have been given safely to children 2 years after HSCT if they do not have chronic GVHD or receipt of ongoing immunosuppressive medication.[35,44,45] While these recommendations are set forward, some experts believe that rather than having one guideline for all HSCT recipients, recommendations should be individualized based on the ability of a particular recipient to mount a response.

SUMMARY

In summary, children undergoing SOT and HSCT are at risk of developing infectious complications following these procedures. Although these children may experience similar types and timing of infections as adults undergoing transplantation, their younger age, lack of immunologic experience, and potential increased likelihood of exposure to community-acquired pathogens require careful attention to the differences in infectious diseases seen in pediatric transplant recipients compared with adults undergoing these procedures.

REFERENCES

1. Available at: http://www.optn.transplant.hrsa.gov/latestData/rptData.asp. Accessed August 30, 2009.
2. Boucek MM, Aurora P, Edwards LB, et al. Registry of the international society for heart and lung transplantation: tenth official pediatric heart transplantation report—2007. J Heart Lung Transplant 2007;8:796–807.
3. Available at: http://www.ustransplant.org/csr/current/nationalViewer.aspx?o=KI&t=11. Accessed January 9, 2009.
4. Fishman JA. Infection in solid organ transplant recipients. N Engl J Med 2007; 357:2601.
5. Green M, Michaels MG. Infections in solid organ transplant recipients. In: Long SS, Prober CG, Pickering LK, editors. Principles & practice of pediatric infectious diseases. 3rd edition. New York: Churchill Livingstone; 2008. p. 551–7.
6. Keough WL, Michaels MG. Infectious complications in pediatric solid organ transplantation. Pediatr Clin North Am 2003;50(6):1451–69.
7. Fishman JA, Rubin RH. Infection in organ-transplant recipients. N Engl J Med 1998;338(24):1741–51.

8. Green M, Michaels MG. Infectious complications of immunosuppressive medications in organ transplant recipients. Pediatr Infect Dis J 2007;26:443–4.
9. Green M, Michaels MG, Webber SA, et al. The management of Epstein-Barr virus associated post-transplant lymphoproliferative disorders in pediatric solid organ transplant recipients. Pediatr Transplant 1999;3(4):271–81.
10. Boyle GJ, Michaels MG, Webber SA, et al. Post-transplant lymphoproliferative disorders in pediatric thoracic organ recipients. J Pediatr 1997;131:309–13.
11. Stovall SH, Ainley KA, Mason EO Jr, et al. Invasive pneumococcal infections in pediatric cardiac transplant patients. Pediatr Infect Dis J 2001;20(10):946–50.
12. Gennery AR, Cant AJ, Baldwin CI, et al. Characterization of the impaired anti-pneumococcal polysaccharide antibody production in immunosuppressed pediatric patients following cardiac transplantation. J Clin Immunol 2001;21:43–50.
13. Pohl C, Green M, Wald ER, et al. Respiratory syncytial virus infections in pediatric liver transplant recipients. J Infect Dis 1992;165(1):166–9.
14. Apalsch AM, Green M, Ledesma-Medina J, et al. Parainfluenza and influenza virus infections in pediatric organ transplant recipients. Clin Infect Dis 1995;20(2):394–9.
15. Green M, Michaels MG. Community-acquired respiratory viruses. Amer J Transplantation 2004;4:S105–9.
16. Burroughs M, Moscona A. Immunization of pediatric solid organ transplant candidates and recipients. Clin Infect Dis 2000;30(6):857–69.
17. Campbell AL, Herold BC. Immunization of pediatric solid organ transplantation candidates: immunizations in transplant candidates. Pediatr Transplant 2005;9(5):652–61.
18. Avery RK, Michaels MG. Update on immunizations in solid organ transplant recipients: what clinicians need to know. Amer J Transplantation 2008;1:9–14.
19. Benden C, Danziger-Isakov LA, Astor T, et al. Variability in immunization guidelines in children before and after lung transplantation. Pediatr Transplant 2007;11:882–7.
20. Webber SA, Fricker FJ, Michaels M, et al. Orthotopic heart transplantation in children with congenital heart disease. Ann Thorac Surg 1994;58:1664–9.
21. Doelling NR, Kanter KR, Sullivan KM, et al. Medium-term results of pediatric patients undergoing orthotopic heart transplantation. J Heart Lung Transpl 1997;16(12):1225–30.
22. Green M, Bueno J, Sigurdsson L, et al. Unique aspects of the infectious complications of intestinal transplantation. Curr Opin Organ Transplant 1999;4:361–7.
23. Breinig MK, Zitelli B, Starzl TE, et al. Epstein-Barr virus, cytomegalovirus, and other viral infections in children after liver transplantation. J Infect Dis 1987;156(2):273–9.
24. Paya CV, Fung JJ, Nalesnik MA, et al. Epstein-Barr virus-induced post-transplant lymphoproliferative disorders. ASTS/ASTP EBV-PTLD Task Force and The Mayo Clinic Organized International Consensus Development Meeting. Transplantation 1999;68(10):1517–25.
25. Allen U, Herbert D, Moore D, et al. Canadian PTLD Survey Group--1998. Epstein Barr virus-related post-transplant lymphoproliferative disease in solid organ transplant recipients, 1988–97: a Canadian multi-center experience. Pediatr Transplant 2001;5(3):198–203.
26. Danziger-Isakov LA, Worley S, Michaels MG, et al. The risk, prevention & outcome of cytomegalovirus after pediatric lung transplantation. Transplantation 2009;87(10):1541–8.

27. Bowman JS, Green M, Scantlebury VP. OKT3 and viral disease in pediatric liver transplant recipients. Clin Transplant 1991;5:294–300.
28. Preiksaitis JK, Brennan DC, Fishman J, et al. Canadian society of transplantation consensus workshop on cytomegalovirus management in solid organ transplantation final report. Amer J Transpl 2005;5(2):218–27.
29. Green M, Michaels MG. Pre-emptive therapy of CMV disease in pediatric transplant recipients. Pediatr Infect Dis J 2000;19:875–7.
30. Blumberg EA, Brozena SC, Stutman P, et al. Immunogenicity of pneumococcal vaccine in heart transplant recipients. Clin Infect Dis 2001;32(2):307–10.
31. McCashland TM, Preheim LC, Gentry MJ. Pneumococcal vaccine response in cirrhosis and liver transplantation. J Infect Dis 2000;181(2):757–60.
32. Blumberg EA, Albano C, Pruett T, et al. The immunogenicity of influenza virus vaccine in solid organ transplant recipients. Clin Infect Dis 1996;22(2): 295–302.
33. Kumar D, Welsh B, Siegal D, et al. Immunogenicity of pneumococcal vaccine in renal transplant recipients—three-year follow-up of a randomized trial. Am J Transplant 2007;7(3):633–8.
34. Lin PL, Michaels MG, Green M, et al. Safety and immunogenicity of the American Academy of Pediatrics—recommended sequential pneumococcal conjugate and polysaccharide vaccine schedule in pediatric solid organ transplant recipients. Pediatrics 2005;116(1):160–7.
35. American Academy of Pediatrics. Immunizations. In: Pickering LK, editor. Red book: 2009 report of the Committee on Infectious Diseases. 28th editon. Elk Grove Village (IL): American Academy of Pediatrics; 2009. p. 68–104.
36. Weinberg A, Horslen SP, Kaufman SS, et al. Safety and immunogenicity of varicella-zoster virus vaccine in pediatric liver and intestine transplant recipients. Am J Transplant 2006;6(3):565–8.
37. Khan S, Erlichman J, Rand EB. Live virus immunization after orthotopic liver transplantation. Pediatr Transplant 2006;10(1):78–82.
38. Kraft JN, Shaw JC. Varicella infection caused by Oka strain vaccine in a heart transplant recipient. Arch Dermatol 2006;142(7):943–5.
39. Levitsky J, Te HS, Faust TW, et al. Varicella infection following varicella vaccination in a liver transplant recipient. Am J Transplant 2002;2(9):880–2.
40. Humar A, Siegal D, Moussa G, et al. A prospective assessment of valganciclovir for the treatment of cytomegalovirus infection and disease in transplant recipients. J Infect Dis 2005;192(7):1154–7.
41. Danziger-Isakov LA, Faro A, Sweet S, et al. Variability in standard care for cytomegalovirus prevention in pediatric lung transplantation: survey of eight pediatric lung transplant programs. Pediatr Transplant 2003;7:469–73.
42. Green M, Webber SA. EBV viral load monitoring: unanswered questions. Am J Transplant 2002;2:894–5.
43. Lee TC, Savoldo B, Rooney CM, et al. Quantitative EBV viral loads and immunosuppression alterations can decrease PTLD incidence in pediatric liver transplant recipients. Am J Transplant 2005;5(9):2222–8.
44. Lujan-Zibermann L. Infections in hematopoietic stem cell transplant recipients. In: Long SS, Prober CG, Pickering LK, editors. Principles & practice of pediatric infectious diseases. 3rd edition. New York: Churchill Livingstone; 2008. p. 558–62.
45. Patrick CC. Opportunistic infections in hematopoietic stem cell transplantation. In: Feigin R, Cherry JD, Demmler G, et al, editors. Textbook of pediatric infectious diseases. 6th edition. Philadelphia: WB Saunders; 2009. p. 1037–47.

46. Centers for Disease Control and Prevention (CDC). Guidelines for preventing opportunistic infections among hematopoietic stem cell transplant recipients. MMWR Recomm Rep 2000;49:1–125.
47. Mullen CA, Nair J, Sandesh S, et al. Fever and neutropenia in pediatric hematopoietic stem cell transplant patients. Bone Marrow Transplant 2000;25: 59–65.
48. Champlin RE, Whimbey E. Community respiratory virus infections in bone marrow transplant recipients: the M.D. Anderson Cancer Center experience. Biol Blood Marrow Transplant 2001;7(Suppl):8S.
49. Couch RB, Englund JA, Whimbey E. Respiratory viral infections in immunocompetent and immunocompromised persons. Am J Med 1997;102:2.
50. Bowden RA. Respiratory virus infections after marrow transplantation: The Fred Hutchison Cancer Research Center Experience. Am J Med 1997;102:27.
51. Ljungman P. Respiratory virus infections in bone marrow transplant recipients: the European perspective. Am J Med 1997;102:44.
52. Bochud PY, Calandra T, Francioli P. Bacteremia due to viridans streptococci in neutropenic patients: a review. Am J Med 1994;97:256.
53. Meyers JD. Fungal infections in bone marrow transplant patients. Semin Oncol 1990;17:10.
54. Zollner-Schwetz I, Auner HW, Paulitsch A, et al. Oral and intestinal *Candida* colonization in patients undergoing hematopoietic stem-cell transplantation. J Infect Dis 2008;198:150.
55. Boutati EI, Anaissie EJ. Fusarium, a significant emerging pathogen in patients with hematologic malignancy: ten years' experience at a cancer center and implications for management. Blood 1997;90:999.
56. Morrison VA, Haake RJ, Weisdorf DJ. Non-*Candida* fungal infections after bone marrow transplantation: risk factors and outcome. Am J Med 1994;96: 497.
57. Wingard JR. Infections in allogeneic bone marrow transplant recipients. Semin Oncol 1993;20:80.
58. Wasserman R, August CS, Plotkin SA. Viral infections in pediatric bone marrow transplant patients. Pediatr Infect Dis J 1988;7:109.
59. Shields AF, Hackman RC, Fife KH, et al. Adenovirus infections in patients undergoing bone-marrow transplantation. N Engl J Med 1985;312:529.
60. Hale GA, Helsop HE, Krance RA, et al. Adenovirus infection after pediatric bone marrow transplantation. Bone Marrow Transplant 1999;23:277–82.
61. De Castro N, Neuville S, Sarfati C, et al. Occurrence of *Pneumocystis jiroveci* pneumonia after allogeneic stem cell transplantation: a 6-year retrospective study. Bone Marrow Transplant 2005;36:879.
62. Klingspor L, Stintzing G, Fasth A, et al. Deep *Candida* infection in children receiving allogeneic bone marrow transplants: incidence, risk factors and diagnosis. Bone Marrow Transplant 1996;17:1043–9.
63. Slavin MA, Meyers JD, Remington JS, et al. *Toxoplasma gondii* infection in marrow transplant recipients: a 20-year experience. Bone Marrow Transplant 1994;13(5):549–57.
64. Boeckh M, Bowden RA, Goodrich JM, et al. Cytomegalovirus antigen detection in peripheral blood leukocytes after allogeneic marrow transplantation. Blood 1992; 80:1358.
65. Enright H, Haake R, Weisdorf D, et al. Cytomegalovirus pneumonia after bone marrow transplantation. Risk factors and response to therapy. Transplantation 1993;55:1339.

66. Meyers JD, Ljungman P, Fisher LD. Cytomegalovirus excretion as a predictor of cytomegalovirus disease after marrow transplantation: importance of cytomegalovirus viremia. J Infect Dis 1990;162:373.
67. Schmidt GM, Horak DA, Niland JC, et al. Randomized controlled trial of prophylactic ganciclovir for cytomegalovirus pulmonary infection in recipients of allogeneic bone marrow transplants. N Engl J Med 1991;324(15):1005–11.
68. Goodrich JM, Bowden RA, Fisher L, et al. Ganciclovir prophylaxis to prevent cytomegalovirus disease after allogeneic marrow transplant. Ann Intern Med 1993; 118(3):173–8.
69. Erard V, Wald A, Corey L, et al. Use of long-term suppressive acyclovir after hematopoietic stem-cell transplantation: impact on herpes simplex virus (HSV) disease and drug-resistant HSV disease. J Infect Dis 2007;196:266.
70. Boeckh M, Leisenring W, Riddell SR, et al. Late cytomegalovirus disease and mortality in recipients of allogeneic hematopoietic stem cell transplants: importance of viral load and T-cell immunity. Blood 2003;101:407.
71. Marr KA, Siedel K, Slavin MA, et al. Prolonged fluconazole propylaxis is associated with persistent protection against candidiasis-related death in allogeneic marrow transplant recipients: long-term follow-up of a randomized, placebo-controlled trial. Blood 2000;96:2055.
72. Slavin MA, Osborne B, Adams R, et al. Efficacy and safety of fluconazole prophylaxis for fungal infections after marrow transplantation—a prospective, randomized, double-blind study. J Infect Dis 1995;171:1545.

Cytomegalovirus in Hematopoietic Stem Cell Transplant Recipients

Per Ljungman, MD, PhD[a,b,*], Morgan Hakki, MD[c],
Michael Boeckh, MD[d,e]

KEYWORDS

- Adoptive immunotherapy • Antiviral therapy • Cytomegalovirus
- Hematopoietic stem cell transplantation

Human cytomegalovirus (CMV) is a betaherpesvirus in the same family as human herpesvirus-6 and -7. CMV is a large virus including approximately 200 proteins. CMV has been found in a wide range of cells, including endothelial cells, epithelial cells, blood cells including neutrophils, and smooth muscle cells.[1] The presence of CMV in these cells may be caused by active replication within the cell, phagocytosis of CMV proteins, or abortive (incomplete) replication, and likely contributes to dissemination and transmission. As the other herpesviruses, CMV remains in the human body after primary infection for life. Little is known about the site or mechanisms of CMV latency and persistence. Several studies indicate that cells of the granulocyte-monocyte lineage carry CMV[2–4] and these might be one site for latency and persistence. Transplantation of solid organs clearly can transmit CMV, so it is possible that cells other than those mentioned can harbor and transmit the virus. Whether the infected cell type in these organs is blood cells, macrophages, or other cell types, however, has not been clarified.

T-cell mediated cellular immunity is the most important factor in controlling CMV replication. CMV induces a strong CD8+ cytotoxic T-lymphocyte (CTL) response,

Per Ljungman had support from the Karolinska Institute research funds, the European Leukemia Net, and the Swedish Children's Cancer Fund. Michael Boeckh had support from the National Institute of Health (NIH CA 18029).

[a] Department of Hematology, Karolinska University Hospital, S-14186 Stockholm, Sweden
[b] Divison of Hematology, Department of Medicine Huddinge, Karolinska Institutet, S-14186 Stockholm, Sweden
[c] Division of Infectious Diseases, Oregon Health and Science University, Portland, OR, USA
[d] University of Washington, Seattle, WA, USA
[e] Vaccine and Infectious Disease Institute, Fred Hutchinson Cancer Research Center, 1100 Fairview Avenue N, Seattle, WA 98109–4417, USA
* Corresponding author. Division of Hematology, Department of Medicine Huddinge, Karolinska Institutet, S-14186 Stockholm, Sweden.
E-mail address: Per.Ljungman@ki.se

Infect Dis Clin N Am 24 (2010) 319–337
doi:10.1016/j.idc.2010.01.008 id.theclinics.com
0891-5520/10/$ – see front matter © 2010 Elsevier Inc. All rights reserved.

and the proportion of circulating CD8+ T cells in healthy individuals that are specific for CMV antigens ranges from 10% to 40% increasing with age.[5–10] Several CMV proteins are targeted by the CD8+ T-cell response including IE-1, IE-2, and pp65.[7,10–16] Lack of CMV-specific CD8+ CTL responses predisposes to CMV infection, whereas reconstitution of CMV-specific CD8+ CTL responses after hematopoietic cell transplantation correlates with protection from CMV and improved outcome of CMV disease.[17–21] After hematopoietic stem cell transplantation (HSCT), CMV-specific CD4+ responses are associated with protection from CMV disease.[17,22–24] The lack of CMV-specific CD4+ cells is associated with late CMV disease and death in patients who have undergone HSCT.[25] The role of humoral immunity in controlling CMV replication is not clear. Although antibodies to gB and gH can neutralize the virus in cell culture, they do not seem to prevent primary infection in adults, but rather may function to limit disease severity.[26,27]

The innate immune system also seems to be involved in controlling CMV replication. CMV triggers cellular inflammatory cytokine production on binding to the target cell, mediated in part by the interaction of gB and gH with toll-like receptor 2.[28–30] Polymorphisms in toll-like receptor 2 have been associated with CMV infection after liver transplantation.[31] In humans, natural killer cell responses increase during CMV infection after renal transplantation, and a deficiency in natural killer cells is associated with severe CMV infection (among other herpesviruses).[32,33] The genotype of the donor-activating killer immunoglobulin-like receptor, which regulates NK cell function, has recently been demonstrated to influence the development of CMV infection after allogeneic HSCT.[34–36] Finally, polymorphisms in chemokine receptor 5 and interleukin-10 have been associated with CMV disease, whereas polymorphisms in monocyte chemoattractant protein 1 are associated with reactivation after allogeneic HSCT.[37]

DIAGNOSTIC METHODS

The serologic determination of CMV-specific antibodies (IgG and IgM) is important for determining a patient's risk for CMV infection after transplantation but cannot be used for the diagnosis of CMV infection or disease. Growth of CMV in tissue culture takes several weeks, making this technique obsolete for diagnosis of CMV in HSCT recipients. The shell vial (rapid culture/DEAFF) technique, in which monoclonal antibodies are used to detect CMV immediate-early proteins in cultured cells, is not sensitive enough to use for routine blood monitoring,[38] but is highly useful on bronchoalveolar lavage (BAL) fluid in the diagnosis of CMV pneumonia.[39]

The detection of the CMV pp65 in peripheral blood leukocytes (antigenemia) is a rapid and semiquantitative method of diagnosing CMV infection. A positive CMV pp65 assay is predictive for the development of invasive disease in transplant patients.[40,41]

Polymerase chain reaction (PCR) is the most sensitive method for detecting CMV.[42] Quantitative PCR (qPCR) relies on the amplification and quantitative measurement of CMV DNA, while at the same time maintaining high specificity. High levels of DNA in blood (whole blood or plasma) is a good predictor of CMV disease in HSCT recipients.[25,43–46] Although PCR has been used on BAL fluid,[47] viral-load cut-offs have not been defined, and although the sensitivity and negative predictive values are very high, the specificity and positive predictive values are not known.

The detection of CMV mRNA by nucleic acid sequence-based amplification on blood samples is similarly useful as DNA qPCR or pp65 antigenemia for guiding preemptive therapy after HSCT.[48,49] This method is less frequently used, however, compared with the other techniques.

The presence of characteristic CMV "owl's eye" nuclear inclusions in histopathology specimens is useful in the diagnosis of invasive CMV disease. This method has relatively low sensitivity, but can be enhanced by use of immunohistochemical techniques.

CLINICAL MANIFESTATIONS

CMV infection is defined as the detection of CMV, typically by DNA PCR, pp65 antigenemia, or mRNA nucleic acid sequence-based amplification, from plasma or whole blood in a CMV-seronegative patient (primary infection) or a CMV-seropositive patient (reactivation of latent or persistent virus or superinfection with another strain of CMV).[50,51] International definitions of CMV disease, requiring the presence of symptoms and signs compatible with CMV end-organ involvement together with the detection of CMV using a validated method in the appropriate clinical specimen, have been published.[52] Almost any organ can be involved in CMV disease. Fever is a common manifestation, but may be absent in patients receiving high-dose immunosuppression.

CMV pneumonia is the most serious manifestation of CMV in HSCT recipients with a mortality of more than 50%.[53–55] CMV pneumonia often manifests with fever, nonproductive cough, hypoxia, and infiltrates commonly interstitial on radiography. The diagnosis of CMV pneumonia is established by detection of CMV by shell-vial, culture, or histology in BAL or lung biopsy specimens, in the presence of compatible clinical signs and symptoms. Pulmonary shedding of CMV is common, and CMV detection in BAL from asymptomatic patients who underwent routine BAL screening at day 35 after HSCT was predictive of subsequent CMV pneumonia in only approximately two thirds of cases.[56] The presence of CMV in a BAL specimen in the absence of clinical evidence of CMV disease is not proof of CMV pneumonia, but the patient needs to be carefully followed. The relevance of PCR testing on BAL fluid is doubtful because there are little data correlating CMV DNA detection by PCR in BAL fluid with CMV pneumonia. Because of the high negative predictive value afforded by its high sensitivity, however, a negative PCR result can be used to rule out the diagnosis of CMV pneumonia.[47] It is possible that qPCR on BAL might provide additional information, allowing this technique to be used for the diagnosis of CMV pneumonia in the future.

CMV can affect the entire gastrointestinal (GI) tract. Ulcers extending deep into the submucosal layers are seen on endoscopy, but can be macroscopically confused with other disorders including graft-versus-host disease (GVHD) and adenovirus disease. The diagnosis of GI disease relies on detection of CMV in biopsy specimens by culture or histology and can occur in the absence of CMV detection in the blood, even by PCR.[57,58] CMV and GVHD are also frequently seen concomitantly, making the assessment of each disorder's contribution to the symptomatology difficult.

Retinitis is relatively uncommon after transplantation, although its incidence seems to be increasing.[59–62] Decreased visual acuity and blurred vision are early symptoms, and approximately 60% of patients have involvement of both eyes.[60] Untreated, the risk for loss of vision on the affected eye is high. Other manifestations including hepatitis and encephalitis do occur, but are rare.

RISK FACTORS

Allogeneic HSCT Recipients

In allogeneic HSCT recipients, the most important risk factors for CMV disease are the serologic status of the donor and recipient. CMV-seronegative patients receiving stem cells from a CMV-seronegative donor (D-/R-) have a very low risk of primary infection if CMV-safe blood products are used. Approximately 30% of seronegative recipients transplanted from a seropositive donor (D+/R-) develop primary CMV infection. Although the risk of CMV disease is low because of preemptive treatment of CMV infection, mortality caused by bacterial and fungal infections in these patients is higher than in similarly matched D-/R- transplants (18.3% vs 9.7%, respectively),[63] possibly because of the immunosuppressive effects of CMV or its therapy.

Without prophylaxis, approximately 80% of CMV-seropositive patients experience CMV infection after allogeneic HSCT. Current preventive strategies have decreased the incidence of CMV disease, which had historically occurred in 20% to 35% of these patients.[64] Although a CMV-seropositive recipient is at higher risk for transplant-related mortality than a seronegative recipient,[65,66] the impact of donor serostatus on nonrelapse mortality and survival when the recipient is seropositive remains controversial.[67–78] This combination, however, has been reported as a risk factor for delayed CMV-specific immune reconstitution,[79–82] repeated CMV reactivations,[80,83] late CMV recurrence,[84] and development of CMV disease.[46,80,85]

Other risk factors for CMV infection after allogeneic HSCT include the use of high-dose corticosteroids, T-cell depletion, acute and chronic GVHD, and the use of mismatched or unrelated donors.[43,46,85–89] The use of sirolimus for GVHD prophylaxis seems to have a protective effect against CMV infection, possibly because of the inhibition of cellular signaling pathways that are co-opted by CMV during infection for synthesis of viral proteins.[85,90] The use of nonmyeloablative conditioning regimens generally has been reported to result in a lower rate of CMV infection and disease early after HSCT compared with standard myeloablative regimens.[87,91] By 1 year after HSCT, however, the risks of CMV infection and disease are comparable.[91,92] Umbilical cord blood transplantation (CBT) is an increasingly used technology for HSCT.[93] Because most infants are born without CMV infection, the transplanted allograft is almost always CMV-negative. Among CMV-seropositive recipients who do not receive antiviral prophylaxis, the rate of CMV infection after CBT is 40% to 80%, with one study reporting 100%.[94–98] When patients receive prophylaxis with high-dose valacyclovir after CBT, it does not seem that CBT entails a significantly greater risk of CMV infection and disease than does peripheral blood stem cell or bone marrow transplantation.[89]

Alemtuzumab is an anti-CD52 monoclonal antibody that results in CD4+ and CD8+ lymphopenia that can last for up to 9 months after administration. Patients who received alemtuzumab experienced a higher rate of CMV infection compared with matched controls not receiving alemtuzumab.[99,100]

Late CMV Infection After Allogeneic HSCT

Today, with the use of preemptive ganciclovir therapy, CMV disease has become a more significant problem after day 100 following allogeneic HSCT.[25,84,101] The risk varies a lot between different centers, presumably because of factors related to patient and donor selection and the choices of transplantation modalities used at the different centers (stem cell source, GVHD prophylaxis and treatment, conditioning regimens). Late CMV infection is strongly associated with nonrelapse mortality.[84] Several factors predict the development of late CMV disease[17,23,25,84,86] and extended monitoring and antiviral therapy are warranted in patients with risk factors to reduce the risk.[25,91,102]

Autologous HSCT

After autologous HSCT, approximately 40% of seropositive patients develop CMV infection.[53,103] Although CMV disease is rare after autologous HSCT,[104–107] the outcome of CMV pneumonia is similar to that after allogeneic HSCT.[53,108,109] Risk factors for CMV disease after autologous HSCT include CD34+ selection, high-dose corticosteroids, and the use of total-body irradiation or fludarabine as part of the conditioning regimen.[106]

PREVENTION OF CMV INFECTION AND DISEASE

CMV serology should be assessed as early as possible when a patient is considered a candidate for HSCT and safe blood products should be used in CMV-seronegative candidates to reduce the risk for primary CMV infection. To reduce the risk for transmission of CMV, blood products from CMV-seronegative donors or leukocyte-reduced, filtered blood products should be used.[110–112] Recipients who are CMV seronegative before allogeneic HSCT should ideally receive a graft from a CMV-negative donor. Weighing the factor of donor CMV serostatus compared with other relevant donor factors, such as HLA-match, is difficult. No data exist indicating whether HLA-matching is more important compared with CMV serostatus in affecting a good outcome for the patient. For lesser degrees of mismatch, (allele-mismatches or mismatches on HLA-C, DQ, or DP), the CMV serostatus of the donor should be considered in the selection process.

Intravenous immunoglobulin (IVIG) is not reliably effective as prophylaxis against primary CMV infection. Likewise, the effect of immunoglobulin on reducing CMV infection in seropositive patients is modest.[113–118] The prophylactic use of immunoglobulin is not recommended. Future possibilities for prevention might include a CMV vaccine, and different vaccines are currently in development.[119]

Antiviral Prophylaxis and Preemptive Therapy

Antiviral prophylaxis is defined as the routine administration of an antiviral agent to all patients at risk. Preemptive therapy is initiated when CMV infection is detected, but before the development of CMV-associated symptoms. Both strategies have their benefits and drawbacks (**Table 1**). If an effective antiviral is used for prophylaxis, it could be argued that monitoring would not be required. Additionally, prophylaxis may potentially prevent the indirect effects associated with CMV infection. Prophylaxis by definition results in some patients receiving the drug unnecessarily, however, exposing them to potential drug-related toxicities. The success of the preemptive treatment strategy is largely dependent on the early detection of CMV in blood. By allowing a limited amount of viral replication, preemptive therapy may stimulate immune responses and thereby promote CMV-specific immune reconstitution.[17] Because both strategies are equally effective in preventing CMV disease,[120] most transplant centers have moved toward preemptive strategies as pp65 antigenemia and DNA PCR-based assays have become readily available.[121–123]

More recently, there has been great interest in using methods to determine CMV-specific immune reconstitution after HSCT as an additional means to determine the risk of CMV infection and disease. The usefulness of measuring T-cell responses as a guide for withholding therapy was evaluated in a small pilot study involving HSCT recipients more than 100 days after transplant.[79] Although promising, this strategy requires validation in larger, randomized trials.

Antiviral Agents

High-dose acyclovir reduces the risk for CMV infection and possibly disease.[124,125] Valacyclovir is the prodrug of acyclovir and is better absorbed, resulting in higher serum-concentration. High-dose valacyclovir is more effective than acyclovir in

Table 1
Strategies for preemptive therapy and prophylaxis after HCT

Prevention Strategy	Patient Population	Timing Post-HCT	Initiation	First-line Choice: Induction	First-line Choice: Maintenance	Alternatives	Duration
Preemptive	Allogeneic HSCT recipients	<100 d	At first detection of CMV infection	GCV 5 mg/kg IV bid × 7–14 d and declining viral load	GCV 5 mg/kg IV qd	Foscarnet Valganciclovir Cidofovir	Indicator test negative and minimum 2–3 wk
	Allogeneic HSCT or GVHD requiring steroid therapy or Early CMV infection	>100 d	pp65 Ag ≥5 cells/slide or ≥2 consecutively positive PCR/viremia	GCV 5 mg/kg IV bid × 7–14 d and declining viral load	GCV 5 mg/kg IV qd	Valganciclovir Foscarnet	Until indicator assay negative and minimum 2–3 wk therapy
	Autologous HSCT and CMV seropositive and at high risk[a]	<100 d	pp65 Ag ≥5 cells/slide (or at any level if CD34 ± selected graft)	GCV 5 mg/kg IV bid × 7 d and declining viral load	GCV 5 mg/kg IV qd	Foscarnet Valganciclovir Cidofovir	Until indicator assay negative and minimum 2 wk therapy
Prophylaxis	Allogeneic HSCT recipients	<100 d	At engraftment	GCV 5 mg/kg IV bid × 5–7 d	GCV 5 mg/kg IV qd	Foscarnet Acyclovir[b] Valacyclovir[b]	Day 100 after HCT

Abbreviations: CMV, cytomegalovirus; GCV, ganciclovir; GVHD, graft-versus-host disease; HSCT, hematopoietic stem cell transplantation; PCR, polymerase chain reaction.

[a] Includes use of TBI in conditioning, recent fludarabine, or 2-chlorodeoxyadenosine, high-dose corticosteroids.

[b] Must be combined with active surveillance for CMV infection.

reducing CMV infection and the need for preemptive therapy with ganciclovir after HSCT, although there is no impact on survival.[126] Routine monitoring for CMV infection is required if valacyclovir or acyclovir prophylaxis is used.

Ganciclovir is currently the first-line agent for CMV prophylaxis and preemptive treatment. Intravenous ganciclovir has been demonstrated to reduce the risk of CMV infection and disease compared with placebo, but does not improve overall survival.[120,127–129] Neutropenia occurs in up to 30% of HSCT recipients during ganciclovir therapy[130] increasing the risk of invasive bacterial and fungal infections.[120,127,130] Therapeutic drug monitoring can be helpful to guide therapy and reduce the risk for toxicity, especially in the situation of pre-existing renal impairment.

Valganciclovir is an orally available prodrug of ganciclovir and administration achieves serum concentrations at least equivalent to intravenous ganciclovir.[131–133] The results of several uncontrolled studies suggest that valganciclovir is comparable with intravenous ganciclovir in terms of efficacy and safety when used as preemptive therapy after allogeneic HSCT.[131,134–136] Preliminary data from a randomized trial have been presented indicating little or no difference in efficacy or toxicity compared with intravenous ganciclovir.[137] Until more data are available, however, caution should be exercised when choosing valganciclovir as preemptive therapy.

Foscarnet is as effective as ganciclovir for preemptive therapy after allogeneic transplantation.[138] The commonly encountered toxicities of foscarnet make this drug a second-line agent, most appropriate when ganciclovir is contraindicated or not tolerated.

Cidofovir is a "broad-spectrum" antiviral with a long half-life allowing a once-per-week dosing schedule. The major toxicity with cidofovir, acute renal tubular necrosis, limits its use after HSCT.[139]

Monitoring for CMV Infection and Initiation of Preemptive Therapy

qPCR assays for CMV DNA are increasingly used because of their performance characteristics allowing the development of institution-specific viral load thresholds for initiation of preemptive treatment, thereby avoiding unnecessary treatment of patients who are at low risk of progression to disease. It has been reported that the initial viral load and the viral load kinetics are important as risk factors for CMV disease.[140] Currently, several different variations are used, making it difficult to establish validated universal viral load thresholds because of differences in assay performance and testing material (whole blood vs plasma).[141]

If the preemptive therapy strategy is used, all patients who have undergone allogeneic HSCT should be monitored up to day 100 posttransplant on a weekly basis for CMV infection. Although CMV infection is rare in D-/R- patients, routine monitoring was effective in identifying CMV infection and preventing disease in a large cohort.[112] The ideal duration and frequency of CMV monitoring later after HSCT have not been determined.[91,102]

Various durations of preemptive antiviral treatment have been explored. Most centers now continue antiviral treatment until the designated viral marker is negative and the patient has received at least 2 weeks of antiviral therapy. If an assay less sensitive than DNA PCR, such as the pp65 antigenemia assay, is used, then preemptive therapy should be continued until two negative results are obtained.[138] If a patient is still positive by PCR or pp65 antigenemia assay after 2 weeks of therapy, treatment should be extended until clearance is achieved. It has been shown that a low rate of viral load decrease is a risk factor for later-occurring CMV disease.[46]

Special Populations

Patients with CMV disease occurring before planned allogeneic HSCT have a very high risk of mortality.[142] After transplantation, a patient with documented pretransplant CMV disease should either be monitored for CMV very closely (ie, twice weekly), or be given prophylaxis with ganciclovir or foscarnet.

The optimal approach to CMV after CBT is not clear. One study described successful preemptive treatment with ganciclovir,[98] whereas another combined high-dose valacyclovir prophylaxis with continued monitoring and preemptive therapy.[89]

ANTIVIRAL RESISTANCE

Risk factors for drug resistance include prolonged (months) antiviral therapy, intermittent low-level viral replication in the presence of drug caused by profound immunosuppression or suboptimal drug levels, and lack of prior immunity to CMV.[143] Drug resistance should be suspected in patients who have increasing quantitative viral loads for more than 2 weeks despite antiviral therapy. After start of antiviral therapy in treatment-naive patients, an increase in the viral load occurs in approximately one third of patients and is likely caused by the underlying immunosuppression (clinical resistance), not true drug resistance caused by mutations in the target genes for the antiviral agent used.[41] If the viral load increases in patients who have received previous antiviral therapy, drug resistance should, however, be suspected.

Ganciclovir resistance most often is caused by mutations in the UL97 gene, but mutations in the UL54-encoded DNA polymerase can also occur. Several UL97 mutations that confer resistance have been described.[144] Because different UL97 mutations confer varying degrees of ganciclovir resistance, however, some cases of genotypically defined ganciclovir-resistant CMV may still respond to therapy.[145]

If ganciclovir resistance is documented or suspected, foscarnet is generally the second-line agent of choice. Unlike ganciclovir, foscarnet activity is not dependent on phosphorylation by the UL97 gene product.[146] Resistance to foscarnet can occur and is caused by mutations in UL54. Because cidofovir is not phosphorylated by the CMV UL97 gene product, it is also active against ganciclovir-resistant UL97 mutants. Certain UL54 mutations, however, can confer cross-resistance between ganciclovir and cidofovir.[146,147] Additional genotype testing of UL54 is indicated to evaluate for potential cross-resistance conferring mutations.

Drugs under evaluation, such as maribavir, may provide therapeutic options in the future. Maribavir inhibits the CMV UL97 kinase and is active against wild-type and ganciclovir-resistant CMV strains[148] and has shown promising results in a small series of patients failing therapy with other antiviral agents either because of toxicity or resistance. Other drugs with possible anti-CMV activity include the arthritis drug leflunomide and the antimalaria compound artesunate.[149–151]

MANAGEMENT OF CMV DISEASE

Several studies established the current standard of care for CMV pneumonia, which is treatment with ganciclovir (or foscarnet as an alternative agent) in combination with IVIG.[152–155] These studies showed improved survival rates compared with historical controls. There does not seem to be a specific advantage of CMV-specific immunoglobulin (CMV-Ig) compared with pooled immunoglobulin.[153] In specific clinical situations, however, such as volume overload, CMV-Ig may be preferred. Several studies have raised doubt regarding the beneficial effect of concomitant IVIG,[156,157] but it is still considered as standard-of-care at most centers.

For GI disease, the standard therapy is most often intravenous ganciclovir for 3 to 4 weeks followed by several weeks of maintenance. Shorter courses of induction therapy (2 weeks) are not as effective.[158] There is no role for concomitant IVIG in the treatment of GI disease.[159] Recurrence may occur in approximately 30% of patients in the setting of continued immunosuppression and such patients may benefit from secondary prophylaxis until immunosuppression has been reduced. Foscarnet can be used as an alternative if neutropenia is present. Valganciclovir as maintenance treatment for GI disease has not been well studied.

CMV retinitis is typically treated with systemic ganciclovir, foscarnet, or cidofovir, with or without intraocular ganciclovir injections or implants.[60,160–162] Fomivirsen is an antisense RNA molecule that targets mRNA encoded by CMV and is approved as second-line therapy for CMV retinitis in patients with AIDS.[163]

Other manifestations of CMV disease, such as hepatitis and encephalitis, are uncommon and are typically managed with intravenous ganciclovir. The duration of therapy for these manifestations has not been well-established and should be tailored to the individual patient.

ADOPTIVE IMMUNOTHERAPY

CMV-specific T cells can be generated by several different mechanisms to restore cellular immunity passively after transplantation.[5] Several groups have reported a beneficial impact of adoptive immunotherapy on CMV viral loads in patients who had undergone HSCT.[164] Despite these seemingly promising results, scientific questions remain unanswered (eg, the optimal cell type and dose for infusion) and technical hurdles persist (availability of clinical grade reagents) that preclude adoptive immunotherapy from becoming a routine clinical procedure at the current time.

REFERENCES

1. Sinzger C, Digel M, Jahn G. Cytomegalovirus cell tropism. Curr Top Microbiol Immunol 2008;325:63–83.
2. Bolovan-Fritts CA, Mocarski ES, Wiedeman JA. Peripheral blood CD14(+) cells from healthy subjects carry a circular conformation of latent cytomegalovirus genome. Blood 1999;93(1):394–8.
3. Kondo K, Kaneshima H, Mocarski ES. Human cytomegalovirus latent infection of granulocyte-macrophage progenitors. Proc Natl Acad Sci U S A 1994;91(25): 11879–83.
4. Taylor-Wiedeman J, Sissons JG, Borysiewicz LK, et al. Monocytes are a major site of persistence of human cytomegalovirus in peripheral blood mononuclear cells. J Gen Virol 1991;72(Pt 9):2059–64.
5. Crough T, Khanna R. Immunobiology of human cytomegalovirus: from bench to bedside. Clin Microbiol Rev 2009;22(1):76–98 [table of contents].
6. Gillespie GM, Wills MR, Appay V, et al. Functional heterogeneity and high frequencies of cytomegalovirus-specific CD8(+) T lymphocytes in healthy seropositive donors. J Virol 2000;74(17):8140–50.
7. Khan N, Cobbold M, Keenan R, et al. Comparative analysis of CD8+ T cell responses against human cytomegalovirus proteins pp65 and immediate early 1 shows similarities in precursor frequency, oligoclonality, and phenotype. J Infect Dis 2002;185(8):1025–34.
8. Khan N, Hislop A, Gudgeon N, et al. Herpesvirus-specific CD8 T cell immunity in old age: cytomegalovirus impairs the response to a coresident EBV infection. J Immunol 2004;173(12):7481–9.
9. Ouyang Q, Wagner WM, Wikby A, et al. Large numbers of dysfunctional CD8+ T lymphocytes bearing receptors for a single dominant CMV epitope in the very old. J Clin Immunol 2003;23(4):247–57.

10. Sylwester AW, Mitchell BL, Edgar JB, et al. Broadly targeted human cytomegalovirus-specific CD4+ and CD8+ T cells dominate the memory compartments of exposed subjects. J Exp Med 2005;202(5):673–85.
11. Elkington R, Walker S, Crough T, et al. Ex vivo profiling of CD8+-T-cell responses to human cytomegalovirus reveals broad and multispecific reactivities in healthy virus carriers. J Virol 2003;77(9):5226–40.
12. Kern F, Bunde T, Faulhaber N, et al. Cytomegalovirus (CMV) phosphoprotein 65 makes a large contribution to shaping the T cell repertoire in CMV-exposed individuals. J Infect Dis 2002;185(12):1709–16.
13. Kern F, Surel IP, Faulhaber N, et al. Target structures of the CD8(+)-T-cell response to human cytomegalovirus: the 72-kilodalton major immediate-early protein revisited. J Virol 1999;73(10):8179–84.
14. Khan N, Best D, Bruton R, et al. T cell recognition patterns of immunodominant cytomegalovirus antigens in primary and persistent infection. J Immunol 2007; 178(7):4455–65.
15. Khan N, Bruton R, Taylor GS, et al. Identification of cytomegalovirus-specific cytotoxic T lymphocytes in vitro is greatly enhanced by the use of recombinant virus lacking the US2 to US11 region or modified vaccinia virus Ankara expressing individual viral genes. J Virol 2005;79(5):2869–79.
16. Kondo E, Akatsuka Y, Kuzushima K, et al. Identification of novel CTL epitopes of CMV-pp65 presented by a variety of HLA alleles. Blood 2004;103(2):630–8.
17. Li CR, Greenberg PD, Gilbert MJ, et al. Recovery of HLA-restricted cytomegalovirus (CMV)-specific T-cell responses after allogeneic bone marrow transplant: correlation with CMV disease and effect of ganciclovir prophylaxis. Blood 1994;83(7):1971–9.
18. Polic B, Hengel H, Krmpotic A, et al. Hierarchical and redundant lymphocyte subset control precludes cytomegalovirus replication during latent infection. J Exp Med 1998;188(6):1047–54.
19. Quinnan GV Jr, Kirmani N, Rook AH, et al. Cytotoxic t cells in cytomegalovirus infection: HLA-restricted T-lymphocyte and non-T-lymphocyte cytotoxic responses correlate with recovery from cytomegalovirus infection in bone-marrow-transplant recipients. N Engl J Med 1982;307(1):7–13.
20. Reusser P, Cathomas G, Attenhofer R, et al. Cytomegalovirus (CMV)-specific T cell immunity after renal transplantation mediates protection from CMV disease by limiting the systemic virus load. J Infect Dis 1999;180(2):247–53.
21. Reusser P, Riddell SR, Meyers JD, et al. Cytotoxic T-lymphocyte response to cytomegalovirus after human allogeneic bone marrow transplantation: pattern of recovery and correlation with cytomegalovirus infection and disease. Blood 1991;78(5):1373–80.
22. Hebart H, Daginik S, Stevanovic S, et al. Sensitive detection of human cytomegalovirus peptide-specific cytotoxic T-lymphocyte responses by interferon-gamma-enzyme-linked immunospot assay and flow cytometry in healthy individuals and in patients after allogeneic stem cell transplantation. Blood 2002;99(10):3830–7.
23. Krause H, Hebart H, Jahn G, et al. Screening for CMV-specific T cell proliferation to identify patients at risk of developing late onset CMV disease. Bone Marrow Transplant 1997;19(11):1111–6.
24. Ljungman P, Aschan J, Azinge JN, et al. Cytomegalovirus viraemia and specific T-helper cell responses as predictors of disease after allogeneic marrow transplantation. Br J Haematol 1993;83(1):118–24.
25. Boeckh M, Leisenring W, Riddell SR, et al. Late cytomegalovirus disease and mortality in recipients of allogeneic hematopoietic stem cell transplants: importance of viral load and T-cell immunity. Blood 2003;101(2):407–14.

26. Boppana SB, Britt WJ. Antiviral antibody responses and intrauterine transmission after primary maternal cytomegalovirus infection. J Infect Dis 1995; 171(5):1115–21.
27. Jonjic S, Pavic I, Lucin P, et al. Efficacious control of cytomegalovirus infection after long-term depletion of CD8+ T lymphocytes. J Virol 1990;64(11):5457–64.
28. Boehme KW, Guerrero M, Compton T. Human cytomegalovirus envelope glycoproteins B and H are necessary for TLR2 activation in permissive cells. J Immunol 2006;177(10):7094–102.
29. Compton T, Kurt-Jones EA, Boehme KW, et al. Human cytomegalovirus activates inflammatory cytokine responses via CD14 and Toll-like receptor 2. J Virol 2003;77(8):4588–96.
30. Juckem LK, Boehme KW, Feire AL, et al. Differential initiation of innate immune responses induced by human cytomegalovirus entry into fibroblast cells. J Immunol 2008;180(7):4965–77.
31. Kijpittayarit S, Eid AJ, Brown RA, et al. Relationship between Toll-like receptor 2 polymorphism and cytomegalovirus disease after liver transplantation. Clin Infect Dis 2007;44(10):1315–20.
32. Biron CA, Byron KS, Sullivan JL. Severe herpesvirus infections in an adolescent without natural killer cells. N Engl J Med 1989;320(26):1731–5.
33. Venema H, van den Berg AP, van Zanten C, et al. Natural killer cell responses in renal transplant patients with cytomegalovirus infection. J Med Virol 1994;42(2): 188–92.
34. Chen C, Busson M, Rocha V, et al. Activating KIR genes are associated with CMV reactivation and survival after non-T-cell depleted HLA-identical sibling bone marrow transplantation for malignant disorders. Bone Marrow Transplant 2006;38(6):437–44.
35. Cook M, Briggs D, Craddock C, et al. Donor KIR genotype has a major influence on the rate of cytomegalovirus reactivation following T-cell replete stem cell transplantation. Blood 2006;107(3):1230–2.
36. Zaia JA, Sun JY, Gallez-Hawkins GM, et al. The effect of single and combined activating killer immunoglobulin-like receptor genotypes on cytomegalovirus infection and immunity after hematopoietic cell transplantation. Biol Blood Marrow Transplant 2009;15(3):315–25.
37. Loeffler J, Steffens M, Arlt EM, et al. Polymorphisms in the genes encoding chemokine receptor 5, interleukin-10, and monocyte chemoattractant protein 1 contribute to cytomegalovirus reactivation and disease after allogeneic stem cell transplantation. J Clin Microbiol 2006;44(5):1847–50.
38. Einsele H, Ehninger G, Hebart H, et al. Polymerase chain reaction monitoring reduces the incidence of cytomegalovirus disease and the duration and side effects of antiviral therapy after bone marrow transplantation. Blood 1995; 86(7):2815–20.
39. Crawford SW, Bowden RA, Hackman RC, et al. Rapid detection of cytomegalovirus pulmonary infection by bronchoalveolar lavage and centrifugation culture. Ann Intern Med 1988;108(2):180–5.
40. Boeckh M, Bowden RA, Goodrich JM, et al. Cytomegalovirus antigen detection in peripheral blood leukocytes after allogeneic marrow transplantation. Blood 1992;80(5):1358–64.
41. Nichols WG, Corey L, Gooley T, et al. Rising pp65 antigenemia during preemptive anticytomegalovirus therapy after allogeneic hematopoietic stem cell transplantation: risk factors, correlation with DNA load, and outcomes. Blood 2001; 97(4):867–74.

42. Boeckh M, Huang M, Ferrenberg J, et al. Optimization of quantitative detection of cytomegalovirus DNA in plasma by real-time PCR. J Clin Microbiol 2004; 42(3):1142–8.
43. Einsele H, Hebart H, Kauffmann-Schneider C, et al. Risk factors for treatment failures in patients receiving PCR-based preemptive therapy for CMV infection. Bone Marrow Transplant 2000;25(7):757–63.
44. Emery VC, Griffiths PD. Prediction of cytomegalovirus load and resistance patterns after antiviral chemotherapy. Proc Natl Acad Sci U S A 2000;97(14):8039–44.
45. Gor D, Sabin C, Prentice HG, et al. Longitudinal fluctuations in cytomegalovirus load in bone marrow transplant patients: relationship between peak virus load, donor/recipient serostatus, acute GVHD and CMV disease. Bone Marrow Transplant 1998;21(6):597–605.
46. Ljungman P, Perez-Bercoff L, Jonsson J, et al. Risk factors for the development of cytomegalovirus disease after allogeneic stem cell transplantation. Haematologica 2006;91(1):78–83.
47. Cathomas G, Morris P, Pekle K, et al. Rapid diagnosis of cytomegalovirus pneumonia in marrow transplant recipients by bronchoalveolar lavage using the polymerase chain reaction, virus culture, and the direct immunostaining of alveolar cells. Blood 1993;81(7):1909–14.
48. Gerna G, Lilleri D, Baldanti F, et al. Human cytomegalovirus immediate-early mRNAemia versus pp65 antigenemia for guiding pre-emptive therapy in children and young adults undergoing hematopoietic stem cell transplantation: a prospective, randomized, open-label trial. Blood 2003;101(12):5053–60.
49. Hebart H, Ljungman P, Klingebiel T, et al. Prospective comparison of PCR-based versus late mRNA-based preemptive antiviral therapy for HCMV infection in patients after allogeneic stem cell transplantation. Blood 2003;102(11):195a.
50. Collier AC, Chandler SH, Handsfield HH, et al. Identification of multiple strains of cytomegalovirus in homosexual men. J Infect Dis 1989;159(1):123–6.
51. Manuel O, Pang XL, Humar A, et al. An assessment of donor-to-recipient transmission patterns of human cytomegalovirus by analysis of viral genomic variants. J Infect Dis 2009;199(11):1621–8.
52. Ljungman P, Griffiths P, Paya C. Definitions of cytomegalovirus infection and disease in transplant recipients. Clin Infect Dis 2002;34(8):1094–7.
53. Boeckh M, Stevens-Ayers T, Bowden RA. Cytomegalovirus pp65 antigenemia after autologous marrow and peripheral blood stem cell transplantation. J Infect Dis 1996;174(5):907–12.
54. Konoplev S, Champlin RE, Giralt S, et al. Cytomegalovirus pneumonia in adult autologous blood and marrow transplant recipients. Bone Marrow Transplant 2001;27(8):877–81.
55. Ljungman P. Cytomegalovirus pneumonia: presentation, diagnosis, and treatment. Semin Respir Infect 1995;10(4):209–15.
56. Schmidt GM, Horak DA, Niland JC, et al. A randomized, controlled trial of prophylactic ganciclovir for cytomegalovirus pulmonary infection in recipients of allogeneic bone marrow transplants. The City of Hope-Stanford-Syntex CMV Study Group. N Engl J Med 1991;324(15):1005–11.
57. Jang EY, Park SY, Lee EJ, et al. Diagnostic performance of the cytomegalovirus (CMV) antigenemia assay in patients with CMV gastrointestinal disease. Clin Infect Dis 2009;48(12):e121–4.
58. Mori T, Okamoto S, Matsuoka S, et al. Risk-adapted pre-emptive therapy for cytomegalovirus disease in patients undergoing allogeneic bone marrow transplantation. Bone Marrow Transplant 2000;25(7):765–9.

59. Coskuncan NM, Jabs DA, Dunn JP, et al. The eye in bone marrow transplantation. VI. Retinal complications. Arch Ophthalmol 1994;112(3):372–9.
60. Crippa F, Corey L, Chuang EL, et al. Virological, clinical, and ophthalmologic features of cytomegalovirus retinitis after hematopoietic stem cell transplantation. Clin Infect Dis 2001;32(2):214–9.
61. Eid AJ, Bakri SJ, Kijpittayarit S, et al. Clinical features and outcomes of cytomegalovirus retinitis after transplantation. Transpl Infect Dis 2008;10(1):13–8.
62. Larsson K, Lonnqvist B, Ringden O, et al. CMV retinitis after allogeneic bone marrow transplantation: a report of five cases. Transpl Infect Dis 2002;4(2):75–9.
63. Nichols WG, Corey L, Gooley T, et al. High risk of death due to bacterial and fungal infection among cytomegalovirus (CMV)-seronegative recipients of stem cell transplants from seropositive donors: evidence for indirect effects of primary CMV infection. J Infect Dis 2002;185(3):273–82.
64. Boeckh M. Current antiviral strategies for controlling cytomegalovirus in hematopoietic stem cell transplant recipients: prevention and therapy. Transpl Infect Dis 1999;1(3):165–78.
65. Broers AE, van Der Holt R, van Esser JW, et al. Increased transplant-related morbidity and mortality in CMV- seropositive patients despite highly effective prevention of CMV disease after allogeneic T-cell-depleted stem cell transplantation. Blood 2000;95(7):2240–5.
66. Craddock C, Szydlo RM, Dazzi F, et al. Cytomegalovirus seropositivity adversely influences outcome after T- depleted unrelated donor transplant in patients with chronic myeloid leukaemia: the case for tailored graft-versus-host disease prophylaxis. Br J Haematol 2001;112(1):228–36.
67. Behrendt CE, Rosenthal J, Bolotin E, et al. Donor and recipient CMV serostatus and outcome of pediatric allogeneic HSCT for acute leukemia in the era of CMV-preemptive therapy. Biol Blood Marrow Transplant 2009;15(1):54–60.
68. Boeckh M, Nichols WG. The impact of cytomegalovirus serostatus of donor and recipient before hematopoietic stem cell transplantation in the era of antiviral prophylaxis and preemptive therapy. Blood 2004;103(6):2003–8.
69. Bordon V, Bravo S, Van Renterghem L, et al. Surveillance of cytomegalovirus (CMV) DNAemia in pediatric allogeneic stem cell transplantation: incidence and outcome of CMV infection and disease. Transpl Infect Dis 2008;10(1):19–23.
70. Cwynarski K, Roberts IA, Iacobelli S, et al. Stem cell transplantation for chronic myeloid leukemia in children. Blood 2003;102(4):1224–31.
71. Erard V, Guthrie KA, Riddell S, et al. Impact of HLA A2 and cytomegalovirus serostatus on outcomes in patients with leukemia following matched-sibling myeloablative allogeneic hematopoietic cell transplantation. Haematologica 2006;91(10):1377–83.
72. Grob JP, Grundy JE, Prentice HG, et al. Immune donors can protect marrow-transplant recipients from severe cytomegalovirus infections. Lancet 1987;1(8536):774–6.
73. Jacobsen N, Badsberg JH, Lonnqvist B, et al. Graft-versus-leukaemia activity associated with CMV-seropositive donor, post-transplant CMV infection, young donor age and chronic graft-versus-host disease in bone marrow allograft recipients. The Nordic Bone Marrow Transplantation Group. Bone Marrow Transplant 1990;5(6):413–8.
74. Kollman C, Howe CW, Anasetti C, et al. Donor characteristics as risk factors in recipients after transplantation of bone marrow from unrelated donors: the effect of donor age. Blood 2001;98(7):2043–51.

75. Ljungman P, Einsele H, Frassoni F, et al. Donor CMV serological status influences the outcome of CMVseropositive recipients after unrelated donor stem cell transplantation. An EBMT Megafile analysis. Blood 2003;102:4255–60.
76. Nachbaur D, Clausen J, Kircher B. Donor cytomegalovirus seropositivity and the risk of leukemic relapse after reduced-intensity transplants. Eur J Haematol 2006;76(5):414–9.
77. Ringden O, Schaffer M, Le Blanc K, et al. Which donor should be chosen for hematopoietic stem cell transplantation among unrelated HLA-A, -B, and -DRB1 genomically identical volunteers? Biol Blood Marrow Transplant 2004;10(2):128–34.
78. Gustafsson Jernberg A, Remberger M, Ringden O, et al. Risk factors in pediatric stem cell transplantation for leukemia. Pediatr Transplant 2004;8(5):464–74.
79. Avetisyan G, Aschan J, Hagglund H, et al. Evaluation of intervention strategy based on CMV-specific immune responses after allogeneic SCT. Bone Marrow Transplant 2007;40(9):865–9.
80. Ganepola S, Gentilini C, Hilbers U, et al. Patients at high risk for CMV infection and disease show delayed CD8+ T-cell immune recovery after allogeneic stem cell transplantation. Bone Marrow Transplant 2007;39(5):293–9.
81. Lilleri D, Fornara C, Chiesa A, et al. Human cytomegalovirus-specific CD4+ and CD8+ T-cell reconstitution in adult allogeneic hematopoietic stem cell transplant recipients and immune control of viral infection. Haematologica 2008;93(2):248–56.
82. Moins-Teisserenc H, Busson M, Scieux C, et al. Patterns of cytomegalovirus reactivation are associated with distinct evolutive profiles of immune reconstitution after allogeneic hematopoeitic stem cell transplantation. J Infect Dis 2008;198(6):818–26.
83. Lin TS, Zahrieh D, Weller E, et al. Risk factors for cytomegalovirus reactivation after CD6+ T-cell-depleted allogeneic bone marrow transplantation. Transplantation 2002;74(1):49–54.
84. Ozdemir E, Saliba R, Champlin R, et al. Risk factors associated with late cytomegalovirus reactivation after allogeneic stem cell transplantation for hematological malignancies. Bone Marrow Transplant 2007;40(2):125–36.
85. Marty FM, Bryar J, Browne SK, et al. Sirolimus-based graft-versus-host disease prophylaxis protects against cytomegalovirus reactivation after allogeneic hematopoietic stem cell transplantation: a cohort analysis. Blood 2007;110(2):490–500.
86. Ljungman P, Aschan J, Lewensohn-Fuchs I, et al. Results of different strategies for reducing cytomegalovirus-associated mortality in allogeneic stem cell transplant recipients. Transplantation 1998;66(10):1330–4.
87. Martino R, Rovira M, Carreras E, et al. Severe infections after allogeneic peripheral blood stem cell transplantation: a matched-pair comparison of unmanipulated and CD34+ cell-selected transplantation. Haematologica 2001;86(10):1075–86.
88. Miller W, Flynn P, McCullough J, et al. Cytomegalovirus infection after bone marrow transplantation: an association with acute graft-v-host disease. Blood 1986;67(4):1162–7.
89. Walker CM, van Burik JA, De For TE, et al. Cytomegalovirus infection after allogeneic transplantation: comparison of cord blood with peripheral blood and marrow graft sources. Biol Blood Marrow Transplant 2007;13(9):1106–15.
90. Kudchodkar SB, Yu Y, Maguire TG, et al. Human cytomegalovirus infection alters the substrate specificities and rapamycin sensitivities of raptor- and rictor-containing complexes. Proc Natl Acad Sci U S A 2006;103(38):14182–7.

91. Junghanss C, Boeckh M, Carter RA, et al. Incidence and outcome of cytomegalovirus infections following nonmyeloablative compared with myeloablative allogeneic stem cell transplantation: a matched control study. Blood 2002; 99(6):1978–85.
92. Nakamae H, Kirby KA, Sandmaier BM, et al. Effect of conditioning regimen intensity on CMV infection in allogeneic hematopoietic cell transplantation. Biol Blood Marrow Transplant 2009;15(6):694–703.
93. Schoemans H, Theunissen K, Maertens J, et al. Adult umbilical cord blood transplantation: a comprehensive review. Bone Marrow Transplant 2006;38(2): 83–93.
94. Albano MS, Taylor P, Pass RF, et al. Umbilical cord blood transplantation and cytomegalovirus: posttransplantation infection and donor screening. Blood 2006;108(13):4275–82.
95. Matsumura T, Narimatsu H, Kami M, et al. Cytomegalovirus infections following umbilical cord blood transplantation using reduced intensity conditioning regimens for adult patients. Biol Blood Marrow Transplant 2007;13(5):577–83.
96. Saavedra S, Sanz GF, Jarque I, et al. Early infections in adult patients undergoing unrelated donor cord blood transplantation. Bone Marrow Transplant 2002;30(12):937–43.
97. Takami A, Mochizuki K, Asakura H, et al. High incidence of cytomegalovirus reactivation in adult recipients of an unrelated cord blood transplant. Haematologica 2005;90(9):1290–2.
98. Tomonari A, Takahashi S, Ooi J, et al. Preemptive therapy with ganciclovir 5 mg/kg once daily for cytomegalovirus infection after unrelated cord blood transplantation. Bone Marrow Transplant 2008;41(4):371–6.
99. Delgado J, Pillai S, Benjamin R, et al. The effect of in vivo T cell depletion with alemtuzumab on reduced-intensity allogeneic hematopoietic cell transplantation for chronic lymphocytic leukemia. Biol Blood Marrow Transplant 2008;14(11): 1288–97.
100. Martin SI, Marty FM, Fiumara K, et al. Infectious complications associated with alemtuzumab use for lymphoproliferative disorders. Clin Infect Dis 2006;43(1): 16–24.
101. Nguyen Q, Champlin R, Giralt S, et al. Late cytomegalovirus pneumonia in adult allogeneic blood and marrow transplant recipients. Clin Infect Dis 1999;28(3): 618–23.
102. Peggs KS, Preiser W, Kottaridis PD, et al. Extended routine polymerase chain reaction surveillance and pre-emptive antiviral therapy for cytomegalovirus after allogeneic transplantation. Br J Haematol 2000;111(3):782–90.
103. Hebart H, Schroder A, Loffler J, et al. Cytomegalovirus monitoring by polymerase chain reaction of whole blood samples from patients undergoing autologous bone marrow or peripheral blood progenitor cell transplantation. J Infect Dis 1997;175(6):1490–3.
104. Bilgrami S, Aslanzadeh J, Feingold JM, et al. Cytomegalovirus viremia, viruria and disease after autologous peripheral blood stem cell transplantation: no need for surveillance. Bone Marrow Transplant 1999;24(1):69–73.
105. Boeckh M, Gooley TA, Reusser P, et al. Failure of high-dose acyclovir to prevent cytomegalovirus disease after autologous marrow transplantation. J Infect Dis 1995;172(4):939–43.
106. Holmberg LA, Boeckh M, Hooper H, et al. Increased incidence of cytomegalovirus disease after autologous CD34-selected peripheral blood stem cell transplantation. Blood 1999;94(12):4029–35.

107. Singhal S, Powles R, Treleaven J, et al. Cytomegaloviremia after autografting for leukemia: clinical significance and lack of effect on engraftment. Leukemia 1997;11(6):835–8.
108. Enright H, Haake R, Weisdorf D, et al. Cytomegalovirus pneumonia after bone marrow transplantation: risk factors and response to therapy. Transplantation 1993;55(6):1339–46.
109. Reusser P, Fisher LD, Buckner CD, et al. Cytomegalovirus infection after autologous bone marrow transplantation: occurrence of cytomegalovirus disease and effect on engraftment. Blood 1990;75(9):1888–94.
110. Bowden R, Cays M, Schoch G, et al. Comparison of filtered blood (FB) to seronegative blood products (SB) for prevention of cytomegalovirus (CMV) infection after marrow transplant. Blood 1995;86:3598–603.
111. Ljungman P, Larsson K, Kumlien G, et al. Leukocyte depleted, unscreened blood products give a low risk for CMV infection and disease in CMV seronegative allogeneic stem cell transplant recipients with seronegative stem cell donors. Scand J Infect Dis 2002;34(5):347–50.
112. Nichols WG, Price TH, Gooley T, et al. Transfusion-transmitted cytomegalovirus infection after receipt of leukoreduced blood products. Blood 2003;101(10): 4195–200.
113. Bass E, Powe N, Goodman S, et al. Efficacy of immune globulin in preventing complications of bone marrow transplantation: a meta-analysis. Bone Marrow Transplant 1993;12:179–83.
114. Messori A, Rampazzo R, Scroccaro G, et al. Efficacy of hyperimmune anti-cytomegalovirus immunoglobulins for the prevention of cytomegalovirus infection in recipients of allogeneic bone marrow transplantation: a meta analysis. Bone Marrow Transplant 1994;13:163–8.
115. Raanani P, Gafter-Gvili A, Paul M, et al. Immunoglobulin prophylaxis in patients undergoing haematopoietic stem cell transplantation: systematic review and meta-analysis [abstract O267]. Bone Marrow Transplant 2008;41(S1):S46.
116. Sullivan KM, Kopecky KJ, Jocom J, et al. Immunomodulatory and antimicrobial efficacy of intravenous immunoglobulin in bone marrow transplantation. N Engl J Med 1990;323(11):705–12.
117. Winston DJ, Ho WG, Lin CH, et al. Intravenous immune globulin for prevention of cytomegalovirus infection and interstitial pneumonia after bone marrow transplantation. Ann Intern Med 1987;106(1):12–8.
118. Zikos P, Van Lint MT, Lamparelli T, et al. A randomized trial of high dose polyvalent intravenous immunoglobulin (HDIgG) vs. cytomegalovirus (CMV) hyperimmune IgG in allogeneic hemopoietic stem cell transplants (HSCT). Haematologica 1998;83(2):132–7.
119. Wloch MK, Smith LR, Boutsaboualoy S, et al. Safety and immunogenicity of a bivalent cytomegalovirus DNA vaccine in healthy adult subjects. J Infect Dis 2008;197(12):1634–42.
120. Boeckh M, Gooley TA, Myerson D, et al. Cytomegalovirus pp65 antigenemia-guided early treatment with ganciclovir versus ganciclovir at engraftment after allogeneic marrow transplantation: a randomized double-blind study. Blood 1996;88(10):4063–71.
121. Avery RK, Adal KA, Longworth DL, et al. A survey of allogeneic bone marrow transplant programs in the United States regarding cytomegalovirus prophylaxis and pre-emptive therapy. Bone Marrow Transplant 2000;26(7):763–7.
122. Ljungman P. CMV infections after hematopoietic stem cell transplantation. Bone Marrow Transplant 2008;42(Suppl 1):S70–2.

123. Ljungman P, Reusser P, de la Camara R, et al. Management of CMV infections: recommendations from the infectious diseases working party of the EBMT. Bone Marrow Transplant 2004;33(11):1075–81.
124. Meyers JD, Reed EC, Shepp DH, et al. Acyclovir for prevention of cytomegalovirus infection and disease after allogeneic marrow transplantation. N Engl J Med 1988;318(2):70–5.
125. Prentice HG, Gluckman E, Powles RL, et al. Impact of long-term acyclovir on cytomegalovirus infection and survival after allogeneic bone marrow transplantation. European Acyclovir for CMV Prophylaxis Study Group. Lancet 1994; 343(8900):749–53.
126. Ljungman P, de la Camara R, Milpied N, et al. Randomized study of valacyclovir as prophylaxis against cytomegalovirus reactivation in recipients of allogeneic bone marrow transplants. Blood 2002;99(8):3050–6.
127. Goodrich JM, Bowden RA, Fisher L, et al. Ganciclovir prophylaxis to prevent cytomegalovirus disease after allogeneic marrow transplant. Ann Intern Med 1993;118(3):173–8.
128. Winston DJ, Ho WG, Bartoni K, et al. Ganciclovir prophylaxis of cytomegalovirus infection and disease in allogeneic bone marrow transplant recipients: results of a placebo- controlled, double-blind trial. Ann Intern Med 1993; 118(3):179–84.
129. Winston DJ, Yeager AM, Chandrasekar PH, et al. Randomized comparison of oral valacyclovir and intravenous ganciclovir for prevention of cytomegalovirus disease after allogeneic bone marrow transplantation. Clin Infect Dis 2003; 36(6):749–58.
130. Salzberger B, Bowden RA, Hackman RC, et al. Neutropenia in allogeneic marrow transplant recipients receiving ganciclovir for prevention of cytomegalovirus disease: risk factors and outcome. Blood 1997;90(6):2502–8.
131. Busca A, de Fabritiis P, Ghisetti V, et al. Oral valganciclovir as preemptive therapy for cytomegalovirus infection post allogeneic stem cell transplantation. Transpl Infect Dis 2007;9(2):102–7.
132. Einsele H, Reusser P, Bornhauser M, et al. Oral valganciclovir leads to higher exposure to ganciclovir than intravenous ganciclovir in patients following allogeneic stem cell transplantation. Blood 2006;107(7):3002–8.
133. Winston DJ, Baden LR, Gabriel DA, et al. Pharmacokinetics of ganciclovir after oral valganciclovir versus intravenous ganciclovir in allogeneic stem cell transplant patients with graft-versus-host disease of the gastrointestinal tract. Biol Blood Marrow Transplant 2006;12(6):635–40.
134. Allice T, Busca A, Locatelli F, et al. Valganciclovir as pre-emptive therapy for cytomegalovirus infection post-allogenic stem cell transplantation: implications for the emergence of drug-resistant cytomegalovirus. J Antimicrob Chemother 2009;63(3):600–8.
135. Ayala E, Greene J, Sandin R, et al. Valganciclovir is safe and effective as preemptive therapy for CMV infection in allogeneic hematopoietic stem cell transplantation. Bone Marrow Transplant 2006;37(9):851–6.
136. Takenaka K, Eto T, Nagafuji K, et al. Oral valganciclovir as preemptive therapy is effective for cytomegalovirus infection in allogeneic hematopoietic stem cell transplant recipients. Int J Hematol 2009;89(2):231–7.
137. Volin L, Barkholt L, Nihtinen A, et al. An open-label randomised study of oral valganciclovir versus intravenous ganciclovir for pre-emptive therapy of cytomegalovirus infection after allogeneic stem cell transplantation. Bone Marrow Transplant 2008;42(Suppl 1):S47.

138. Reusser P, Einsele H, Lee J, et al. Randomized multicenter trial of foscarnet versus ganciclovir for preemptive therapy of cytomegalovirus infection after allogeneic stem cell transplantation. Blood 2002;99(4):1159–64.
139. Ljungman P, Deliliers GL, Platzbecker U, et al. Cidofovir for cytomegalovirus infection and disease in allogeneic stem cell transplant recipients. The Infectious Diseases Working Party of the European Group for Blood and Marrow Transplantation. Blood 2001;97(2):388–92.
140. Emery VC, Sabin CA, Cope AV, et al. Application of viral-load kinetics to identify patients who develop cytomegalovirus disease after transplantation. Lancet 2000;355(9220):2032–6.
141. Pang XL, Fox JD, Fenton JM, et al. Interlaboratory comparison of cytomegalovirus viral load assays. Am J Transplant 2009;9(2):258–68.
142. Fries BC, Riddell SR, Kim HW, et al. Cytomegalovirus disease before hematopoietic cell transplantation as a risk for complications after transplantation. Biol Blood Marrow Transplant 2005;11(2):136–48.
143. Chou SW. Cytomegalovirus drug resistance and clinical implications. Transpl Infect Dis 2001;3(Suppl 2):20–4.
144. Chou S. Cytomegalovirus UL97 mutations in the era of ganciclovir and maribavir. Rev Med Virol 2008;18(4):233–46.
145. Iwasenko JM, Scott GM, Rawlinson WD, et al. Successful valganciclovir treatment of post-transplant cytomegalovirus infection in the presence of UL97 mutation N597D. J Med Virol 2009;81(3):507–10.
146. Prichard MN, Britt WJ, Daily SL, et al. Human cytomegalovirus UL97 kinase is required for the normal intranuclear distribution of pp65 and virion morphogenesis. J Virol 2005;79(24):15494–502.
147. Chou S, Lurain NS, Thompson KD, et al. Viral DNA polymerase mutations associated with drug resistance in human cytomegalovirus. J Infect Dis 2003;188(1):32–9.
148. Drew WL, Miner RC, Marousek GI, et al. Maribavir sensitivity of cytomegalovirus isolates resistant to ganciclovir, cidofovir or foscarnet. J Clin Virol 2006;37(2):124–7.
149. Avery RK, Bolwell BJ, Yen-Lieberman B, et al. Use of leflunomide in an allogeneic bone marrow transplant recipient with refractory cytomegalovirus infection. Bone Marrow Transplant 2004;34(12):1071–5.
150. Battiwalla M, Paplham P, Almyroudis NG, et al. Leflunomide failure to control recurrent cytomegalovirus infection in the setting of renal failure after allogeneic stem cell transplantation. Transpl Infect Dis 2007;9(1):28–32.
151. Efferth T, Romero M, Wolf D, et al. The antiviral activities of artemisinin and artesunate. Clin Infect Dis 2008;47:804–11.
152. Emanuel D, Cunningham I, Jules-Elysee K, et al. Cytomegalovirus pneumonia after bone marrow transplantation successfully treated with the combination of ganciclovir and high-dose intravenous immune globulin. Ann Intern Med 1988;109(10):777–82.
153. Ljungman P, Engelhard D, Link H, et al. Treatment of interstitial pneumonitis due to cytomegalovirus with ganciclovir and intravenous immune globulin: experience of European Bone Marrow Transplant Group. Clin Infect Dis 1992;14(4):831–5.
154. Reed EC, Bowden RA, Dandliker PS, et al. Treatment of cytomegalovirus pneumonia with ganciclovir and intravenous cytomegalovirus immunoglobulin in patients with bone marrow transplants. Ann Intern Med 1988;109(10):783–8.
155. Schmidt GM, Kovacs A, Zaia JA, et al. Ganciclovir/immunoglobulin combination therapy for the treatment of human cytomegalovirus-associated interstitial pneumonia in bone marrow allograft recipients. Transplantation 1988;46(6):905–7.

156. Erard V, Gutherie KA, Smith J, et al. Cytomegalovirus pneumonia (CMV-IP) after hematopoeitic cell transplantation (HCT): outcomes and factors associated with mortality [abstract V-1379]. 47th interscience conference on antimicrobial agents and chemotherapy; September 17–20; Chicago (IL) 2007.
157. Machado CM, Dulley FL, Boas LS, et al. CMV pneumonia in allogeneic BMT recipients undergoing early treatment of pre-emptive ganciclovir therapy. Bone Marrow Transplant 2000;26(4):413–7.
158. Reed EC, Wolford JL, Kopecky KJ, et al. Ganciclovir for the treatment of cytomegalovirus gastroenteritis in bone marrow transplant patients: a randomized, placebo-controlled trial. Ann Intern Med 1990;112(7):505–10.
159. Ljungman P, Cordonnier C, Einsele H, et al. Use of intravenous immune globulin in addition to antiviral therapy in the treatment of CMV gastrointestinal disease in allogeneic bone marrow transplant patients: a report from the European Group for Blood and Marrow Transplantation (EBMT). Infectious Diseases Working Party of the EBMT. Bone Marrow Transplant 1998;21(5):473–6.
160. Chang M, Dunn JP. Ganciclovir implant in the treatment of cytomegalovirus retinitis. Expert Rev Med Devices 2005;2(4):421–7.
161. Okamoto T, Okada M, Mori A, et al. Successful treatment of severe cytomegalovirus retinitis with foscarnet and intraocular infection of ganciclovir in a myelosuppressed unrelated bone marrow transplant patient. Bone Marrow Transplant 1997;20(9):801–3.
162. Ganly PS, Arthur C, Goldman JM, et al. Foscarnet as treatment for cytomegalovirus retinitis following bone marrow transplantation. Postgrad Med J 1988; 64(751):389–91.
163. Biron KK. Antiviral drugs for cytomegalovirus diseases. Antiviral Res 2006; 71(2-3):154–63.
164. Einsele H, Kapp M, Grigoleit GU. CMV-specific T cell therapy. Blood Cells Mol Dis 2008;40(1):71–5.

Viral Impact on Long-term Kidney Graft Function

Ilkka Helanterä, MD, PhD[a,b], Adrian Egli, MD, PhD[c,d], Petri Koskinen, MD, PhD[b], Irmeli Lautenschlager, MD, PhD[a,e], Hans H. Hirsch, MD, MS[c,f,*]

KEYWORDS

- BK virus • JC virus • Cytomegalovirus • Adenovirus
- Parvovirus • HHV6 • Kidney transplantation • Pathogenesis

In the past 2 decades, novel potent immunosuppressive regimens have helped to significantly reduce graft lost caused by acute rejection from 30% to 15% across HLA- and ABO-mismatches. However, in the same time period, infectious complications have steadily increased.[1] Viral infections 6 months after transplant have significantly increased from 10% to 30%.[2,3] Immunosuppression unspecifically blocks the function of immune effectors including those needed to control microbes and their infectious complications.[4] In addition, virus replication may trigger long-term effects through inflammation with cytokine release and induction of fibrosis.[5,6] These factors may contribute to reduced graft function and survival. In kidney transplant recipients, early cytomegalovirus (CMV) reactivation has been associated with reduced graft function in the following years.[6]

Reactivation of latent virus infection and uncontrolled viral replication following transplantation is common, especially in the classic high-risk situation of transplanting

I.H. and A.E. equally contributed to this article.

[a] Transplant Unit Research Laboratory, Transplantation and Liver Surgery Clinic, Helsinki University Hospital, and University of Helsinki, Meilahti, PL 340, Helsinki, FI-00029 HUS, Finland
[b] Department of Medicine, Division of Nephrology, Helsinki University Hospital, and University of Helsinki, PL 263, Helsinki, FI-00029 HUS, Finland
[c] Department of Biomedicine, Transplantation Virology, Institute for Medical Microbiology, University of Basel, Petersplatz 10, CH-4003 Basel, Switzerland
[d] Department of Medicine, University Hospital Basel, Petersgraben 4, CH-4031 Basel, Switzerland
[e] Department of Virology, Helsinki University Hospital, and University of Helsinki, PL 400, Helsinki, FI-00029 HUS, Finland
[f] Department of Internal Medicine, Infectious diseases and Hospital Epidemiology, University Hospital Basel, Petersgraben 4, CH-4031 Basel, Switzerland
* Corresponding author. Department of Biomedicine, Transplantation Virology, Institute for Medical Microbiology, University of Basel, Petersplatz 10, CH-4003 Basel, Switzerland.
E-mail address: Hans.Hirsch@unibas.ch

Infect Dis Clin N Am 24 (2010) 339–371
doi:10.1016/j.idc.2010.02.003
id.theclinics.com
0891-5520/10/$ – see front matter © 2010 Elsevier Inc. All rights reserved.

the graft of a seropositive donor (D+) into a seronegative recipient (R−). Despite receiving (val)ganciclovir prophylaxis, 40% of CMV D+R− patients seroconvert within the first 6 months after solid-organ transplantation (SOT).[7] For polyomavirus BK (BKV), low-level BK viruria of less than 5 log10 genome equivalents (geq)/mL is found in 5% to 10% of immunocompetent healthy blood donors, but high-level BKV viruria of more than 7 log10 geq/mL is observed in up to 60% of urine samples from SOT recipients.[8–12] On the one hand, the procedure of transplantation is associated with stress signals resulting from brain death, ischemia, inflammatory mediators, catecholamines, and drugs. Intracellular transduction may activate transcription factor sites shared by host and virus genes such as NFkB, AP1, glucocorticoid regulatory elements that among others stimulate virus reactivation and replication.[11,13,14]

On the other hand, virus replication is kept in check by virus-specific cellular immune surveillance mediating deletion of infected cells in immunocompetent individuals.[4,15–20] Current immunosuppressive protocols unspecifically reduce the quality (function) and quantity (frequency) of the virus-specific immune response. Accordingly, CMV-specific T cells are low or absent early after transplantation when CMV replication is observed.[16,20–24] Calcineurin inhibitors interfering with signal 1 of T-cell activation cause a dose-dependent decrease of interferon gamma (IFNγ) releasing BKV- and CMV-specific T cells, whereas antiproliferative drugs such as mycophenolic acid leave IFN production unaffected, but interfere with antigen-specific T-cell expansion.[25,26] Particularly in the first 3 months after transplant, when immunosuppression is more intense, BKV-specific killing function is inhibited.[27,28] Thus, immunosuppression interferes with the quality and quantity of virus-specific immune effectors thereby disturbing the balance of virus replication and control (**Fig. 1**).

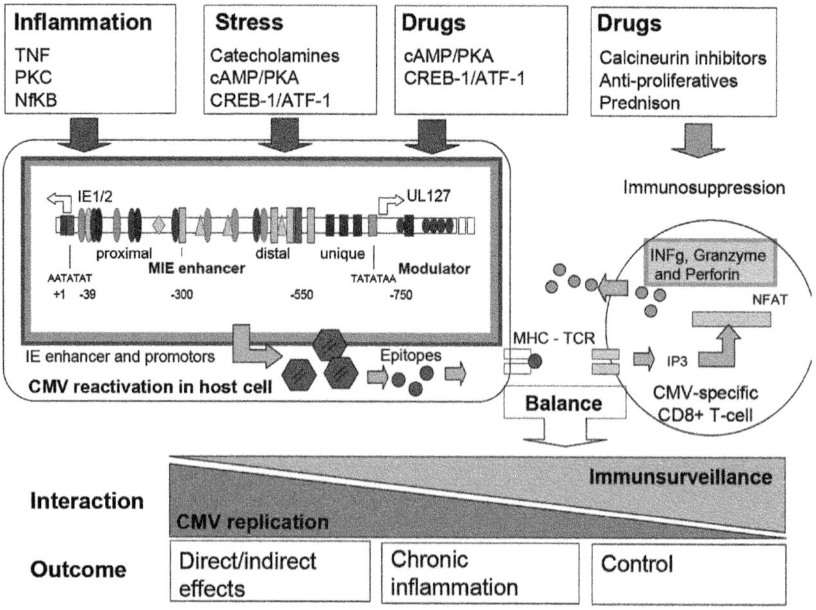

Fig. 1. Reactivation and control of virus. The binding of stress factors leading to an intracellular reactivation of CMV is shown. In parallel, CMV-specific T cells controlling the amount of virus epitope expressing host cells are suppressed by drugs. The balance between replication and control defines the patient's outcome.

The pathogenic consequences of uncontrolled virus replication after transplant have been classified as direct and indirect effects.[29,30] Direct effects result from viral cytopathic damage of host cells through cell lysis, inflammation and functio leasa of the respective organ such as CMV colitis, parvovirus B19 (PVB19) anemia, or adenovirus (ADV) nephritis. Indirect effects could result from immunomodulatory effects mediated by viral proteins (eg, CMV interleukin (IL)-10–like protein resulting in local immunosuppression and impaired antibacterial or antifungal immune clearance) or from effects compromising organ function through the release of proinflammatory and profibrotic factors (eg, CMV-triggered acute rejection or accelerated allograft nephropathy) (**Table 1**).[4,11] However, the detection of smoldering low-grade replication of CMV and BKV in cases of accelerated graft dysfunction has challenged the traditional divide of direct and indirect short-term effects.[6,31–33]

Reducing the impact of direct and indirect viral effects both short- and long-term is key to improving graft survival and function in the future. However, specific antiviral drugs are limited and whether prophylactic or preemptive treatment strategy is superior remains controversial. In principle, antiviral prophylaxis inhibits reactivation, replication, and virus-associated diseases at the cost of developing antiviral immunity, whereas preemptive treatment allows replication and antigen exposure visible to the immune system, but prevents virus-associated disease. Both strategies are largely successful,[34–36] but recent data suggested that prophylaxis may be superior in also reducing long-term indirect effects. Kliem and colleagues[33] reported that CMV replication within the first 3 months after transplant may lead to a significantly reduced long-term outcome within 4 years follow-up, most likely as a result of indirect effects. Similar processes may be caused by BKV replication in kidney allografts, because fibrogenic factors are induced at least in vitro.[37–39] Despite the prototypic effects of CMV and BKV, similar effects of other viruses on long-term graft function are less clear. This review focuses on the short-term and potential long-term effects of important viruses after kidney transplantation and summarizes current data on pathophysiology, diagnostics, and treatment.

ADENOVIRUS

Virological Aspects

Adenoviruses (ADV) have a nonenveloped icosahedral shell that harbors the linear double-stranded DNA of about 35 kB. The viral DNA genome encodes for more than 30 structural and nonstructural proteins. Nonstructural proteins regulate the human cell cycle and various aspects of the host's immune response (eg, ADV-E1 and -E3 regions).[40,41] Fifty-one ADV serotypes are described and divided into 6 subgroups A to F based on hemagglutination properties, oncogenic potential, and DNA homology (**Fig. 2**).[42,43] All subgroups except for B use the Coxsackie-adenovirus receptor, abbreviated CAR for cell entry. Coreceptors are $\alpha_V\beta_3$ and $\alpha_V\beta_5$ integrins.[44] Whether or not persistence of ADV may occur (eg, in lymphocytes and other cells) is not conclusively resolved.[45,46] However, transmission of ADV from seropositive donors (D+) to seronegative recipients (R−) after SOT has been reported, as well as ADV reactivation following profound T-cell depletion, both arguing for longer-term persistence, if not latency.[41,47]

Immunologic Aspects

The ADV hexon and fiber antigens harbor dominant epitopes recognized by neutralizing antibodies. ADV-type specific antibodies conferred by the fiber are measured by hemagglutination inhibition and by serum neutralization assays.[48] ADV-induced

Table 1
Direct and indirect effects of virus replication in solid-organ transplant recipients

	Adenovirus	Polyomavirus BK and JC	Cytomegalovirus	Human Herpesvirus-6 and -7	Parvovirus B19
Direct	Nephritis Cystitis Hepatitis	PyVAN Cystitis Ureter stenosis PML	Colitis Hepatitis Pneumonitis Nephritis Retinitis	Encephalitis Hepatitis Pneumonitis Colitis?	Anemia Enteritis Nephritis Collapsing glomerulopathy
Indirect	Bronchiolitis obliterans	Acute rejection?	Graft rejection Coinfection Allograft nephropathy Cardiac allograft vasculopathy Vanishing bile duct syndrome Bronchiolitis obliterans Posttransplant lymphoproliferative disorder Chorioretinitis uveitis	Graft rejection Coinfection Allograft nephropathy?	Glumerulonephritis Chronic allograft nephropathy Acute rejection?

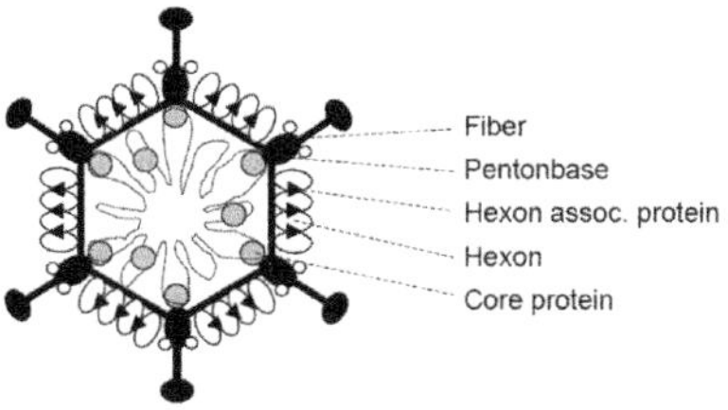

Subgroups	Serotypes	Clinical Presentation	Occurrence in SOT
A	12, 18, 31	Gastroenteritis	Liver: 31
B	3, 7, 16, 21, 50, 11, 14, 34, 35	Pneumonia Haemorrh. Cystitis Myocarditis	Kidney: 11, 34, 35 Liver: 7
C	1, 2, 5, 6	Pharyngitis Hepatitis	Liver: 1, 2, 5 Lung: 2, 5
D	8, 9, 10, 13, 15, 17, 19, 22, 23, 24, 26, 27, 30, 32, 33, 36, 37, 38, 39, 42, 43, 44,45, 46, 47, 48, 49, 51	Kerato-conjunctivitis Gastroenteritis	
E	4	Pneumonia	
F	40, 41	Gastroenteritis	

Fig. 2. ADV and disease. A scheme of ADV is shown, as well as ADV subgroups and serotypes with associated disease in solid-organ transplant recipients.

innate immunity has been primarily studied in murine pneumonia models and is mediated mainly by monocytes and particularly natural killer cells releasing IL-1, IL-6, and tumor necrosis factor α (TNFα).[49] In humans, increased levels of these cytokines seem to correlate with the severity of replication.[50] As a correlate of the adaptive cellular immune response, ADV-specific CD4+ but also CD8+ T-cell activity can be assessed in the peripheral blood.[51] Studies of ADV-specific T-cell responses have revealed a significant cross-reactivity among the different serotypes, especially based on shared epitope homologies of the hexon protein.[41] An age-related decrease of ADV-specific T-cell responses has been noted in healthy individuals and kidney transplant recipients, suggesting that immunosenescence may be a risk factor for ADV-associated disease.[52,53] Some ADV proteins provide immunosuppressive effects: Early gene 3 (E3) transcripts code for several immune regulatory proteins; for example, E3-gp19K retains major histocompatibility complex class I molecules in the endoplasmic reticulum for epitope presentation, E3-RIDa/b inhibits TNFα Fas and TRAIL induced cell apoptosis. Also TNFα-triggered cytokine levels such as IL-8, MCP1, and IP10 are modulated.[48,54,55] These and other immunomodulatory mechanisms may be responsible for smoldering ADV replication and indirect effects.

Clinical Aspects

Data on ADV seroprevalence are limited because there are more than 50 serotypes. Most symptomatic ADV are observed in children between 6 months and 5 years of age. Group C ADV-1, -2, and -5 primarily cause acute respiratory tract infections, group B ADV-7, -11, -14, -34, and -36, the urinary tract infections, group D ADV-8, -17, -19, and -37 keratoconjunctivitis, and group F ADV-40 and -41 gastrointestinal tract infections, with some overlaps. ADV replication is frequently detectable in transplant patients, but significant disease primarily affects children. Given the numerous serotypes, primary infection with a given subtype can still occur during adult life and run a more severe course in some patients. Severe ADV-associated diseases have been reported after SOT, hemopoietic stem cell transplantation (HSCT), AIDS, malignancies, and primary immunodeficiencies. The highest incidence and most fatal outcomes have been observed 1 to 3 months after allogeneic HSCT, in pediatric patients, in combination with acute graft-versus-host-disease (GVHD), T-cell depleting antibodies, and cord-blood HSCT.[56] In HSCT, hemorrhagic colitis (ADV-1, -5, -7, -8, -11, -31, -34, -35, -40, and -41), hemorrhagic cystitis and nephritis (ADV-11, -34, and -35), and pneumonitis (ADV-1, -2, -5, -29, -31, and -35) are associated with high morbidity and mortality.[57] In SOT recipients, the site of ADV disease manifestation shows a predilection for the transplanted organ; for example, renal transplants develop nephritis[58] and liver transplants develop hepatitis.[59,60] This highlights the importance of organ-specific HLA mismatches and thereby reduced viral epitope recognition through virus-specific T cells as well as the necessity for more intense immunosuppression as a contributing risk factor.

Role in Kidney Transplantation

As most patients have been exposed to ADV before transplantation, ADV replication and disease are not frequent problems after SOT. In a survey, ADV disease in kidney transplant recipients occurs in 1% and is less frequent than in lung (20%) or liver transplant recipients (3.4%). However, ADV replication can be detected in up to 11% of urine samples.[61] Little systematic information is available on ADV detection in blood. In a large study of (val)ganciclovir prophylaxis in CMV D+/R− SOT, low-level ADV DNA was detected in plasma in 0.2% to 3% of patients, mostly after 3 months, corresponding to mostly asymptomatic replication.[62] If occurring months after kidney transplantation, ADV (re)exposure or ADV reactivation is possible. However, pretransplant neutralizing antibodies to ADV-11 were not detectable in recipients who developed ADV-11 replication and cystitis soon after transplantation, suggesting that primary infection can be acquired from the donor kidney.[57]

The rate of ADV-associated disease is difficult to enumerate.[58,61] Hemorrhagic cystitis and (less commonly) nephritis are the major ADV diseases described in kidney transplant patients.[58] Estimates of ADV-associated hemorrhagic cystitis are about 2%, most of which occurred within the first year after transplant, with prolonged periods of low-grade fever, pain, and hematuria more than grade II.[58,63] If measured, ADV load in urine is often greater than 7 log geq/m, and viremia is also detected. Increases in serum creatinine level may be caused by postrenal obstruction from clots, but undiagnosed nephritis may also be present.[64,65] Most commonly, serotypes ADV-11, -34, and -35 are detected. ADV pneumonitis, hepatitis, and disseminated disease are rarely diagnosed after kidney transplantation, but may be responsible for a case fatality rate as high as 18%.[66] Screening is not commonly used, hence diagnosis is usually delayed. However, this may change as more intense immunosuppressive regimens are combined with lymphocyte-depleting therapies for induction and rejection, such as thymoglobulin, alemtuzumab, and rituximab. The long-term effects of early graft replication and immunomodulatory effects on kidney allograft function have been only marginally examined so far.[57]

Therapeutic Aspects

ADV replication should be suspected in kidney transplant patients with profound immunosuppression and hematuria, cystitis, low-grade fever, and small increases in serum creatinine levels, when other more frequent diagnoses have been excluded.

Urine and plasma viral loads may be helpful, but allograft biopsy demonstrating cytopathic changes in renal tubular epithelial cells and specific immunohistochemistry is required for a definitive diagnosis. ADV-specific treatment with antiviral agents is not established. The use of ribavirin, cidofovir, and ganciclovir has been reported in small case series.[67–69] However, the outcomes are variable and may in part be ADV-type specific. For example, ribavirin may only be effective for hemorrhagic cystitis with ADV type C. Cidofovir is limited by its risk of nephrotoxicity, especially in the context of kidney transplantation. Moreover, exact dosage and duration of treatment remains to be clarified; Either 5 mg/kg bodyweight intravenously once a week or so-called low-dose 1 mg/kg 3 times per week has been used. With antiviral treatment, with a judicious reduction of immunosuppression, patients may mount ADV-specific immune control. Adoptive transfer of ADV-specific T cells have been explored after HSCT, but not after kidney transplantation.[43]

POLYOMAVIRUS BK AND JC

Virological Aspects

Five polyomaviruses have been consistently detected in human specimens and include BK (BKV), JC (JCV), KI virus (KIV), WU virus (WUV), and Merckel cell carcinoma virus (MCV). Current studies have focused on the direct and indirect effects of polyomaviruses (PyV), or in combination with other agents.[70,71] PyV particles are nonenveloped and harbor a circular double-stranded DNA of about 5.2 kB. The viral genome encodes for early proteins (small T and large T antigen) and for late proteins (viral capsid protein [VP] 1 to 3 and agno protein). An overview of the replication cycle of BKV is shown in **Fig. 3**. Besides α2-3 and α2-6 glycosylated surface structures, gangliosides GD1b and GT1b serve for cell entry of BKV and the serotonergic 5HT2A receptor for JCV.[72,73] The receptors of KIV, WUV, and MCV are not yet known.

BKV and JCV cause polyomavirus-associated nephropathy (PyVAN) and PyV-associated multifocal leukoencephalopathy (PyVML), in kidney transplant recipients. The role of KIV and WUV in immunocompetent individuals and in transplant patients is only now becoming understood. The route of natural transmission is not known for

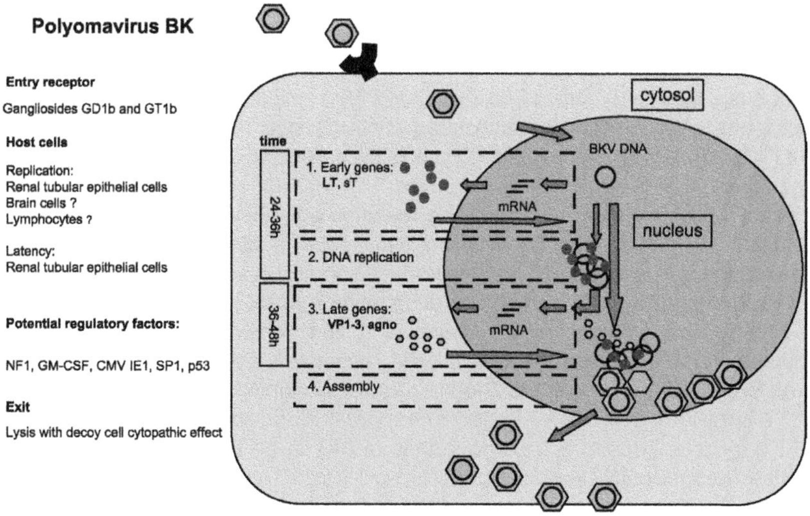

Fig. 3. BKV replication in host cell.

BKV or JCV, but may be respiratory or oral. For KIV and WUV, respiratory transmission is strongly implicated.[74] Screening of immunocompetent individuals with respiratory tract infection detected KIV and WUV in 1% to 7%, without pronounced seasonality, but with a predilection for pediatric patients.[75,76] MCV has been detected in 38% of forehead skin swabs from otherwise healthy individuals.[77] Therefore, the development of Merkel cell carcinoma is likely to require cofactors besides MCV infection, such as UV-light exposure in immunocompromised patients. In a retrospective polymerase chain reaction (PCR) study of respiratory secretions from 200 immunocompromised patients from France, KIV and WUV were detected in 8% and 1%, respectively.[78] KIV was significantly more frequent (18%) among 45 allogeneic HSCT patients tested. In several of these patients, stool samples were positive for KIV.[78] Thus, the data suggest that WUV and KIV may play a role in respiratory tract pathologies, but it is not clear whether this is reactivation or reinfection. The association with respiratory and gastrointestinal disease requires further study.[79] Thus, because SV40, KIV, WUV, and MCV have no known role in kidney transplant deterioration, this article focuses on BKV and JCV.

Immunologic Aspects

The BKV seroprevalence increases to 80% to 90% during childhood, whereas JCV seroprelavence reaches 58% during adult life.[12,80] For KIV, WUV, and MCV, the average seroprevalence has been determined as 55%, 69%, and 42%, respectively.[81] For BKV and JCV, neutralizing antibodies inhibit host cell infection by targeting the major capsid protein VP1.[82] Several studies have confirmed that the amount of antibody activity measured by enzyme-linked immunosorbent assays seems to correspond more to recent BKV antigen exposure rather than protection from polyomavirus replication.[12,83–85] In healthy individuals JCV-specific immunoglobulin (Ig) G has been linked to more antigen exposure.[12] Subclinical infection may also contribute to an increase of BKV-specific IgG and IgA.[86] The role of BKV serology in kidney transplantation to assess potential risk of infection is controversial. Bohl and colleagues[87] screened 198 transplant recipients and found that the relative risk of developing a BKV infection was highest for the D+R+ group. The likelihood of developing viruria in 1 year was associated with donor serostatus and increased stepwise with increasing donor BKV antibody titers.

The primary humoral immune response is followed by an adaptive PyV-specific humoral and cellular response.[27,84,85] The importance of the PyV-specific immune control is highlighted by studies on BKV in kidney transplant patients. BKV replication and progression to disease are associated with older age, male gender,[88] seropositive donor,[87,89] seronegative recipient,[83,89] lack of BKV-specific cellular immune memory,[17] use of potent immunosuppressive regimens,[90–95] HLA C7 negative donor or negative recipients,[87] HLA mismatches,[8,94,96] and rejection episodes followed by antirejection treatment.[8,94,96,97] Control of BKV replication is mainly achieved through BKV-specific IFNγ-producing T cells. Low BKV-specific T-cell control is associated with higher BKV loads in plasma and graft, and risk of developing PyVAN.[17,28,84,98–102] T-cell control over BKV replication appeared to be linked to responses against the BKV large T antigen, and only to a lesser extent to VP1 responses. Patients with a decrease of plasma BKV loads by more than 2 log10 showed a significant increase to more than 69 IFNγ spot-forming units per million peripheral blood mononuclear cells for BKV large T antigen epitopes.[102] The importance of BKV large T antigen–specific immune responses has recently been elaborated to cytotoxic T-cell responses clearing BKV replication.[27] Other antigens such as BKV cell lysates, different staining techniques with flow cytometry or tetramer staining, and even different stimulation protocols with BKV-pulsed dendritic cells are in line with the important role of BKV-specific T-cell control[27,28,84,98,102,103] (for review see ref.[25]). The role of inflammatory damage mediated through BKV-specific CD8+ T cells has been described, as well as single cases of immune reconstitution syndrome-like diseases, but these cases are rare and somewhat controversial.[103,104]

Clinical Aspects

BKV and JCV infect up to 80% of the human population[12,80,105,106] and establish a latent state in the renourinary tract.[107,108] In healthy donors, BKV is detectable in 10% of urine samples with a median viral load of 3.5 log geq/mL, whereas JCV is found in about 20% with median viral load of 5 log geq/mL.[12,109,110] BKV or JCV viremia is typically absent in immunocompetent individuals.[12,111]

After kidney transplantation, BKV detection increases to 20% to 60% of urine samples with about 1000-fold higher BKV loads compared with healthy individuals. JCV can be detected in 20% to 50% of urine samples with similar fold increase.[8,112,113] A third of patients with BKV viruria also develop BKV viremia and progression to PyVAN.[8,114] The negative predictive value for PyVAN without BKV viremia is almost 100% and the positive predictive value is about 50% to 90%.[8,115–117] BKV plasma loads of more than 4 log10 geq/mL are associated with a high sensitivity and specificity (>95%) to PyVAN.[115,116,118] Up to 5% of all PyVAN cases could be associated with JCV replication.[112] In kidney transplant patients with JCV-mediated PyVAN, JCV viremia is rarely detected and then only with lower viral loads (14.2%, mean 2000 cells/mL).[112] Up to 5% of all PyVAN cases could be associated with JCV replication.[112]

Current recommendations for screening propose a urinary screening strategy for high-level PyV replication by demonstrating either decoy cells by urine cytology, viral particles by electron microscopy, or BKV loads of greater than 7 log geq/mL by quantitative PCR. The screening test has a high negative predictive value and lead time to PyVAN of approximately 6 to 12 weeks. In kidney transplant patients with high-level viruria, plasma BKV loads should be measured.[119]

Role in Kidney Transplantation

Prolonged BKV replication has been associated with reduced graft function. Histopathology studies indicate that viral replication starts focally with little inflammation (PyVAN stage A) and progresses to pronounced inflammation in response to extensive tubular cell necrosis, denudation of the basement membrane (PyVAN stage B), and finally to a state of tubular atrophy and extensive chronic fibrotic graft changes (PyVAN stage C). The histologic stages A, B, and C correlate with the risk of subsequent graft lost of less than 10% to 50% and greater than 80%.[115,116,118,120,121] As the disease starts with a focal pattern, sampling errors yielding false negative biopsy results are estimated to occur in at least 10% to 30% of cases. Therefore, in line with the Banff recommendation, at least 2 biopsy cores should be analyzed.[122] Prolonged BKV replication leads to accumulation of rearrangements in the virus noncoding control region (NCCR), which harbors major transcription sites. Deletions and insertions into the NCCR are associated with increased early BKV gene expression and more pronounced cytopathic effects in vitro and in vivo. BKV variants with rearranged NCCRs are associated with 20-fold higher plasma loads (median 440,000 geq/mL vs 20,000 geq/mL), and a faster progression to PyVAN B.[106] The role of JCV NCCR for PyVAN is not defined, but so far, no rearrangements have been observed in renal allografts with JCV-mediated PyVAN.[112] Despite inflammatory infiltrates, the clinical course of JCV-PyVAN seems to run a more benign course, but larger studies are lacking.[112] BKV replication has been demonstrated to selectively induce not only genes involved in cell division and DNA replication but also those down-regulating immune and defense genes in vitro.[123] Further studies reported that BKV replication activated profibrotic cytokines such as tumor growth factor β (TGFβ) and induced proliferation of fibroblasts that might play a role in chronic graft fibrosis observed in PyVAN C.[37–39,124,125] Expression profiling of kidney biopsies support the notion that BKV replication may induce proinflammatory and profibrotic changes in vivo.[126] Thus, changes consistent with TA/IF and chronic allograft nephropathy after BKV replication and PyVAN may result from acute virus-mediated tubular epithelial cell injury and the strong inflammatory response, by virus-induced exhaustion of tubular regeneration, and/or by virus-induced profibrotic host cell response that persists and accumulates during chronic low-grade BKV replication in the kidney allograft. Moreover, sensitization to the allograft may occur in this microenvironment contributing by chronic rejection, especially when treatment of BKV replication is largely based on reduced immunosuppression. Clearly, further studies are needed to unravel the most important factors of BKV-mediated long-term contribution to kidney transplant loss and the most appropriate intervention.

Therapeutic Aspects

Treatment of BKV replication has been reviewed in several previous publications.[11,25,26,127] The key intervention is the reduction of immunosuppression. This can be performed by reducing the calcineurin inhibitor to lower trough levels of less than 6 ng/mL for tacrolimus, and less than 125 ng/mL for cyclosporine, or by reducing the dose of mycophenolate by 50%.[128] However, there are no randomized controlled trials evaluating one strategy versus another. The authors recently described a dose-dependent correlation between calcineurin inhibitors and BKV-specific T-cell function which would advocate reducing calcineurin inhibitors to lower levels of 3 ng/mL for tacrolimus, and 100 ng/mL for cyclosporine.[25,26] No specific antiviral treatment is available. Switching to leflunomide has been proposed based on the belief that a combination of immunosuppressive and antiviral activities could resolve the double-bind situation of PyVAN by replacing a stronger immunosuppressive drug mycophenolate, an antiproliferative purine antagonist, with leflunomide, a pyrimidine antagonist. Both drugs have been shown to interfere with BKV replication in vitro via host cell proliferation, although a direct comparison is lacking. Even though cidofovir and leflunomide may interfere with BKV replication by inhibiting viral and cellular DNA replication and possibly additional mechanisms related to viral egress,[129–131] the optimal setting in which to add these agents to reduced immunosuppression is not defined.[132–135] Newer compounds, such as CMX001, a lipid-derivative of cidofovir, which has reduced toxicity, might be a promising option.[136]

CYTOMEGALOVIRUS

Virological Aspects

Cytomegalovirus (CMV) is the fifth of the 8 known human herpesviruses. The linear double-stranded DNA genome with 235 kb is protected by a viral capsid, matrix, and envelope and encodes for at least 59 proteins.[137,138] CMV latency and replication is tightly regulated with coordinated expression of immediate-early (IE), early, and late genes. **Fig. 4** shows the replication cycle of CMV. CMV is transmitted via saliva, body fluids, cells, and tissues.[11]

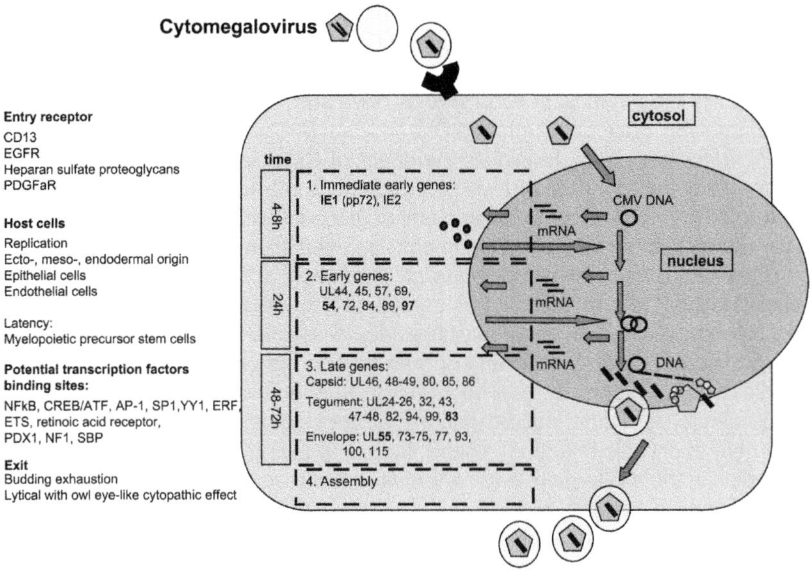

Fig. 4. CMV replication in host cell.

Clinical Aspects

Primary CMV infection occurring in healthy individuals usually during the first 2 decades of life, leads to a life-long latency. The seroprevalence of CMV varies in different populations, and is estimated to be between 40% and 95%.[139] In immunocompromised individuals the activation of CMV is common, and CMV remains one of the most important pathogens causing morbidity and costs after organ transplantation. Despite antiviral medications, CMV infections continue to represent an increasing threat to transplant recipients, especially with the use of new and more potent immunosuppressive medications to prevent chronic allograft loss.

Most of the CMV infections in transplant recipients are caused by reactivation of latent virus of either recipient or donor origin. In recipients with no previous history of CMV infection, primary infection is often more severe compared with a reactivation of the virus in a seropositive host. CMV infection in organ transplant recipients manifests commonly as fever, malaise, leucopenia, or thrombocytopenia, but can also cause organ-specific manifestations, such as hepatitis, gastrointestinal symptoms, renal dysfunction, and CMV pneumonitis, which still has a high fatality rate despite effective antiviral medication. After kidney transplantation, approximately 10% to 20% of recipients suffer from symptomatic CMV infection.[140,141] CMV seronegative recipients of a kidney from a seropositive donor (R+/D−) are at highest risk of symptomatic CMV infection; symptomatic activation of the virus can be detected in up to 60% of these recipients.[142]

Role in Kidney Transplantation

The first reports of the association of CMV with the kidney allograft rejection process and decreased graft survival were published in the 1970s and the 1980s.[143] The association of CMV and acute rejection has since been shown in many studies,[144–147] although opposite evidence exists as well.[148] Some studies have found an association of only symptomatic CMV infection (CMV disease) with acute rejection.[147,149,150]

CMV has also been associated with glomerulopathic changes in the allograft.[151–153] The earliest reports about the association of CMV infection with inferior graft survival came from the 1980s.[154–156] Even in the current era of immunosuppression and molecular CMV diagnostics, several studies have shown inferior kidney graft function in recipients with past CMV infection[157–159] or CMV replication after transplantation.[35,160] In some studies, however, the effect of CMV replication and disease was scored for a combined end point with graft loss and mortality (graft loss uncensored for death).[161,162] A recent randomized study of oral ganciclovir prophylaxis or preemptive therapy in kidney transplant recipients showed increased graft survival in the prophylaxis group with fewer episodes of CMV replication.[33] Although the general impression is that CMV replication has an overall detrimental effect on graft outcome, the sequence of events can either start from acute rejection to CMV replication or vice versa, both impacting on the decline of graft function to premature failure.[148,163,164]

The role of CMV on chronic renal allograft dysfunction has been discussed since the 1980s. Evidence from other solid-organ transplants indicates that CMV enhances the development of chronic rejection in heart, lung, and liver transplantations.[165–172] Only a few studies in the modern era have addressed the association of CMV with histopathology changes in the renal allograft, in particular with what was earlier called chronic allograft rejection but is now referred to as chronic allograft nephropathy, or according to the most recent guidelines, interstitial fibrosis and tubular atrophy (IF/TA).[173] A study by Humar and colleagues[174] reported an association of CMV replication with biopsy-proved chronic rejection only in the presence of previous acute rejection episodes. In a recent analysis of 3-month protocol biopsies in patients with CMV replication after transplantation, Reischig and colleagues[150] reported increased interstitial fibrosis and tubular atrophy only in patients with CMV viral loads of 2000 geq/mL or more, but not in all patients with CMV infection. In a study from Finland, histopathologic changes were systematically analyzed in 6-month protocol biopsies, but previous CMV replication was not associated with significant histopathologic changes.[175] However, in patients with CMV pp65 antigen or DNA detected in the biopsy, together with a previous history of acute rejection, increased vascular changes were demonstrated.

CMV is able to infect most cell types of the kidney in cell cultures, including glomerular, tubular, and endothelial cells.[176–178] After kidney transplantation, CMV has been detected in the allograft in several studies.[179–183] CMV is able to persist in the kidney allograft for months after viremia with active infection associated with chronic changes in the graft.[182] Similar findings of persistent CMV DNA in the allograft and increased histopathologic changes have been described after liver transplantation.[167,170] Persistent CMV in the kidney allograft, as detected by a positive pp65 antigen or CMV DNA by in situ hybridization in an allograft biopsy more than 30 days after the last positive CMV finding in blood or urine, was associated with reduced graft function and reduced graft survival, compared with patients with no intragraft CMV.[6] CMV was detected in various tubular, glomerular, and vascular structures of the graft for some time after CMV replication when blood or urine were already negative for several weeks or months.

In addition to the direct injury to the allograft caused by CMV and the respective inflammatory response, there are several other mechanisms through which CMV could indirectly enhance alloresponses and intragraft pathologies. CMV can directly or indirectly induce the production of several proinflammatory cytokines such as IL-1, IL-2, TNFα,[184–186] adhesion molecules such as intercellular adhesion molecule (ICAM)-1, vascular cell adhesion molecule (VCAM)-1,[187–189] and profibrotic and vasculopathic growth factors such as TGFβ, platelet-derived growth factor (PDGF), connective tissue growth factor (CTGF), vascular endothelial growth factor.[190–192] These molecules are known to have a key role in acute allograft rejection as well as in chronic allograft nephropathy. In rat models of chronic kidney allograft rejection, CMV increased inflammation, the development of vascular changes, and the generation of fibrosis.[193–196] In addition, CMV increased expression of adhesion molecules (ICAM-1, VCAM-1) and growth factors (TGFβ, PDGF, CTGF).[193,194,196,197]

The inflammatory cytokines involved in T-cell activation and induction of adhesion molecules, especially TNFα, are suggested to play a central role in the augmentation of the rejection process. TNFα is also believed to be a key molecule in activation of CMV from latency during an alloresponse,[13,14] and it is a central molecule for the activation of adhesion molecules, synthesis, and release of growth factors TGFβ and PDGF,[198,199] which induce smooth muscle proliferation in the vascular wall and collagen synthesis by fibroblasts. CTGF, up-regulated by TGFβ,[200] is especially important in the generation of fibrosis. CMV induces the production of TNFα,[186] but may also directly induce TGFβ and PDGF.[201–203] These cytokines participate in the profibrotic and vasculopathic cascades in direct and indirect ways. CMV also enhances the development of tubular atrophy, which is characteristic for chronic allograft damage.[173,204] This may be a result of CMV increased tubular apoptosis, which was found to be mediated through the TNFα -TNF-R1 pathway.[205]

In addition to up-regulating the production of several chemokines during infections, the CMV genome encodes chemokine analogs (UL146 and UL147)[206] and chemokine receptor analogs (UL33, UL78, US 27, US28), through which the virus is able to further modify the immune response and stimulate cellular responses.[207,208] The chemokine receptor analogs US28 and R33 have been associated with smooth muscle cell migration and development of transplant vasculopathy in experimental models.[209,210] Experimental data also indicate that CMV up-regulates several genes involved in the processes of wound repair and angiogenesis, important also for chronic allograft injury.[210,211] Recent experimental data suggest that CMV infection in the allograft may also disrupt the development of graft acceptance and inhibit tolerogenic responses, and contribute to the continuous damage in the graft.[212] Clinical data point to persistent CMV infection in the allograft as a risk factor of kidney allograft dysfunction and impaired survival.[5,6] The results from Helantera and Lautenschlager[5] further suggest that the persistence of CMV in the graft is associated with an inferior outcome after transplantation by provoking an excess inflammatory response but also by persistent expression of adhesion molecules and production of cytokines inducing premature chronic changes in the graft with subsequent deterioration of graft function. Accordingly, profibrotic and vasculopathic growth factors TGFβ and PDGF, and adhesion molecules like ICAM-1 are increased in biopsies with persistent intragraft CMV replication. These concepts are summarized in **Fig. 5**.

Interaction of CMV with other viruses has been of interest, because occasionally CMV and BKV replication can be simultaneously observed in kidney transplant patients, raising the question of mutual interaction. In vitro studies indicate that the homologous large T antigen of SV40 can activate CMV promoters,[213] and, on the other hand, CMV and BKV expression is activated under common conditions (eg, via activating similar transcription factor pathways such as NF-kappa B or AP1). However, despite this overlap, it is not very likely that BKV and CMV coinfection of the same renal tubular epithelial cells can occur to such an extent that would support persistent coreplication with synergistically increasing viral loads of viruses. It is clear that intense immunosuppression unspecifically paralyses immune effectors not only to alloantigens but also to CMV and BKV.[214] Currently, most studies are confounded by the use of ganciclovir prophylaxis, and uncorrected differences in CMV and BKV

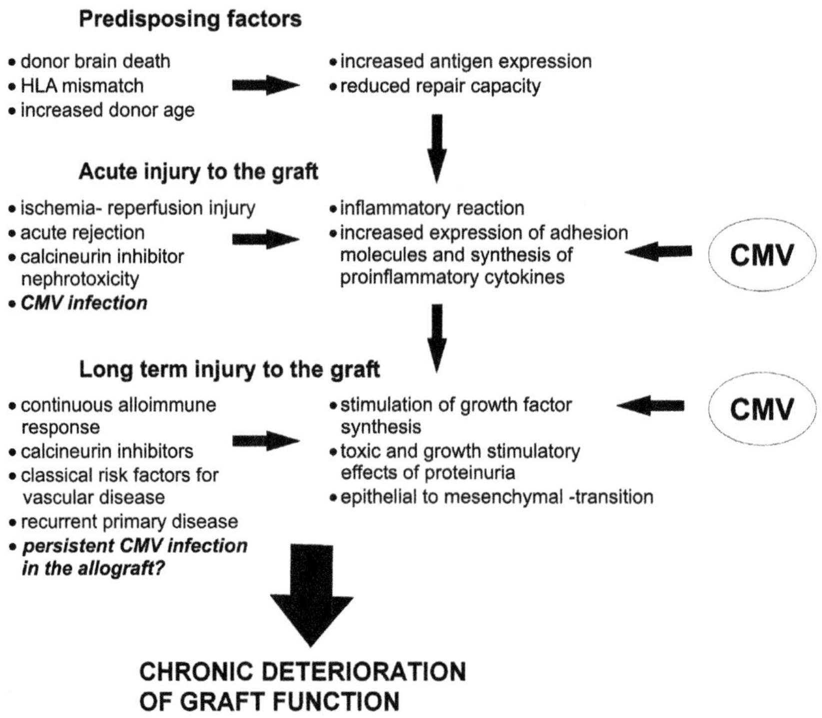

Fig. 5. The suggested role of CMV in the process of chronic deterioration of graft function (previously referred to as chronic allograft nephropathy).

serostatus of donor and recipient. In the prospective study by Hirsch and colleagues,[8] no universal prophylaxis to CMV was used and the serostatus to both viruses was known. The results demonstrated that in patients seropositive for CMV and BKV, the onset of CMV antigenemia and BKV high-level viruria measured by decoy cells was not related. Thus, despite an overlap in risk factors, both viruses seem to reactivate independently, but if occurring together, could result in worse graft outcomes.

HUMAN HERPESVIRUS-6 AND -7

Virological Aspects

Human herpesvirus-6 and -7 (HHV-6, HHV-7) are members of the *Roseolavirus* genus of the betaherpesvirus subfamily. HHV-6 was first isolated from the peripheral blood lymphocytes of immunocompromised patients.[215] Like all herpesviruses, it is a large DNA virus of 200 nm in diameter consisting of a linear double-stranded DNA of approximately 160 to 162 kb inside an icosahedral nucleocapsid.[215] There are 2 variants of HHV-6, variants A and B, of which HHV-6B is the most common.[216] The HHV-6B genome contains 119 open reading frames (ORFs), 9 of which are absent in HHV-6A.[216] The overall nucleotide sequence identity between HHV-6A and -B variants is 90%. HHV-6 is a close relative to CMV, and the genetic homology is as high as 67%, and 21% with all other herpesviruses.[217,218] HHV-7 was isolated from CD4+ T cells of a healthy adult in 1990[219] and is closely related to HHV-6 and CMV.[220] HHV-7 has a linear double-stranded DNA with a size of 140 to 160 kb, and is genetically most closely related to the 2 HHV-6 variants.[220] HHV-6 and HHV-7 are lymphotropic viruses; HHV-7 primarily infects T cells and uses CD4 as a cellular receptor,[221] but HHV-6 uses the CD46 molecule as its receptor[222] and may also infect monocytes/macrophages, endothelial, and epithelial cells.

Clinical Aspects

HHV-6 and HHV-7 have both been associated with roseola infantum in early childhood. Seroprevalence of HHV-6 and HHV-7 is globally high, about 90% to 95%, and primary infections among adults are rare. Of the 2 variants of HHV-6, HHV-6B is the most common and known to cause exanthema subitum in infants but the clinical significance of HHV-6A is less clear.[216,223] The characteristic features of exanthema subitum are fever and skin rash, and the clinical course of the primary HHV-6 infection is usually benign, but some complications such as encephalitis or febrile seizures may occur. Mild liver dysfunction is also occasionally associated with HHV-6 infection, but cases of fulminant hepatitis are rare. Little is known about the clinical characteristics of primary HHV-7 infection, but it has been associated with roseola infantum, hepatitis and neurologic complications.[224–226] After primary infection, HHV-6 and HHV-7 persist in the host for life, and may reactivate during immunosuppression.

HHV-6 and HHV-7 are commonly reactivated after organ transplantation with an incidence of up to approximately 50% depending on the patient population.[227–229] In organ transplant recipients most of the HHV-6 reactivations are caused by the variant HHV-6B, and appear 2 to 4 weeks after transplantation and are asymptomatic. However, HHV-6 may cause fever, leukopenia and other clinical symptoms, such as neurologic disorders, encephalitis, rash, graft dysfunction, pneumonitis, gastrointestinal infection, and hepatitis.[228,230–236]

Role in Kidney Transplantation

In addition to the direct effect of HHV-6, indirect effects have been suggested. HHV-6 is considered an immunomodulatory virus stimulating inflammatory pathways.[237] Akin to CMV, HHV-6 induces the release of inflammatory cytokines, such as TNFα and IL-1, which are important mediators in the early phase of the rejection cascade. HHV-6 seems to be involved in immunologic processes of the transplant that promote acute or chronic rejection.[227,233] Like CMV, HHV-6 is associated with intragraft lymphoid activation and adhesion molecule induction in vascular endothelium in liver transplants.[238] In renal transplantation, HHV-6 has been associated with acute rejection and in the development of chronic allograft nephropathy.[157,239–242] Data from Finland demonstrated that HHV-6 may persist in renal allografts,[243] but the significance for allograft function remains to be shown. Analyzing 22 kidney transplant biopsies of patients with previous CMV infection, HHV-6 antigens were found in the biopsies of 7 patients, with biopsies taken 30 to 1484 days after transplantation. Patients with intragraft HHV-6 had a slightly higher frequency of acute rejection episodes, but no differences were seen in graft function or survival, possibly in part because of the small sample size. As a potential confounder, HHV-6 reactivations frequently occurred as a coinfection with CMV, but only 1 patient showed the presence of both viruses in the graft.[243]

The significance of HHV-7 in transplantation is even less clear. The incidence of HHV-7 reactivation has been reported to reach 46% in this patient population,[244] but symptomatic disease has not been documented. HHV-7 has been found together with CMV and might be a cofactor for the progression of CMV disease.[245] HHV-7 uses the CD4 molecule as its receptor and is more strictly lymphotrophic than HHV-6. However, the virus may also have similar indirect effects as CMV. HHV-7 has been associated with increased acute rejection of renal transplants,[244] graft dysfunction, and chronic allograft nephropathy.[157,229] In conclusion, reactivation of beta herpesvirus replication is common after kidney transplantation and associated with significant morbidity and costs in the case of CMV. More studies in kidney transplant recipients are needed to identify the pathologic role of HHV-6 and HHV-7.

PARVOVIRUS B19

Virological Aspects

Parvovirus B19 (PVB19) encodes 2 nonstructural proteins, NS-1 and NS-2, as well as 3 viral capsid proteins (VP1–3) which form the nonenveloped icosahedral viral particle harboring the single-stranded DNA of 5 kb. The blood-group P antigen is the viral receptor for cell entry into erythroid progenitor cells.[246] Lack of P antigen has been associated with resistance to PVB19 infections. The $\alpha5\beta1$ integrins probably acts as coreceptors.[247] Cell entry is further supported by a phospholipase A2 activity of the capsid VP1 protein.[248,249]

PVB19-specific Immune Response

After primary infection with lysis of infected cells, virus-specific IgM antibodies are detectable about 12 days later, followed by an IgG response with neutralizing activities, mainly targeting the VP1 protein.[250,251] After primary infection, PVB19-specific CD8+ T cells seem to persist for several months.[252] Increased levels of IL-2, IL-12 and IL-15, but not IFNγ, are present at time of the primary PVB19 peak viral load. Subsequently, patients maintain sustained Th1 cytokine responses for almost 2 years. Patients with persistent PVB19 replication showed no imbalance of their cytokine pattern, except for an increased INFγ response.[253] TGFβ might also be up-regulated during PVB19 replication, similar to BKV.[254] Certain HLA alleles have been associated with symptomatic infection: HLA-DRB1*01, *04, *07, and B49. Single nucleotide polymorphisms in genes that are linked to apoptosis, cell cycle, and growth were also associated with symptomatic infection.[255]

PVB19 Infection and Replication

Seroprevalence of PVB19 ranges from 30% to 90% in the adult population.[248,249,256] Transmission normally occurs through droplets and smear inoculation, but vertical transmission with hydrops fetalis during pregnancy and transmission through blood products,[257] SOT, and HSCT have been described.[258,259]

Primary infection during childhood presents as erythema infectiosum, also known as the fifth disease. In immunocompetent adults, PVB19 may cause arthopathy and even arthritis, preferentially in women, and myocarditis (**Table 2**). Glomerular disease with nephritis and proteinuria, hypocomplementemia, pancytopenia, and hypocomplementemia has been described in several case reports of previously healthy individuals.[260–263] In some cases, the histologic features were endocapillary and/or mesangial proliferation often with subendothelial deposits together with granular deposition of C3 and IgG along capillary walls and mesangium, which is consistent with a postinfectious glomerulonephritis.

Role in Kidney Transplantation

PVB19 was first discovered in 1975 by Cossart and colleagues,[264] but the first report of PVB19 infection after transplant was described in1986 in a kidney transplant patient with stable graft function.[265] Overall, PVB19 replication appeared more severe and prolonged with anemia as the predominant clinical manifestation. In addition, PVB19 replication after transplant has also been associated with hepatitis, myocarditis, pneumonitis, and allograft dysfunction.[248,249] A single case of PVB19-associated

Table 2
Complications during parvovirus B19 infection

Established Syndromes	Potential Associations
Erythema infectiosum	Renal: proliferative glomerulonephrititis, collapsing glomerulopathy, focal segmental glomerulo sclerosis, thrombotic microangiopathy, renal transplant function, acute allograft rejection
Arthropathy	Rheumatic: rheumatoid arthritis, systemic lupus erythematosus, dermatomyosisits, systemic sclerosis
Hydrops fetalis	Cardiac: myocarditis, cardiomyopathy
Transient aplastic crisis	Hepatobiliary: hepatitis, fulminant liver failure
Chronic pure red blood cell aplasia	Hematologic: hemophagocytic syndrome, idiopathic thrombocytopenia, hemolytic uremic syndrome
	Dermatologic: Gianotti-Crosti syndrome, erythema nodosum
	Vasculitis: Kawasaki disease, Henoch-Schönlein purpura, microscopic polyarteritis nodosa
	Neurologic: encephalopathy, Guillain-Barré syndrome
	Pulmonary: idiopathic pulmonary fibrosis, lymphocytic interstitital pneumonitis

encephalitis occurred 5 days after renal transplantation in a 9-year-old boy, and was successfully treated with reduced immunosuppression.[266] PVB19 replication has also been associated with diarrhea.[267] Although no systematic screening for PVB19 is performed, the incidence of PVB19 complications was estimated to range from 1% to 12%, occurring mainly during the first year after kidney transplantation.[268,269] Ki and colleagues[268] reported that the median onset to PVB19 disease was relatively early, at 7 weeks after transplantation. In kidney transplant recipients, the onset was 5 weeks after transplant, suggesting that significant amounts of PVB19 had been transferred with the renal tissues, although the onset at 64 weeks in heart and lung transplant recipients suggested that only a low copy of PVB19 was present in the transplant, or that infection was community acquired. PVB19 DNA can be found in the blood of almost one-third of kidney transplant patients with anemia.[268,270] Eid and colleagues[269] summarized 98 published cases of PVB19 infection in transplant recipients up to 2006 (24 HSCT; 74 SOT including 53 kidney transplants). Among kidney transplant recipients, anemia was present in 98.1%, leucopenia in 34%, thrombocytopenia in 19.1%, fever in 23.9%, rash in 4.4%, arthralgia in 4.4%, and hepatitis in 6.5%. In a prospective study of 143 kidney transplant recipients with 6 sampling time points in the first 20 weeks after transplant, Park and colleagues[271] detected at least 1 positive PCR in 58.7%. In 11.1% of kidney transplant recipients (n = 16), sustained severe anemia was observed with hemoglobin lower than 7.0 g/dL. The incidence of severe anemia correlated with a PVB19 load greater than 8 log geq/mL whole blood (positive predictive value 84.6%, negative predictive value 96.2%), whereas low or negative viral load had little clinical consequences.

Thrombotic microangiopathy in kidney allografts and intrarenal small- and medium-sized vasculitits after PVB19 infection have been detected in 8 renal transplant recipients.[272] Kidney transplant failure despite a negative cross-match was reported for a case of PVB19 infection with hyporegenerative anemia following transplantation from a viremic donor. However, the effect of PVB19 on renal allograft function is controversial. Ki and colleagues[268] did not observe a difference in graft function in 52/167 (31.1%) patients with a positive PVB19 PCR compared with negative patients. Eid and colleagues[269] observed a PVB19 recurrence rate of 34%, which was associated with significant graft dysfunction and loss in 52/167 (31.1%) patients. More recently, Barzon and colleagues analyzed kidney biopsies before transplantation and 3, 6, and 12 months after transplant for the presence of different herpesviruses, polyomavirus, and PVB19 DNA by PCR and found a positive PVB19 PCR in around 30% of cases. PVB19 and HHV-6 were frequently already detectable in the donor kidneys. The intrarenal persistence of PVB19 DNA and PVB19 DNAemia was associated with the development of chronic allograft injury (hazard ratio 1.94, $P = .08$), whereas human CMV DNAemia was a risk factor for acute rejection. The persistence of PVB19 DNA might be an important confounder. Its role in allograft failure needs to be better understood by investigating immunohistochemistry as independent evidence.

PVB19-specific Treatment and Outcome

PVB19 treatment relies mainly on intravenous immunoglobulin (IVIG) and, if necessary, also reduction of immunosuppression.[273] However, IVIG may lead to nephrotoxic side effects in 11.6% of SOT patients, most likely resulting from the osmotic effects of carbohydrate preservatives.[269] The response to IVIG is typically only transient with an increase in reticulocytes and increasing hemoglobin values. Patients with anemia less than 10 g/dL usually require red blood cell transfusions. In the study by Cavallo and colleagues,[270] 3/11 (27%) patients recovered spontaneously from anemia, whereas 8/11 (73%) patients required blood transfusion and/or erythropoietin (4000 U subcutaneously 3 times). Relapsing anemia is frequently observed in patients with primary PVB19 infections or in patients with lymphocyte-depleting induction treatment.[274] This supports the importance of sufficient PVB19-specific T-cell control. The effect of reduction of immunosuppression has not been systematically examined. No PBV19 attributable mortality has been reported, but 1.3% of nonkidney SOT recipients and 8.3% of HSCT patients died.[269]

SUMMARY

Viral infections after transplant have emerged as important modifiers of graft function and survival in the current era of increased efficacy of newer immunosuppressive regimens. Whereas the role of ADV, BKV, and CMV in acute and chronic injury is clearly recognized, other suspects such as HHV-6 and PBV19 require further studies with regard to direct and indirect viral effects. Antiviral prophylaxis and screening and intervention algorithms have been found valuable for CMV and BKV, but similar approaches are largely lacking for ADV, HHV-6, and PVB19, because the significance of viral DNA detection and pathology is less well understood. Future studies need to combine molecular genetic testing with sensitive and specific immunohistochemistry and clinical studies to resolve these issues.

REFERENCES

1. Meier-Kriesche HU, Li S, Gruessner RW, et al. Immunosuppression: evolution in practice and trends, 1994–2004. Am J Transplant 2006;6(5 Pt 2):1111–31.
2. Dharnidharka VR, Stablein DM, Harmon WE. Post-transplant infections now exceed acute rejection as cause for hospitalization: a report of the NAPRTCS. Am J Transplant 2004;4(3):384–9.

3. Dharnidharka VR, Caillard S, Agodoa LY, et al. Infection frequency and profile in different age groups of kidney transplant recipients. Transplantation 2006; 81(12):1662–7.
4. Fishman JA. Infection in solid-organ transplant recipients. N Engl J Med 2007; 357(25):2601–14.
5. Helantera I, Loginov R, Koskinen P, et al. Persistent cytomegalovirus infection is associated with increased expression of TGF-beta1, PDGF-AA and ICAM-1 and arterial intimal thickening in kidney allografts. Nephrol Dial Transplant 2005; 20(4):790–6.
6. Helantera I, Koskinen P, Finne P, et al. Persistent cytomegalovirus infection in kidney allografts is associated with inferior graft function and survival. Transpl Int 2006;19(11):893–900.
7. Humar A, Mazzulli T, Moussa G, et al. Clinical utility of cytomegalovirus (CMV) serology testing in high-risk CMV D+/R– transplant recipients. Am J Transplant 2005;5(5):1065–70.
8. Hirsch HH, Knowles W, Dickenmann M, et al. Prospective study of polyomavirus type BK replication and nephropathy in renal-transplant recipients. N Engl J Med 2002;347(7):488–96.
9. Munoz P, Fogeda M, Bouza E, et al. Prevalence of BK virus replication among recipients of solid organ transplants. Clin Infect Dis 2005;41(12):1720–5.
10. Randhawa P, Uhrmacher J, Pasculle W, et al. A comparative study of BK and JC virus infections in organ transplant recipients. J Med Virol 2005;77(2):238–43.
11. Egli A, Binggeli S, Bodaghi S, et al. Cytomegalovirus and polyomavirus BK post-transplant. Nephrol Dial Transplant 2007;22(Suppl 8):viii72–82.
12. Egli A, Infanti L, Dumoulin A, et al. Prevalence of polyomavirus BK and JC infection and replication in 400 healthy blood donors. J Infect Dis 2009;199:837–46.
13. Fietze E, Prosch S, Reinke P, et al. Cytomegalovirus infection in transplant recipients. The role of tumor necrosis factor. Transplantation 1994;58(6):675–80.
14. Reinke P, Prosch S, Kern F, et al. Mechanisms of human cytomegalovirus (HCMV) (re)activation and its impact on organ transplant patients. Transpl Infect Dis 1999;1(3):157–64.
15. Fishman JA, Rubin RH. Infection in organ-transplant recipients. N Engl J Med 1998;338(24):1741–51.
16. Sester M, Sester U, Gartner B, et al. Levels of virus-specific CD4 T cells correlate with cytomegalovirus control and predict virus-induced disease after renal transplantation. Transplantation 2001;71(9):1287–94.
17. Comoli P, Azzi A, Maccario R, et al. Polyomavirus BK-specific immunity after kidney transplantation. Transplantation 2004;78(8):1229–32.
18. Klenerman P, Hill A. T cells and viral persistence: lessons from diverse infections. Nat Immunol 2005;6(9):873–9.
19. Comoli P, Hirsch HH, Ginevri F. Cellular immune responses to BK virus. Curr Opin Organ Transplant 2008;13(6):569–74.
20. Egli A, Binet I, Binggeli S, et al. Cytomegalovirus-specific T-cell responses and viral replication in kidney transplant recipients. J Transl Med 2008;6(1):29.
21. Lacey SF, Gallez-Hawkins G, Crooks M, et al. Characterization of cytotoxic function of CMV-pp65-specific CD8+ T-lymphocytes identified by HLA tetramers in recipients and donors of stem-cell transplants. Transplantation 2002;74(5): 722–32.
22. Sester U, Gartner BC, Wilkens H, et al. Differences in CMV-specific T-cell levels and long-term susceptibility to CMV infection after kidney, heart and lung transplantation. Am J Transplant 2005;5(6):1483–9.

23. Lacey SF, La Rosa C, Zhou W, et al. Functional comparison of T cells recognizing cytomegalovirus pp65 and intermediate-early antigen polypeptides in hematopoietic stem-cell transplant and solid organ transplant recipients. J Infect Dis 2006;194(10):1410–21.
24. Lilleri D, Zelini P, Fornara C, et al. Inconsistent responses of cytomegalovirus-specific T cells to pp65 and IE-1 versus infected dendritic cells in organ transplant recipients. Am J Transplant 2007;7(8):1997–2005.
25. Egli A, Dumoulin A, Köhli S, et al. Polyomavirus BK after kidney transplantation – role of molecular and immunological markers. Trends in Transplantation 2009;3:85–102.
26. Egli A, Koehli S, Dickenmann M, et al. Inhibition of polyomavirus BK- and cytomegalovirus-specific T-cell responses by immunosuppressive drugs. Transplantation 2009;88(10):1161–8.
27. Ginevri F, Azzi A, Hirsch HH, et al. Prospective monitoring of polyomavirus BK replication and impact of pre-emptive intervention in pediatric kidney recipients. Am J Transplant 2007;7(12):2727–35.
28. Ginevri F, Basso S, Hirsch HH, et al. Reconstitution of BKV-specific immunity through immunosuppression reduction prevents BKV nephropathy in pediatric kidney recipients monitored prospectively. Transpl Int 2007;20:80–80.
29. Preiksaitis JK, Brennan DC, Fishman J, et al. Canadian Society of Transplantation consensus workshop on cytomegalovirus management in solid organ transplantation final report. Am J Transplant 2005;5(2):218–27.
30. Fishman JA, Emery V, Freeman R, et al. Cytomegalovirus in transplantation - challenging the status quo. Clin Transplant 2007;21(2):149–58.
31. Hirsch HH. Polyomavirus BK nephropathy: a (re-)emerging complication in renal transplantation. Am J Transplant 2002;2(1):25–30.
32. Tantravahi J, Womer KL, Kaplan B. Why hasn't eliminating acute rejection improved graft survival? Annu Rev Med 2007;58:369–85.
33. Kliem V, Fricke L, Wollbrink T, et al. Improvement in long-term renal graft survival due to CMV prophylaxis with oral ganciclovir: results of a randomized clinical trial. Am J Transplant 2008;8(5):975–83.
34. Brennan DC. Cytomegalovirus in renal transplantation. J Am Soc Nephrol 2001;12(4):848–55.
35. Schnitzler MA, Lowell JA, Hmiel SP, et al. Cytomegalovirus disease after prophylaxis with oral ganciclovir in renal transplantation: the importance of HLA-DR matching. J Am Soc Nephrol 2003;14(3):780–5.
36. Khoury JA, Storch GA, Bohl DL, et al. Prophylactic versus preemptive oral valganciclovir for the management of cytomegalovirus infection in adult renal transplant recipients. Am J Transplant 2006;6(9):2134–43.
37. Gupta G, Gasper G, Bista BR, et al. High production of TGF-beta increases the risk of development of BK virus allograft nephropathy [abstract 157]. Am J Transplant 2006;6(S2):S119.
38. Gupta G, Ishwad C, Gasper G, et al. BK virus upregulates TGF-beta as well as specific components of the TGF-beta signaling pathway [abstract 158]. Am J Transplant 2006;6(S2):S119–20.
39. Abend JR, Imperiale MJ. Transforming growth factor-beta-mediated regulation of BK virus gene expression. Virology 2008;378(1):6–12.
40. Stewart PL, Fuller SD, Burnett RM. Difference imaging of adenovirus: bridging the resolution gap between X-ray crystallography and electron microscopy. EMBO J 1993;12(7):2589–99.
41. Leen AM, Bollard CM, Myers GD, et al. Adenoviral infections in hematopoietic stem cell transplantation. Biol Blood Marrow Transplant 2006;12(3):243–51.

42. Roelvink PW, Lizonova A, Lee JG, et al. The coxsackievirus-adenovirus receptor protein can function as a cellular attachment protein for adenovirus serotypes from subgroups A, C, D, E, and F. J Virol 1998;72(10):7909–15.
43. Leen AM, Rooney CM. Adenovirus as an emerging pathogen in immunocompromised patients. Br J Haematol 2005;128(2):135–44.
44. Bergelson JM, Cunningham JA, Droguett G, et al. Isolation of a common receptor for Coxsackie B viruses and adenoviruses 2 and 5. Science 1997; 275(5304):1320–3.
45. Horvath J, Palkonyay L, Weber J. Group C adenovirus DNA sequences in human lymphoid cells. J Virol 1986;59(1):189–92.
46. Chu Y, Sperber K, Mayer L, et al. Persistent infection of human adenovirus type 5 in human monocyte cell lines. Virology 1992;188(2):793–800.
47. de Mezerville MH, Tellier R, Richardson S, et al. Adenoviral infections in pediatric transplant recipients: a hospital-based study. Pediatr Infect Dis J 2006;25(9):815–8.
48. Horwitz MS. Adenovirus immunoregulatory genes and their cellular targets. Virology 2001;279(1):1–8.
49. Ginsberg HS, Moldawer LL, Sehgal PB, et al. A mouse model for investigating the molecular pathogenesis of adenovirus pneumonia. Proc Natl Acad Sci U S A 1991;88(5):1651–5.
50. Mistchenko AS, Diez RA, Mariani AL, et al. Cytokines in adenoviral disease in children: association of interleukin-6, interleukin-8, and tumor necrosis factor alpha levels with clinical outcome. J Pediatr 1994;124(5 Pt 1):714–20.
51. Myers GD, Bollard CM, Wu MF, et al. Reconstitution of adenovirus-specific cell-mediated immunity in pediatric patients after hematopoietic stem cell transplantation. Bone Marrow Transplant 2007;39(11):677–86.
52. Castle SC. Clinical relevance of age-related immune dysfunction. Clin Infect Dis 2000;31(2):578–85.
53. Sester M, Sester U, Alarcon Salvador S, et al. Age-related decrease in adenovirus-specific T cell responses. J Infect Dis 2002;185(10):1379–87.
54. Mahr JA, Gooding LR. Immune evasion by adenoviruses. Immunol Rev 1999; 168:121–30.
55. Burgert HG, Ruzsics Z, Obermeier S, et al. Subversion of host defense mechanisms by adenoviruses. Curr Top Microbiol Immunol 2002;269:273–318.
56. Howard DS, Phillips IG, Reece DE, et al. Adenovirus infections in hematopoietic stem cell transplant recipients. Clin Infect Dis 1999;29(6):1494–501.
57. Kojaoghlanian T, Flomenberg P, Horwitz MS. The impact of adenovirus infection on the immunocompromised host. Rev Med Virol 2003;13(3):155–71.
58. Yagisawa T, Nakada T, Takahashi K, et al. Acute hemorrhagic cystitis caused by adenovirus after kidney transplantation. Urol Int 1995;54(3):142–6.
59. Cames B, Rahier J, Burtomboy G, et al. Acute adenovirus hepatitis in liver transplant recipients. J Pediatr 1992;120(1):33–7.
60. Michaels MG, Green M, Wald ER, et al. Adenovirus infection in pediatric liver transplant recipients. J Infect Dis 1992;165(1):170–4.
61. Lecatsas G, van Wyk JA. DNA viruses in urine after renal transplantation. S Afr Med J 1978;53(20):787–8.
62. Humar A. Reactivation of viruses in solid organ transplant patients receiving cytomegalovirus prophylaxis. Transplantation 2006;82(Suppl 2):S9–14.
63. Hofland CA, Eron LJ, Washecka RM. Hemorrhagic adenovirus cystitis after renal transplantation. Transplant Proc 2004;36(10):3025–7.
64. Asim M, Chong-Lopez A, Nickeleit V. Adenovirus infection of a renal allograft. Am J Kidney Dis 2003;41(3):696–701.

65. Hensley JL, Sifri CD, Cathro HP, et al. Adenoviral graft-nephritis: case report and review of the literature. Transpl Int 2009;22(6):672–7.
66. Ardehali H, Volmar K, Roberts C, et al. Fatal disseminated adenoviral infection in a renal transplant patient. Transplantation 2001;71(7):998–9.
67. Wreghitt TG, Gray JJ, Ward KN, et al. Disseminated adenovirus infection after liver transplantation and its possible treatment with ganciclovir. J Infect 1989; 19(1):88–9.
68. Murphy GF, Wood DP Jr, McRoberts JW, et al. Adenovirus-associated hemorrhagic cystitis treated with intravenous ribavirin. J Urol 1993;149(3):565–6.
69. Arav Boger R, Echavarria M, Forman M, et al. Clearance of adenoviral hepatitis with ribavirin therapy in a pediatric liver transplant recipient. Pediatr Infect Dis J 2000;19(11):1097–100.
70. Swaminathan S, Lager DJ, Qian X, et al. Collapsing and non-collapsing focal segmental glomerulosclerosis in kidney transplants. Nephrol Dial Transplant 2006;21(9):2607–14.
71. Thomas LD, Milstone AP, Vilchez RA, et al. Polyomavirus infection and its impact on renal function and long-term outcomes after lung transplantation. Transplantation 2009;88(3):360–6.
72. Elphick GF, Querbes W, Jordan JA, et al. The human polyomavirus, JCV, uses serotonin receptors to infect cells. Science 2004;306(5700):1380–3.
73. Low JA, Magnuson B, Tsai B, et al. Identification of gangliosides GD1b and GT1b as receptors for BK virus. J Virol 2006;80(3):1361–6.
74. Bialasiewicz S, Whiley DM, Lambert SB, et al. A newly reported human polyomavirus, KI virus, is present in the respiratory tract of Australian children. J Clin Virol 2007;40(1):15–8.
75. Dalianis T, Ramqvist T, Andreasson K, et al. KI, WU and Merkel cell polyomaviruses: a new era for human polyomavirus research. Semin Cancer Biol 2009; 19(4):270–5.
76. Sharp CP, Norja P, Anthony I, et al. Reactivation and mutation of newly discovered WU, KI, and Merkel cell carcinoma polyomaviruses in immunosuppressed individuals. J Infect Dis 2009;199(3):398–404.
77. Wieland U, Mauch C, Kreuter A, et al. Merkel cell polyomavirus DNA in persons without Merkel cell carcinoma. Emerg Infect Dis 2009;15:1496–8.
78. Mourez T, Bergeron A, Ribaud P, et al. Polyomaviruses KI and WU in immunocompromised patients with respiratory disease. Emerg Infect Dis 2009;15(1):107–9.
79. Babakir-Mina M, Ciccozzi M, Alteri C, et al. Excretion of the novel polyomaviruses KI and WU in the stool of patients with hematological disorders. J Med Virol 2009;81(9):1668–73.
80. Knowles WA, Pipkin P, Andrews N, et al. Population-based study of antibody to the human polyomaviruses BKV and JCV and the simian polyomavirus SV40. J Med Virol 2003;71(1):115–23.
81. Kean JM, Rao S, Wang M, et al. Seroepidemiology of human polyomaviruses. PLoS Pathog 2009;5(3):e1000363.
82. Knowles WA. Propagation and assay of BK virus. Methods Mol Biol 2001;165: 19–31.
83. Ginevri F, De Santis R, Comoli P, et al. Polyomavirus BK infection in pediatric kidney-allograft recipients: a single-center analysis of incidence, risk factors, and novel therapeutic approaches. Transplantation 2003;75(8):1266–70.
84. Chen Y, Trofe J, Gordon J, et al. Interplay of cellular and humoral immune responses against BK virus in kidney transplant recipients with polyomavirus nephropathy. J Virol 2006;80(7):3495–505.

85. Leuenberger D, Andresen PA, Gosert R, et al. Human polyomavirus type 1 (BK virus) agnoprotein is abundantly expressed but immunologically ignored. Clin Vaccine Immunol 2007;14(8):959–68.
86. Randhawa PS, Gupta G, Vats A, et al. Immunoglobulin G, A, and M responses to BK virus in renal transplantation. Clin Vaccine Immunol 2006;13(9):1057–63.
87. Bohl DL, Storch GA, Ryschkewitsch C, et al. Donor origin of BK virus in renal transplantation and role of HLA C7 in susceptibility to sustained BK viremia. Am J Transplant 2005;5(9):2213–21.
88. Ramos E, Drachenberg CB, Papadimitriou JC, et al. Clinical course of polyoma virus nephropathy in 67 renal transplant patients. J Am Soc Nephrol 2002;13(8):2145–51.
89. Smith JM, McDonald RA, Finn LS, et al. Polyomavirus nephropathy in pediatric kidney transplant recipients. Am J Transplant 2004;4(12):2109–17.
90. Binet I, Nickeleit V, Hirsch HH, et al. Polyomavirus disease under new immunosuppressive drugs: a cause of renal graft dysfunction and graft loss. Transplantation 1999;67(6):918–22.
91. Mengel M, Marwedel M, Radermacher J, et al. Incidence of polyomavirus-nephropathy in renal allografts: influence of modern immunosuppressive drugs. Nephrol Dial Transplant 2003;18(6):1190–6.
92. Brennan DC, Agha I, Bohl DL, et al. Incidence of BK with tacrolimus versus cyclosporine and impact of preemptive immunosuppression reduction. Am J Transplant 2005;5(3):582–94.
93. Hirsch HH, Friman S, Wiecek A, et al. Prospective study of polyomavirus BK viruria and viremia in de novo renal transplantation [abstract 77]. Am J Transplant 2007;7(Suppl 5):150.
94. Dharnidharka VR, Cherikh WS, Abbott KC. An OPTN analysis of national registry data on treatment of BK virus allograft nephropathy in the United States. Transplantation 2009;87(7):1019–26.
95. Manitpisitkul W, Drachenberg C, Ramos E, et al. Maintenance immunosuppressive agents as risk factors for BK virus nephropathy: a case-control study. Transplantation 2009;88(1):83–8.
96. Awadallah Y, Randhawa P, Ruppert K, et al. HLA mismatching increases the risk of BK virus nephropathy in renal transplant recipients. Am J Transplant 2004;4(10):1691–6.
97. Kayler LK, Batal I, Mohanka R, et al. Antirejection treatment in kidney transplant patients with BK viruria. Transplantation 2008;86(6):797–803.
98. Comoli P, Basso S, Azzi A, et al. Dendritic cells pulsed with polyomavirus BK antigen induce ex vivo polyoma BK virus-specific cytotoxic T-cell lines in seropositive healthy individuals and renal transplant recipients. J Am Soc Nephrol 2003;14(12):3197–204.
99. Binggeli S, Egli A, Dickenmann M, et al. BKV replication and cellular immune responses in renal transplant recipients. Am J Transplant 2006;6(9):2218–9.
100. Comoli P, Azzi A, Basso S, et al. Prospective evaluation of BKV-specific cellular immunity after pediatric kidney transplantation [abstract 79]. Am J Transplant 2006;6(S2):S93.
101. Prosser SE, Orentas RJ, Cohen EP, et al. Elispot as a technique for measuring BKV-specific cellular immunity in clinical BKV nephritis [abstract 1859]. Am J Transplant 2006;6(S2):S685.
102. Binggeli S, Egli A, Schaub S, et al. Polyomavirus BK-specific cellular immune response to VP1 and large T-antigen in kidney transplant recipients. Am J Transplant 2007;7(5):1131–9.

103. Hammer MH, Brestrich G, Andree H, et al. HLA type-independent method to monitor polyoma BK virus-specific CD4 and CD8 T-cell immunity. Am J Transplant 2006;6(3):625–31.
104. Schaub S, Mayr M, Egli A, et al. Transient allograft dysfunction from immune reconstitution in a patient with polyoma BK-virus-associated nephropathy. Nephrol Dial Transplant 2007;22(8):2386–90.
105. Stolt A, Sasnauskas K, Koskela P, et al. Seroepidemiology of the human polyomaviruses. J Gen Virol 2003;84(Pt 6):1499–504.
106. Gosert R, Rinaldo CH, Funk GA, et al. Polyomavirus BK with rearranged noncoding control region emerge in vivo in renal transplant patients and increase viral replication and cytopathology. J Exp Med 2008;205(4):841–52.
107. Chesters PM, Heritage J, McCance DJ. Persistence of DNA sequences of BK virus and JC virus in normal human tissues and in diseased tissues. J Infect Dis 1983;147(4):676–84.
108. Dorries K, ter Meulen V. Progressive multifocal leucoencephalopathy: detection of papovavirus JC in kidney tissue. J Med Virol 1983;11(4):307–17.
109. Polo C, Perez JL, Mielnichuck A, et al. Prevalence and patterns of polyomavirus urinary excretion in immunocompetent adults and children. Clin Microbiol Infect 2004;10(7):640–4.
110. Zhong S, Zheng HY, Suzuki M, et al. Age-related urinary excretion of BK polyomavirus by nonimmunocompromised individuals. J Clin Microbiol 2007;45(1):193–8.
111. Ling PD, Lednicky JA, Keitel WA, et al. The dynamics of herpesvirus and polyomavirus reactivation and shedding in healthy adults: a 14-month longitudinal study. J Infect Dis 2003;187(10):1571–80.
112. Drachenberg CB, Hirsch HH, Papadimitriou JC, et al. Polyomavirus BK versus JC replication and nephropathy in renal transplant recipients: a prospective evaluation. Transplantation 2007;84(3):323–30.
113. Funk GA, Gosert R, Comoli P, et al. Polyomavirus BK replication dynamics in vivo and in silico to predict cytopathology and viral clearance in kidney transplants. Am J Transplant 2008;8:2368–77.
114. Nickeleit V, Klimkait T, Binet IF, et al. Testing for polyomavirus type BK DNA in plasma to identify renal-allograft recipients with viral nephropathy. N Engl J Med 2000;342(18):1309–15.
115. Hirsch HH, Drachenberg CB, Steiger J, et al. Polyomavirus-associated nephropathy in renal transplantation: critical issues of screening and management. Adv Exp Med Biol 2006;577:160–73.
116. Hirsch HH, Drachenberg C, Ramos E, et al. BK viremia level strongly correlates with the extent/pattern of viral nephropathy (BKPVN) implications for a diagnostic cut-off value [abstract 1168]. Transplantation 2006;82(1):460.
117. Viscount HB, Eid AJ, Espy MJ, et al. Polyomavirus polymerase chain reaction as a surrogate marker of polyomavirus-associated nephropathy. Transplantation 2007;84(3):340–5.
118. Drachenberg CB, Hirsch HH, Ramos E, et al. Polyomavirus disease in renal transplantation: review of pathological findings and diagnostic methods. Hum Pathol 2005;36(12):1245–55.
119. Hirsch HH, Brennan DC, Drachenberg CB, et al. Polyomavirus-associated nephropathy in renal transplantation: interdisciplinary analyses and recommendations. Transplantation 2005;79(10):1277–86.
120. Drachenberg CB, Papadimitriou JC, Hirsch HH, et al. Histological patterns of polyomavirus nephropathy: correlation with graft outcome and viral load. Am J Transplant 2004;4(12):2082–92.

121. Drachenberg CB, Papadimitriou JC, Ramos E, et al. Histologic versus molecular diagnosis of BK polyomavirus-associated nephropathy: a shifting paradigm? Clin J Am Soc Nephrol 2006;1(3):374–9.
122. Drachenberg CB, Papadimitriou JC. Polyomavirus-associated nephropathy: update in diagnosis. Transpl Infect Dis 2006;8(2):68–75.
123. Grinde B, Gayorfar M, Rinaldo CH. Impact of a polyomavirus (BKV) infection on mRNA expression in human endothelial cells. Virus Res 2007;123(1): 86–94.
124. Cheng O, Abend JR, Imperiale J, et al. The pro-fibriogenic effect of BK polyomavirus infection [abstract 81]. Am J Transplant 2006;6(S2):S93–4.
125. Sporn MB. The early history of TGF-beta, and a brief glimpse of its future. Cytokine Growth Factor Rev 2006;17(1–2):3–7.
126. Mannon RB, Hoffmann SC, Kampen RL, et al. Molecular evaluation of BK polyomavirus nephropathy. Am J Transplant 2005;5(12):2883–93.
127. Rinaldo CH, Hirsch HH. Antivirals for the treatment of polyomavirus BK replication. Expert Rev Anti Infect Ther 2007;5(1):105–15.
128. Trofe J, Hirsch HH, Ramos E. Polyomavirus-associated nephropathy: update of clinical management in kidney transplant patients. Transpl Infect Dis 2006;8(2): 76–85.
129. Farasati NA, Shapiro R, Vats A, et al. Effect of leflunomide and cidofovir on replication of BK virus in an in vitro culture system. Transplantation 2005;79(1): 116–8.
130. Randhawa P, Farasati NA, Shapiro R, et al. Ether lipid ester derivatives of cidofovir inhibit polyomavirus BK replication in vitro. Antimicrob Agents Chemother 2006;50(4):1564–6.
131. Bernhoff E, Gutteberg TJ, Sandvik K, et al. Cidofovir inhibits polyomavirus BK replication in human renal tubular cells downstream of viral early gene expression. Am J Transplant 2008;8:1413–22.
132. Williams JW, Javaid B, Kadambi PV, et al. Leflunomide for polyomavirus type BK nephropathy. N Engl J Med 2005;352(11):1157–8.
133. Josephson MA, Williams JW, Chandraker A, et al. Polyomavirus-associated nephropathy: update on antiviral strategies. Transpl Infect Dis 2006;8(2): 95–101.
134. Faguer S, Hirsch HH, Kamar N, et al. Leflunomide treatment for polyomavirus BK-associated nephropathy after kidney transplantation. Transpl Int 2007; 20(11):962–9.
135. Baumann P, Mandl-Weber S, Volkl A, et al. Dihydroorotate dehydrogenase inhibitor A771726 (leflunomide) induces apoptosis and diminishes proliferation of multiple myeloma cells. Mol Cancer Ther 2009;8(2):366–75.
136. Rinaldo CH, Gosert R, Hirsch HH. Hexadecyloxypropyl-cidofovir (CMX001) BK virus (BKV) replication in primary renal tubular epithelial cells [abstract OP5-8]. J Clin Virol 2009;46(Suppl 1):S12–3.
137. Dunn W, Chou C, Li H, et al. Functional profiling of a human cytomegalovirus genome. Proc Natl Acad Sci U S A 2003;100(24):14223–8.
138. Dolan A, Cunningham C, Hector RD, et al. Genetic content of wild-type human cytomegalovirus. J Gen Virol 2004;85(Pt 5):1301–12.
139. Ho M. Epidemiology of cytomegalovirus infections. Rev Infect Dis 1990; 12(Suppl 7):S701–10.
140. Becker BN, Becker YT, Leverson GE, et al. Reassessing the impact of cytomegalovirus infection in kidney and kidney-pancreas transplantation. Am J Kidney Dis 2002;39(5):1088–95.

141. Sagedal S, Nordal KP, Hartmann A, et al. The impact of cytomegalovirus infection and disease on rejection episodes in renal allograft recipients. Am J Transplant 2002;2(9):850–6.
142. Sagedal S, Nordal KP, Hartmann A, et al. A prospective study of the natural course of cytomegalovirus infection and disease in renal allograft recipients. Transplantation 2000;70(8):1166–74.
143. Rubin RH, Tolkoff-Rubin NE. Viral infection in the renal transplant patient. Proc Eur Dial Transplant Assoc 1983;19:513–26.
144. von Willebrand E, Pettersson E, Ahonen J, et al. CMV infection, class II antigen expression, and human kidney allograft rejection. Transplantation 1986;42(4):364–7.
145. Pouteil-Noble C, Ecochard R, Landrivon G, et al. Cytomegalovirus infection–an etiological factor for rejection? A prospective study in 242 renal transplant patients. Transplantation 1993;55(4):851–7.
146. Reinke P, Fietze E, Ode-Hakim S, et al. Late-acute renal allograft rejection and symptomless cytomegalovirus infection. Lancet 1994;344(8939-8940): 1737–8.
147. Toupance O, Bouedjoro-Camus MC, Carquin J, et al. Cytomegalovirus-related disease and risk of acute rejection in renal transplant recipients: a cohort study with case-control analyses. Transpl Int 2000;13(6):413–9.
148. Dickenmann MJ, Cathomas G, Steiger J, et al. Cytomegalovirus infection and graft rejection in renal transplantation. Transplantation 2001;71(6):764–7.
149. Reischig T, Jindra P, Svecova M, et al. The impact of cytomegalovirus disease and asymptomatic infection on acute renal allograft rejection. J Clin Virol 2006;36(2):146–51.
150. Reischig T, Jindra P, Hes O, et al. Effect of cytomegalovirus viremia on subclinical rejection or interstitial fibrosis and tubular atrophy in protocol biopsy at 3 months in renal allograft recipients managed by preemptive therapy or antiviral prophylaxis. Transplantation 2009;87(3):436–44.
151. Richardson WP, Colvin RB, Cheeseman SH, et al. Glomerulopathy associated with cytomegalovirus viremia in renal allografts. N Engl J Med 1981;305(2): 57–63.
152. Tuazon TV, Schneeberger EE, Bhan AK, et al. Mononuclear cells in acute allograft glomerulopathy. Am J Pathol 1987;129(1):119–32.
153. Rao KV, Hafner GP, Crary GS, et al. De novo immunotactoid glomerulopathy of the renal allograft: possible association with cytomegalovirus infection. Am J Kidney Dis 1994;24(1):97–103.
154. Fryd DS, Peterson PK, Ferguson RM, et al. Cytomegalovirus as a risk factor in renal transplantation. Transplantation 1980;30(6):436–9.
155. Rubin RH, Tolkoff-Rubin NE, Oliver D, et al. Multicenter seroepidemiologic study of the impact of cytomegalovirus infection on renal transplantation. Transplantation 1985;40(3):243–9.
156. Lewis RM, Johnson PC, Golden D, et al. The adverse impact of cytomegalovirus infection on clinical outcome in cyclosporine-prednisone treated renal allograft recipients. Transplantation 1988;45(2):353–9.
157. Tong CY, Bakran A, Peiris JS, et al. The association of viral infection and chronic allograft nephropathy with graft dysfunction after renal transplantation. Transplantation 2002;74(4):576–8.
158. Geddes CC, Church CC, Collidge T, et al. Management of cytomegalovirus infection by weekly surveillance after renal transplant: analysis of cost, rejection and renal function. Nephrol Dial Transplant 2003;18(9):1891–8.

159. Sola R, Diaz JM, Guirado L, et al. Significance of cytomegalovirus infection in renal transplantation. Transplant Proc 2003;35(5):1753–5.
160. Opelz G, Dohler B, Ruhenstroth A. Cytomegalovirus prophylaxis and graft outcome in solid organ transplantation: a collaborative transplant study report. Am J Transplant 2004;4(6):928–36.
161. Sagedal S, Hartmann A, Nordal KP, et al. Impact of early cytomegalovirus infection and disease on long-term recipient and kidney graft survival. Kidney Int 2004;66(1):329–37.
162. Arthurs SK, Eid AJ, Pedersen RA, et al. Delayed-onset primary cytomegalovirus disease and the risk of allograft failure and mortality after kidney transplantation. Clin Infect Dis 2008;46(6):840–6.
163. Akposso K, Rondeau E, Haymann JP, et al. Long-term prognosis of renal transplantation after preemptive treatment of cytomegalovirus infection. Transplantation 1997;63(7):974–6.
164. Ricart MJ, Malaise J, Moreno A, et al. Cytomegalovirus: occurrence, severity, and effect on graft survival in simultaneous pancreas-kidney transplantation. Nephrol Dial Transplant 2005;20(Suppl 2):ii25–32, ii62.
165. Grattan MT, Moreno-Cabral CE, Starnes VA, et al. Cytomegalovirus infection is associated with cardiac allograft rejection and atherosclerosis. JAMA 1989;261(24):3561–6.
166. Loebe M, Schuler S, Zais O, et al. Role of cytomegalovirus infection in the development of coronary artery disease in the transplanted heart. J Heart Transplant 1990;9(6):707–11.
167. Arnold JC, Portmann BC, O'Grady JG, et al. Cytomegalovirus infection persists in the liver graft in the vanishing bile duct syndrome. Hepatology 1992;16(2):285–92.
168. Koskinen PK, Nieminen MS, Krogerus LA, et al. Cytomegalovirus infection and accelerated cardiac allograft vasculopathy in human cardiac allografts. J Heart Lung Transplant 1993;12(5):724–9.
169. Kroshus TJ, Kshettry VR, Savik K, et al. Risk factors for the development of bronchiolitis obliterans syndrome after lung transplantation. J Thorac Cardiovasc Surg 1997;114(2):195–202.
170. Lautenschlager I, Hockerstedt K, Jalanko H, et al. Persistent cytomegalovirus in liver allografts with chronic rejection. Hepatology 1997;25(1):190–4.
171. Evans PC, Coleman N, Wreghitt TG, et al. Cytomegalovirus infection of bile duct epithelial cells, hepatic artery and portal venous endothelium in relation to chronic rejection of liver grafts. J Hepatol 1999;31(5):913–20.
172. Valantine HA, Gao SZ, Menon SG, et al. Impact of prophylactic immediate posttransplant ganciclovir on development of transplant atherosclerosis: a post hoc analysis of a randomized, placebo-controlled study. Circulation 1999;100(1):61–6.
173. Solez K, Colvin RB, Racusen LC, et al. Banff '05 Meeting Report: differential diagnosis of chronic allograft injury and elimination of chronic allograft nephropathy ('CAN'). Am J Transplant 2007;7(3):518–26.
174. Humar A, Gillingham KJ, Payne WD, et al. Association between cytomegalovirus disease and chronic rejection in kidney transplant recipients. Transplantation 1999;68(12):1879–83.
175. Helantera I, Koskinen P, Tornroth T, et al. The impact of cytomegalovirus infections and acute rejection episodes on the development of vascular changes in 6-month protocol biopsy specimens of cadaveric kidney allograft recipients. Transplantation 2003;75(11):1858–64.

176. Heieren MH, Kim YK, Balfour HH. Human cytomegalovirus infection of kidney glomerular visceral epithelial and tubular epithelial cells in culture. Transplantation 1988;46(3):426–32.
177. Heieren MH, van der Woude FJ, Balfour HH. Cytomegalovirus replicates efficiently in human kidney mesangial cells. Proc Natl Acad Sci U S A 1988; 85(5):1642–6.
178. Ustinov JA, Loginov RJ, Mattila PM, et al. Cytomegalovirus infection of human kidney cells in vitro. Kidney Int 1991;40(5):954–60.
179. Ulrich W, Schlederer MP, Buxbaum P, et al. The histopathologic identification of CMV infected cells in biopsies of human renal allografts. An evaluation of 100 transplant biopsies by in situ hybridization. Pathol Res Pract 1986;181(6): 739–45.
180. Andersen CB, Ladefoged SD, Lauritsen HK, et al. Detection of CMV DNA and CMV antigen in renal allograft biopsies by in situ hybridisation and immunohistochemistry. Nephrol Dial Transplant 1990;5(12):1045–50.
181. Lardelli P, Aguilar D, Gomez-Morales M, et al. Presence of cytomegalovirus genome and leucocyte subsets in renal transplant biopsies. Relationship with prognosis. Pathol Res Pract 1994;190(2):142–50.
182. Holma K, Tornroth T, Gronhagen-Riska C, et al. Expression of the cytomegalovirus genome in kidney allografts during active and latent infection. Transpl Int 2000;13(Suppl 1):S363–5.
183. Liapis H, Storch GA, Hill DA, et al. CMV infection of the renal allograft is much more common than the pathology indicates: a retrospective analysis of qualitative and quantitative buffy coat CMV-PCR, renal biopsy pathology and tissue CMV-PCR. Nephrol Dial Transplant 2003;18(2):397–402.
184. Iwamoto GK, Monick MM, Clark BD, et al. Modulation of interleukin 1 beta gene expression by the immediate early genes of human cytomegalovirus. J Clin Invest 1990;85(6):1853–7.
185. Geist LJ, Monick MM, Stinski MF, et al. The immediate early genes of human cytomegalovirus upregulate expression of the interleukin-2 and interleukin-2 receptor genes. Am J Respir Cell Mol Biol 1991;5(3):292–6.
186. Smith PD, Saini SS, Raffeld M, et al. Cytomegalovirus induction of tumor necrosis factor-alpha by human monocytes and mucosal macrophages. J Clin Invest 1992;90(5):1642–8.
187. van Dorp WT, van Wieringen PA, Marselis-Jonges E, et al. Cytomegalovirus directly enhances MHC class I and intercellular adhesion molecule-1 expression on cultured proximal tubular epithelial cells. Transplantation 1993;55(6): 1367–71.
188. Sedmak DD, Knight DA, Vook NC, et al. Divergent patterns of ELAM-1, ICAM-1, and VCAM-1 expression on cytomegalovirus-infected endothelial cells. Transplantation 1994;58(12):1379–85.
189. Craigen JL, Grundy JE. Cytomegalovirus induced up-regulation of LFA-3 (CD58) and ICAM-1 (CD54) is a direct viral effect that is not prevented by ganciclovir or foscarnet treatment. Transplantation 1996;62(8):1102–8.
190. Srivastava R, Curtis M, Hendrickson S, et al. Strain specific effects of cytomegalovirus on endothelial cells: implications for investigating the relationship between CMV and cardiac allograft vasculopathy. Transplantation 1999;68(10):1568–73.
191. Reinhardt B, Mertens T, Mayr-Beyrle U, et al. HCMV infection of human vascular smooth muscle cells leads to enhanced expression of functionally intact PDGF beta-receptor. Cardiovasc Res 2005;67(1):151–60.

192. Reinhardt B, Schaarschmidt P, Bossert A, et al. Upregulation of functionally active vascular endothelial growth factor by human cytomegalovirus. J Gen Virol 2005;86(Pt 1):23–30.
193. Yilmaz S, Koskinen PK, Kallio E, et al. Cytomegalovirus infection-enhanced chronic kidney allograft rejection is linked with intercellular adhesion molecule-1 expression. Kidney Int 1996;50(2):526–37.
194. Lautenschlager I, Soots A, Krogerus L, et al. Effect of cytomegalovirus on an experimental model of chronic renal allograft rejection under triple-drug treatment in the rat. Transplantation 1997;64(3):391–8.
195. van Dam JG, Damoiseaux JG, Christiaans MH, et al. Acute primary infection with cytomegalovirus (CMV) in kidney transplant recipients results in the appearance of a phenotypically aberrant CD8+ T cell population. Microbiol Immunol 2000;44(12):1011–7.
196. Inkinen K, Soots A, Krogerus L, et al. Cytomegalovirus increases collagen synthesis in chronic rejection in the rat. Nephrol Dial Transplant 2002;17(5):772–9.
197. Kloover JS, Soots AP, Krogerus LA, et al. Rat cytomegalovirus infection in kidney allograft recipients is associated with increased expression of intracellular adhesion molecule-1 vascular adhesion molecule-1, and their ligands leukocyte function antigen-1 and very late antigen-4 in the graft. Transplantation 2000; 69(12):2641–7.
198. Phan SH, Gharaee-Kermani M, McGarry B, et al. Regulation of rat pulmonary artery endothelial cell transforming growth factor-beta production by IL-1 beta and tumor necrosis factor-alpha. J Immunol 1992;149(1):103–6.
199. Pintavorn P, Ballermann BJ. TGF-beta and the endothelium during immune injury. Kidney Int 1997;51(5):1401–12.
200. Grotendorst GR. Connective tissue growth factor: a mediator of TGF-beta action on fibroblasts. Cytokine Growth Factor Rev 1997;8(3):171–9.
201. Michelson S, Alcami J, Kim SJ, et al. Human cytomegalovirus infection induces transcription and secretion of transforming growth factor beta 1. J Virol 1994; 68(9):5730–7.
202. Yoo YD, Chiou CJ, Choi KS, et al. The IE2 regulatory protein of human cytomegalovirus induces expression of the human transforming growth factor beta1 gene through an Egr-1 binding site. J Virol 1996;70(10):7062–70.
203. Funayama H, Ikeda U, Takahashi M, et al. Human monocyte-endothelial cell interaction induces platelet-derived growth factor expression. Cardiovasc Res 1998;37(1):216–24.
204. Isoniemi H, Taskinen E, Hayry P. Histological chronic allograft damage index accurately predicts chronic renal allograft rejection. Transplantation 1994; 58(11):1195–8.
205. Krogerus L, Soots A, Loginov R, et al. CMV increases tubular apoptosis through the TNF-alpha-TNF-R1 pathway in a rat model of chronic renal allograft rejection. Transpl Immunol 2008;18(3):232–6.
206. Penfold ME, Dairaghi DJ, Duke GM, et al. Cytomegalovirus encodes a potent alpha chemokine. Proc Natl Acad Sci U S A 1999;96(17):9839–44.
207. Vink C, Beisser PS, Bruggeman CA. Molecular mimicry by cytomegaloviruses. Function of cytomegalovirus-encoded homologues of G protein-coupled receptors, MHC class I heavy chains and chemokines. Intervirology 1999;42(5–6): 342–9.
208. Streblow DN, Vomaske J, Smith P, et al. Human cytomegalovirus chemokine receptor US28-induced smooth muscle cell migration is mediated by focal adhesion kinase and Src. J Biol Chem 2003;278(50):50456–65.

209. Streblow DN, Kreklywich CN, Smith P, et al. Rat cytomegalovirus-accelerated transplant vascular sclerosis is reduced with mutation of the chemokine-receptor R33. Am J Transplant 2005;5(3):436–42.
210. Streblow DN, Kreklywich CN, Andoh T, et al. The role of angiogenic and wound repair factors during CMV-accelerated transplant vascular sclerosis in rat cardiac transplants. Am J Transplant 2008;8(2):277–87.
211. Dumortier J, Streblow DN, Moses AV, et al. Human cytomegalovirus secretome contains factors that induce angiogenesis and wound healing. J Virol 2008; 82(13):6524–35.
212. Cook CH, Bickerstaff AA, Wang JJ, et al. Disruption of murine cardiac allograft acceptance by latent cytomegalovirus. Am J Transplant 2009;9(1):42–53.
213. Moens U, Van Ghelue M, Bendiksen S, et al. Simian virus 40 large T-antigen, but not small T-antigen, trans-activates the human cytomegalovirus major immediate early promoter. Virus Genes 2001;23(2):215–26.
214. Toyoda M, Puliyanda DP, Amet N, et al. Co-infection of polyomavirus-BK and cytomegalovirus in renal transplant recipients. Transplantation 2005;80(2): 198–205.
215. Biberfeld P, Kramarsky B, Salahuddin SZ, et al. Ultrastructural characterization of a new human B lymphotropic DNA virus (human herpesvirus 6) isolated from patients with lymphoproliferative disease. J Natl Cancer Inst 1987;79(5):933–41.
216. Dominguez G, Dambaugh TR, Stamey FR, et al. Human herpesvirus 6B genome sequence: coding content and comparison with human herpesvirus 6A. J Virol 1999;73(10):8040–52.
217. Efstathiou S, Gompels UA, Craxton MA, et al. DNA homology between a novel human herpesvirus (HHV-6) and human cytomegalovirus. Lancet 1988; 1(8575–6):63–4.
218. De Bolle L, Naesens L, De Clercq E. Update on human herpesvirus 6 biology, clinical features, and therapy. Clin Microbiol Rev 2005;18(1):217–45.
219. Frenkel N, Schirmer EC, Wyatt LS, et al. Isolation of a new herpesvirus from human CD4+ T cells. Proc Natl Acad Sci U S A 1990;87(2):748–52.
220. Dominguez G, Black JB, Stamey FR, et al. Physical and genetic maps of the human herpesvirus 7 strain SB genome. Arch Virol 1996;141(12):2387–408.
221. Lusso P, Secchiero P, Crowley RW, et al. CD4 is a critical component of the receptor for human herpesvirus 7: interference with human immunodeficiency virus. Proc Natl Acad Sci U S A 1994;91(9):3872–6.
222. Santoro F, Kennedy PE, Locatelli G, et al. CD46 is a cellular receptor for human herpesvirus 6. Cell 1999;99(7):817–27.
223. Yamanishi K, Okuno T, Shiraki K, et al. Identification of human herpesvirus-6 as a causal agent for exanthem subitum. Lancet 1988;1(8594):1065–7.
224. Tanaka K, Kondo T, Torigoe S, et al. Human herpesvirus 7: another causal agent for roseola (exanthem subitum). J Pediatr 1994;125(1):1–5.
225. Hashida T, Komura E, Yoshida M, et al. Hepatitis in association with human herpesvirus-7 infection. Pediatrics 1995;96(4 Pt 1):783–5.
226. Ward KN. The natural history and laboratory diagnosis of human herpesviruses-6 and -7 infections in the immunocompetent. J Clin Virol 2005;32(3): 183–93.
227. Griffiths PD, Ait-Khaled M, Bearcroft CP, et al. Human herpesviruses 6 and 7 as potential pathogens after liver transplant: prospective comparison with the effect of cytomegalovirus. J Med Virol 1999;59(4):496–501.
228. Ljungman P, Singh N. Human herpesvirus-6 infection in solid organ and stem cell transplant recipients. J Clin Virol 2006;37(Suppl 1):S87–91.

229. Smith JM, McDonald RA. Emerging viral infections in transplantation. Pediatr Transplant 2006;10:1–6.
230. Ward KN, Gray JJ, Efstathiou S. Brief report: primary human herpesvirus 6 infection in a patient following liver transplantation from a seropositive donor. J Med Virol 1989;28(2):69–72.
231. Herbein G, Strasswimmer J, Altieri M, et al. Longitudinal study of human herpesvirus 6 infection in organ transplant recipients. Clin Infect Dis 1996;22(1):171–3.
232. Singh N, Carrigan DR, Gayowski T, et al. Human herpesvirus-6 infection in liver transplant recipients: documentation of pathogenicity. Transplantation 1997; 64(5):674–8.
233. Lautenschlager I, Hockerstedt K, Linnavuori K, et al. Human herpesvirus-6 infection after liver transplantation. Clin Infect Dis 1998;26(3):702–7.
234. Humar A, Kumar D, Raboud J, et al. Interactions between cytomegalovirus, human herpesvirus-6, and the recurrence of hepatitis C after liver transplantation. Am J Transplant 2002;2(5):461–6.
235. Razonable RR, Paya CV. The impact of human herpesvirus-6 and -7 infection on the outcome of liver transplantation. Liver Transpl 2002;8(8):651–8.
236. Halme L, Arola J, Hockerstedt K, et al. Human herpesvirus 6 infection of the gastroduodenal mucosa. Clin Infect Dis 2008;46(3):434–9.
237. Flamand L, Gosselin J, D'Addario M, et al. Human herpesvirus 6 induces interleukin-1 beta and tumor necrosis factor alpha, but not interleukin-6, in peripheral blood mononuclear cell cultures. J Virol 1991;65(9):5105–10.
238. Lautenschlager I, Harma M, Hockerstedt K, et al. Human herpesvirus-6 infection is associated with adhesion molecule induction and lymphocyte infiltration in liver allografts. J Hepatol 2002;37(5):648–54.
239. Morris DJ, Littler E, Arrand JR, et al. Human herpesvirus 6 infection in renal-transplant recipients. N Engl J Med 1989;320(23):1560–1.
240. Okuno T, Higashi K, Shiraki K, et al. Human herpesvirus 6 infection in renal transplantation. Transplantation 1990;49(3):519–22.
241. Hoshino K, Nishi T, Adachi H, et al. Human herpesvirus-6 infection in renal allografts: retrospective immunohistochemical study in Japanese recipients. Transpl Int 1995;8(3):169–73.
242. Sebekova K, Feber J, Carpenter B, et al. Tissue viral DNA is associated with chronic allograft nephropathy. Pediatr Transplant 2005;9(5):598–603.
243. Helantera I, Loginov R, Koskinen P, et al. Demonstration of HHV-6 antigens in biopsies of kidney transplant recipients with cytomegalovirus infection. Transpl Int 2008;21(10):980–4.
244. Kidd IM, Clark DA, Sabin CA, et al. Prospective study of human betaherpesviruses after renal transplantation: association of human herpesvirus 7 and cytomegalovirus co-infection with cytomegalovirus disease and increased rejection. Transplantation 2000;69(11):2400–4.
245. Osman HK, Peiris JS, Taylor CE, et al. Cytomegalovirus disease in renal allograft recipients: is human herpesvirus 7 a co-factor for disease progression? J Med Virol 1996;48(4):295–301.
246. Brown KE, Anderson SM, Young NS, et al. Erythrocyte P antigen: cellular receptor for B19 parvovirus. Science 1993;262(5130):114–7.
247. Brown KE, Hibbs JR, Gallinella G, et al. Resistance to parvovirus B19 infection due to lack of virus receptor (erythrocyte P antigen). N Engl J Med 1994;330(17):1192–6.
248. Anderson LJ. Human parvovirus B19. Pediatr Ann 1990;19(9):509–10, 512–3.
249. Anderson LJ. Human parvoviruses. J Infect Dis 1990;161(4):603–8.

250. Lindner J, Barabas S, Saar K, et al. CD4(+) T-cell responses against the VP1-unique region in individuals with recent and persistent parvovirus B19 infection. J Vet Med B Infect Dis Vet Public Health 2005;52(7–8):356–61.
251. Ogata M, Satou T, Kawano R, et al. Plasma HHV-6 viral load-guided preemptive therapy against HHV-6 encephalopathy after allogeneic stem cell transplantation: a prospective evaluation. Bone Marrow Transplant 2008;41(3):279–85.
252. Norbeck O, Isa A, Pohlmann C, et al. Sustained CD8+ T-cell responses induced after acute parvovirus B19 infection in humans. J Virol 2005;79(18):12117–21.
253. Isa A, Norbeck O, Hirbod T, et al. Aberrant cellular immune responses in humans infected persistently with parvovirus B19. J Med Virol 2006;78(1):129–33.
254. Kerr JR, Cunniffe VS, Kelleher P, et al. Circulating cytokines and chemokines in acute symptomatic parvovirus B19 infection: negative association between levels of pro-inflammatory cytokines and development of B19-associated arthritis. J Med Virol 2004;74(1):147–55.
255. Kerr JR. Pathogenesis of parvovirus B19 infection: host gene variability, and possible means and effects of virus persistence. J Vet Med B Infect Dis Vet Public Health 2005;52(7–8):335–9.
256. Kelly H, Leydon J. Letter to the editor: outbreaks caused by parvovirus B19. Euro Surveill 2005;10(9):E1–2 [author reply: E5–6].
257. Azzi A, Morfini M, Mannucci PM. The transfusion-associated transmission of parvovirus B19. Transfus Med Rev 1999;13(3):194–204.
258. Heegaard ED, Laub Petersen B. Parvovirus B19 transmitted by bone marrow. Br J Haematol 2000;111(2):659–61.
259. Broliden K. Parvovirus B19 infection in pediatric solid-organ and bone marrow transplantation. Pediatr Transplant 2001;5(5):320–30.
260. Murer L, Zacchello G, Bianchi D, et al. Thrombotic microangiopathy associated with parvovirus B 19 infection after renal transplantation. J Am Soc Nephrol 2000;11(6):1132–7.
261. Moudgil A, Nast CC, Bagga A, et al. Association of parvovirus B19 infection with idiopathic collapsing glomerulopathy. Kidney Int 2001;59(6):2126–33.
262. Iwafuchi Y, Morita T, Kamimura A. Acute endocapillary proliferative glomerulonephritis associated with human parvovirus B19 infection. Clin Nephrol 2002;57(3): 246–50.
263. Onguru P, Dede F, Bodur H, et al. Glomerulonephritis associating parvovirus B19 infection. Ren Fail 2006;28(1):85–8.
264. Cossart YE, Field AM, Cant B, et al. Parvovirus-like particles in human sera. Lancet 1975;1(7898):72–3.
265. Neild G, Anderson M, Hawes S, et al. Parvovirus infection after renal transplant. Lancet 1986;2(8517):1226–7.
266. Laurenz M, Winkelmann B, Roigas J, et al. Severe parvovirus B19 encephalitis after renal transplantation. Pediatr Transplant 2006;10(8):978–81.
267. Rodrigues C, Pinto D, Medeiros R. Molecular epidemiology characterization of the urinary excretion of polyomavirus in healthy individuals from Portugal–a Southern European population. J Med Virol 2007;79(8):1194–8.
268. Ki CS, Kim IS, Kim JW, et al. Incidence and clinical significance of human parvovirus B19 infection in kidney transplant recipients. Clin Transplant 2005;19(6): 751–5.
269. Eid AJ, Brown RA, Patel R, et al. Parvovirus B19 infection after transplantation: a review of 98 cases. Clin Infect Dis 2006;43(1):40–8.
270. Cavallo R, Merlino C, Re D, et al. B19 virus infection in renal transplant recipients. J Clin Virol 2003;26(3):361–8.

271. Park JB, Kim DJ, Woo SY, et al. Clinical implications of quantitative real time-polymerase chain reaction of parvovirus B19 in kidney transplant recipients - a prospective study. Transpl Int 2009;22(4):455–62.
272. Ardalan MR, Shoja MM, Tubbs RS, et al. Postrenal transplant hemophagocytic lymphohistiocytosis and thrombotic microangiopathy associated with parvovirus b19 infection. Am J Transplant 2008;8(6):1340–4.
273. Moudgil A, Shidban H, Nast CC, et al. Parvovirus B19 infection-related complications in renal transplant recipients: treatment with intravenous immunoglobulin. Transplantation 1997;64(12):1847–50.
274. Beckhoff A, Steffen I, Sandoz P, et al. Relapsing severe anaemia due to primary parvovirus B19 infection after renal transplantation: a case report and review of the literature. Nephrol Dial Transplant 2007;22(12):3660–3.

Herpes Viruses in Transplant Recipients: HSV, VZV, Human Herpes Viruses, and EBV

Kevin Shiley, MD*, Emily Blumberg, MD

KEYWORDS

- Herpes virus • PTLD • Kaposi sarcoma
- Zoster • HHV-6 • HHV-7

The herpes viruses comprise a large group of enveloped DNA-containing viruses that characteristically cause latent infection in their respective hosts. There are 8 known herpes family viruses associated with human infection: herpes simplex virus (HSV) types 1 and 2, varicella zoster virus (VZV), Epstein-Barr virus (EBV), *Cytomegalovirus* (CMV), *Human herpesvirus 6* (HHV-6), *Human herpesvirus 7* (HHV-7), and *Human herpesvirus 8* (HHV-8). Of these, CMV has received the most attention as a cause of morbidity and mortality among transplant recipients and is discussed separately in articles by Ljungman, Strasfeld, Hirsch, and Einsele in this issue. The remaining herpes viruses are also responsible for significant disease in the transplant patient population. The role of each of these viruses as a cause of disease in the transplant population is discussed in this article.

HSV-1 AND HSV-2

The α-herpes viruses, HSV-1 and HSV-2, are responsible for oral and genital mucocutaneous ulcers in the general population. HSV-2 is generally considered to be sexually transmitted and primarily infects the urogenital mucosa, whereas HSV-1 predominantly affects the oral mucosa and is often transmitted through nonsexual contact.

Dr Shiley has no financial disclosures.
Dr Blumberg receives financial support from Roche Pharmaceuticals for research support and consulting services. She also receives research support from Viropharma as a site investigator in a multicenter trial.
Division of Infectious Diseases, Hospital of the University of Pennsylvania, 3rd Floor Silverstein Pavilion, Suite E, 3400 Spruce Street, Philadelphia, PA 19104, USA
* Corresponding author.
E-mail address: shileyk@uphs.upenn.edu

Infect Dis Clin N Am 24 (2010) 373–393
doi:10.1016/j.idc.2010.01.003
0891-5520/10/$ – see front matter © 2010 Elsevier Inc. All rights reserved.

Both viruses are neurotropic and primarily infect neurons in their latent forms. Reactivation of HSV is common among transplant recipients, and is the second most common cause of viral infection after transplantation.[1–3]

Most HSV-1 and HSV-2 infections occur in the setting of reactivation rather than primary infection, although primary HSV infections are well documented, particularly among younger patients.[4] Primary infection from transplanted tissue is uncommon but has been observed in renal transplant recipients.[5,6] The high percentage of cases attributed to reactivation is undoubtedly a result of a high baseline population seroprevalence of HSV-1 and HSV-2. Seroprevalence increases with age and varies by geographic, racial, socioeconomic, and ethnic characteristics among the general population. Antibodies to HSV-1 were found in 50% to 96% of people in previous seroprevalence studies.[7–9] Analysis of Americans from the National Health and Nutrition Examination Survey showed the seroprevalence of HSV-1 to be 65% and HSV-2 to be 26% by age 49 years.[10] Higher rates of seropositivity were found in women and minorities in the same survey. The greatest risk factor for reactivation of HSV following transplantation is lack of antiviral prophylaxis.[4,11–15]

Before the introduction of acyclovir, reactivation of HSV infection was estimated to occur in up to 80% of patients receiving hematopoetic stem cell transplant.[13–15] Lower, but still substantial, reactivation rates were described in solid-organ transplant recipients in the years before effective antiviral prophylaxis.[5,16–19] The clinical manifestations of HSV infection range from limited mucocutaneous outbreaks to disseminated infections involving visceral organs and the central nervous system (CNS).

The most common manifestations of HSV are mucocutaneous outbreaks, usually involving the oral and genitourinary mucosa.[20] These infections, which can lead to extensive mucosal involvement, typically occur in the first 30 days following transplantation if prophylaxis is not administered.[1,14,15,18,21] Less common manifestations of HSV involving the lungs and viscera are also described. Pneumonia as a result of HSV-1 and HSV-2 is typically preceded by gingivostomatitis, however pulmonary involvement from disseminated infection and airway manipulation may also occur.[22–28] The diagnosis of HSV pneumonia is complicated because viral shedding within the airways is common in immunosuppressed and critically ill adults and does not necessarily reflect true pneumonia.[29–33] The use of acyclovir in critically ill patients with HSV isolated from respiratory secretions has not been shown to influence mortality, ventilator dependence, or length of hospitalization.[33,34] Therefore, caution should be taken in interpreting results from viral cultures, direct fluorescent antibody staining, and nucleic acid assays without associated cytopathic evidence of infection on tissue biopsy.

Hepatitis is an uncommon manifestation of HSV that is described in several case reports and case series.[17,35–40] When HSV presents with hepatitis there is often evidence of disseminated disease with involvement of the skin and mucous membranes.[36,39] Patients may seem well initially, with elevated liver function tests as the only sign of infection.[37] More often, patients present with nonspecific flulike symptoms of fever, malaise, and myalgias. Increasing levels of aspartate aminotransferase and alanine aminotransferase, sometimes 10 to 20 times the upper limit of normal, are often observed. Cross-sectional imaging may appear normal, but in some cases liver infiltration with microabscesses has been observed.[35] Most cases occur within 30 days of transplant, however some cases have occurred years after transplant.[40] Nearly all HSV hepatitis cases in the literature occurred in patients while off antiviral prophylaxis. Diagnosis is made by liver biopsy with culture and antibody staining for HSV-1 and HSV-2. Pathology typically reveals necrotic hepatitis with loss of lobular architecture.[38] Other visceral manifestations of HSV infection in immunosuppressed hosts include esophagitis, gastritis, and colitis.[41–48]

Encephalitis as a result of HSV infection is rare in the transplant population.[49] On presentation, confusion, fever, and behavioral changes are the predominant findings. Up to one-third of patients present with seizure and one-fifth with focal neurologic findings.[50] Cerebrospinal fluid (CSF) typically has a lymphocytic pleocytosis and increased protein level.[50] The diagnosis of HSV encephalitis is now usually made by polymerase chain reaction (PCR) from CSF rather than brain biopsy.[51] In the general population, on which most research on HSV encephalitis has been conducted, significant neurologic compromise is common following HSV encephalitis.[50] The early initiation of high-dose acyclovir was shown to significantly decrease the morbidity and mortality from HSV encephalitis.[52] In a large cohort of immunocompetent and immunosuppressed patients, long-term neurologic deficits were common despite antiviral treatment.[50] There are insufficient data in the era of antiviral prophylaxis to know if outcomes are worse in transplant recipients.

The introduction of oral and intravenous acyclovir in the 1980s markedly decreased the incidence of serious HSV infections following transplantation. Several small randomized trials demonstrated intravenous and oral acyclovir to be safe and effective as a prophylactic regimen against HSV infections.[1,14,15,18,21] Acyclovir appeared to abbreviate viral shedding and expedite healing from mucocutaneous outbreaks in hematopoetic stem cell transplant recipients.[53] Since the introduction of acyclovir, related compounds such as valacyclovir and famciclovir have also been used successfully for treatment of HSV and varicella zoster infections following transplantation. Ganciclovir also has activity against HSV, and its use in the posttransplant population has been shown to significantly decrease rates of reactivation.[11,12] Resistance to acyclovir and its derivatives does occur and typically reflects prolonged exposure to inadequate dosing of acyclovir at the time of viral reactivation. The highest rates of acyclovir resistance are found in allogeneic stem cell transplant recipients with estimates ranging from 1% to 14% of patients with resistant virus.[54–57] Second-line treatment with foscarnet is typically used if acyclovir resistance is detected.[58]

VZV

VZV, the α-herpes virus responsible for chickenpox and shingles, causes symptomatic infection through reactivation or primary infection in approximately 1% to 20% of solid-organ transplant recipients, with lung transplant recipients having the highest rates.[2,59–61] The rate of VZV disease approaches more than 40% in hematopoetic stem cell transplant recipients.[62–66] Reactivation of VZV is the most common route of VZV disease in adult transplant recipients, with more than 90% of adults in the United States estimated to have antibodies against VZV.[67] In previous series, the median time frame for reactivation ranged from 9 to 23 months following solid-organ transplant.[68–70] In hematopoietic cell transplant recipients most cases of VZV disease tends to occur within the first 12 months following transplantation, with up to 26% of transplant recipients developing disease following discontinuation of antiviral prophylaxis.[63] Suggested risk factors for VZV disease in solid-organ transplant include mycophenolate use, recent treatment of rejection, induction therapy, and age greater than 50 years.[69,71] All solid-organ transplant candidates should be tested before transplantation for VZV antibodies in an effort to determine the risk for primary infection. Solid-organ transplant candidates with VZV IgG negative status should undergo vaccination with the live attenuated Oka strain VZV vaccine before solid-organ transplant.[58] The vaccine should not be given after transplant because it is a live vaccine and there are currently insufficient data to determine its safety in immunosuppressed transplant recipients.[72–77] The rate of VZV disease (primary and reactivation) in allogeneic stem cell transplant recipients remains high regardless of VZV serostatus before transplant.[66] An investigational inactivated varicella vaccine was successfully used to prevent disease in autologous hematopoetic stem cell transplant recipients; however it is currently not available.[78]

As with HSV, the clinical manifestations of VZV disease are wide ranging, but can be severe and associated with increased mortality, especially in the early posttransplant period. Primary infection with VZV in the posttransplant setting can be severe, with disseminated infection presenting with skin, lung, and visceral organ involvement.[79–81] Donor-derived VZV infections are rare, but have been reported.[82] The most common presentation of VZV is cutaneous infection, typically with single dermatomal involvement. However, multiple dermatome involvement occurs in a sizable minority of cases. In cases of disseminated disease, typical vesicular skin lesions remain a common marker of disease. It is notable that the rash is not always vesicular in immunosuppressed hosts; consequently biopsy of the skin may be required for viral identification either by direct fluorescence or nucleic acid detection or culture. Patients may present with other symptoms of disseminated disease, including abdominal pain or hepatitis before the onset of rash.[83] CNS involvement with VZV can present with encephalitis, myelitis, or meningoencephalitis. Unlike disseminated cutaneous infections, CNS VZV often presents without skin or other organ involvement.[84] The diagnosis of VZV CNS infection is typically made by detection of VZV in the CSF using nucleic acid testing in conjunction with a compatible clinical presentation.[85,86] CSF typically shows a lymphocyte predominant pleocytosis, moderately increased protein level and normal to low-normal glucose level.[87] All cases of disseminated zoster should be placed in isolation once the diagnosis is suspected in an effort to prevent spread to other immunocompromised patients and susceptible health care workers.

Treatment of VZV disease is generally recommended for all transplant recipients.[58] High-dose acyclovir or its analogues has been successfully used for the treatment of localized and disseminated VZV infections. In cases of disseminated disease and CNS infection, intravenous acyclovir (30 mg/kg/d in 3 divided doses) is preferred as initial therapy. Ganciclovir has not been studied specifically in the treatment of VZV, however it has been used successfully for treatment in several reports.[88] Oral agents, such as valacyclovir (1 g every 8 hours), acyclovir (800 mg 5 times each day) and famciclovir (500 mg every 8 hours) are reasonable choices for localized infections.[58,89] In rare cases where acyclovir resistance occurs, foscarnet can be used.[58]

Several studies have shown acyclovir and ganciclovir to be effective as prophylaxis against VZV reactivation in the posttransplant period.[1,11,12,14,15,18,21,53] Other methods of preventing primary infection in VZV-negative transplant recipients (who were not vaccinated before transplant or failed to mount a detectable VZV antibody titer) include vaccinating household and close contacts at risk for primary infection, preferably before transplant. VZV seronegative patients exposed to persons with active VZV (either chicken pox or shingles) should ideally be given postexposure prophylaxis with intravenous varicella zoster immunoglobulin (VZIG) given within the first 96 hours of exposure.[58,90,91] Unfortunately, VZIG is no longer available in the United States.[92] An intramuscularly dosed formulation of concentrated VZV IgG (VariZIG, Cangene Corp, Winnepeg, Canada) is available through an investigational new drug expanded access protocol from the Food and Drug Administration (http://www.fda.gov/BiologicsBloodVaccines/SafetyAvailability/ucm176029.htm). There are currently insufficient data to support the use of antiviral agents after VZV exposure, and it is currently not recommended by the Centers of Disease Control's Advisory Committee on Immunization Practices.[91]

EBV

EBV is a gammaherpes virus responsible for several clinical entities. In the general population, EBV is the causative agent of infectious mononucleosis, Burkitt lymphoma, and nasopharyngeal carcinoma. The role of EBV as a cause of posttransplant lymphoproliferative disorder (PTLD) is now well established, accounting for 90% of cases of PTLD.[93–95] Other rare disorders attributed to EBV in the posttransplant period include smooth muscle tumors and the hemophagocytic syndrome.[96,97] EBV is ubiquitous, with up to 90% seropositivity observed in the general community.[98] Infection in early childhood is common and often without significant symptoms.[99] The clinical entity of mononucleosis, characterized by pharyngitis, lymphadenopathy, and fatigue, is typically seen with primary infection in young immunocompetent adults. Rarely, neurologic manifestations of EBV infection, including encephalitis and optic neuritis, occur.[100] Like other herpes viruses, EBV is a chronic infection, with latent virus infecting B cells in the blood and lymphoid tissues. The virus is typically transmitted to naive individuals through saliva and respiratory secretions. Transmissions to naive transplant recipients through blood transfusion and organ transplant are also described.[95,101,102]

The clinical entity known as PTLD comprises a spectrum of disease characterized by the abnormal proliferation of lymphocytic cells, often with an invasive component, in patients following transplantation. The clinical manifestations of PTLD vary considerably. In some instances patients are asymptomatic and disease is only suggested by incidental imaging findings. Other cases may present with a mononucleosis-like syndrome, organ dysfunction secondary to tissue infiltration or septic-appearing febrile illness. Tissue infiltration from PTLD may present as extranodal masses, which can involve various organs, including the lungs, liver, spleen, bowels, and CNS.[95,103,104] In some instances, allografts are the primary site of PTLD, with resulting organ dysfunction mimicking rejection.[105] PTLD may present as an infiltrative process rather than a focal mass, mimicking such entities as pneumonia, lymphocele, and colitis.[106–109]

Numerous risk factors for the development of PTLD are described. Host EBV seronegative status has been shown to increase the risk of developing PTLD up to 76-fold, making the issue particularly troublesome for pediatric patients.[110–113] These patients, at risk for primary EBV infection, are most likely to present with disease within only a few months of transplant. Other risk factors in solid-organ transplant recipients, reflect a state of actual or potentially augmented immune suppression and include CMV disease, CMV donor/recipient mismatch, and intensity of pharmacologically mediated immune suppression.[112–116] Risk factors for PTLD in hematopoetic stem cell recipients include unrelated donor HLA mismatch, use of antithymocyte globulin, T-cell depletion, and use of anti-CD3 monoclonal antibodies for graft-versus-host disease prophylaxis.[117]

The initial diagnosis of PTLD is best made with tissue, ideally from an excisional biopsy specimen.[118] High serum levels of EBV DNA may be seen in PTLD, especially in younger recipients, and may precede clinical disease.[119,120] Currently, the incongruity in EBV DNA testing methods between centers and the need for tissue for pathologic grading, argue against the use of EBV viral load testing as replacement for histologic diagnosis, although it is estimated that up to 90% of PTLD is EBV-associated.[93] The Society of Hematopathology classification schema for PTLD divides lesions into 3 general categories: lymphoid hyperplasia (early lesions), polymorphic PTLD, and lymphomatous (monomorphic) PTLD.[121,122] Lymphoid hyperplasia, sometimes referred to as early PTLD, is subcharacterized into posttransplant infectious mononucleosis and reactive plasmacytic hyperplasia. A notable characteristic in both of these groups is the presence of polyclonal cell populations.[94,121] Polymorphic PTLD is characterized by more aggressive lesions that escape the normal lymphatic system boundaries and infiltrate underlying tissue. Although these lesions behave similarly to malignant lymphoma, the cell population involved remains heterogeneous in appearance, although they are all typically monoclonal at the molecular level. The term monomorphic PTLD is used to describe lymphomas in the posttransplant setting. Many are associated with EBV, although some are not. These lesions are generally categorized according to the Revised European American Lymphoma system with the suffix PTLD to note the correlation with transplant status.[121]

Treatment varies considerably depending on which variation of PTLD is diagnosed. A cornerstone of therapy is decreasing the level of immunosuppression whenever possible.[93,123,124] In 1 series of solid-organ transplant recipients treated for PTLD, 63% of patients treated by reducing immunosuppression alone had complete disease remission.[124] Risk factors for failing treatment with reduction of immunosuppression included a high baseline lactate dehydrogenase level, multiorgan involvement, presence of B symptoms, and organ dysfunction from disease.[124] The data for antiviral medications in the treatment of PTLD through suppression of EBV are limited. Although early reports suggested acyclovir and ganciclovir, which have some in vitro activity against EBV, might have a potential role in PTLD treatment there is no compelling clinical data to support their use.[125–128] Treatment with immunomodulatory agents such as anti-CD-20 (rituximab), interleukin 6 (IL-6) and interferon-α is described.[95,127,129–132] Infusions of cytotoxic EBV-specific T cells have also been used as a therapeutic and prophylactic treatment in solid-organ and hematopoetic stem cell transplant recipients.[133–140] As a treatment, results have been mixed and no controlled trials have been published on the subject.[133,136–138,140] The use of cytotoxic EBV-specific T cells as a prophylactic measure in individuals with high levels of circulating EBV DNA were also reported to be beneficial, but data are limited to small uncontrolled series.[133,134,139] In some cases treatment with chemotherapeutic agents used in nontransplant-associated lymphomas are also used, often in conjunction with rituximab.[141–144] Other strategies include resection of localized tumors, radiotherapy, and treatment of other infections, such as CMV, that may act to suppress the immune system further.[127,145] In cases where reduction of immunosuppression has resulted in graft loss, retransplantation can be successful.[146]

The use of antivirals gained some support as a prophylactic measure against EBV based on the results of some uncontrolled studies.[147–149] A randomized controlled trial exploring the use of ganciclovir and acyclovir as a prophylactic strategy for EBV and CMV did not show any decrease in PTLD, however.[150] The use of quantitative EBV viral load monitoring has been advocated as another method to prevent the development of PTLD in high-risk individuals.[93] In this approach regular quantitative EBV viral loads are obtained and immunosuppression is decreased when viral loads reach a predetermined threshold.[119,151]

HHV-6 AND HHV-7

HHV-6, the causative agent of the common childhood disease roseola infantum (exanthem sabitum), has received attention in the past several years as an opportunistic infection in the posttransplant population. The virus, first described in 1986, is a member of the β-herpes virus family, and establishes latency in CD4+ T lymphocytes.[152] Genetic sequencing has demonstrated 2 variants, A and B. The B variant has been linked to most disease in children and in the transplant population.[153] It is estimated that greater than 90% of children are seropositive for HHV-6 by 1 year of age.[154,155] Therefore, most cases of HHV-6 viremia are believed to be caused by viral reactivation, although primary infection following transplantation has been described.[156,157]

Reactivation of HHV-6 is common in the immediate period following hematopoetic stem cell transplant, when immunosuppression is highest. A prospective study by Zerr and colleagues[158] detected HHV-6 viremia in 52 of 110 (47%) patients evaluated during the first 100 days after transplant. Numerous indirect effects have been suggested related to HHV-6 viremia in the hematopoetic stem cell transplant population. These include delayed engraftment, higher rates of graft-versus-host disease, cytomegalovirus disease, and all-cause mortality.[158–162] Estimates of HHV-6 viremia following solid-organ transplant range from 24% to 66%, although this is likely reduced in patients receiving ganciclovir for CMV prophylaxis.[163–167] Reported indirect effects associated with HHV-6 viremia include higher frequencies of allograft rejection, severe CMV disease, and invasive fungal infections.[163,164,168–170] Despite these associations, no causal link has been definitively established between HHV-6 reactivation and indirect effects. A recent prospective cohort study that included 298 solid-organ transplant recipients found no connection between severity or duration of CMV disease and HHV-6 coinfection.[171]

Several case series and reports have linked HHV-6 with encephalitis in solid-organ and hematopoetic stem cell transplant recipients.[156,158,172–176] Most of the cases reported in the literature occurred 30 to 90 days after transplant. Manifestations of neurologic disease include generalized confusion, amnesia, insomnia, seizures (often subclinical), and coma.[172,176,177] Magnetic resonance imaging imaging of the brain often reveals involvement of the basal ganglia.[100,176,177] The detection of HHV-6 in CSF through PCR or culture, in conjunction with compatible neuroradiology and clinical manifestations, is highly suggestive of HHV-6 encephalitis.[178] Nonetheless, other causes of encephalitis should be ruled out as HHV-6 has been detected in the CSF of asymptomatic patients and the symptoms of HHV-6 encephalitis may be strikingly similar to those of immunosuppression leukoencephalopathy.[172,179,180] Other manifestations of HHV-6 disease reported in the literature include gastroenteritis, pneumonitis, hepatitis, and myelosuppression.[181–183]

No prospective clinical trials have evaluated the use of antiviral medications in the treatment of HHV-6 associated disease. In vitro data suggest that HHV-6 is inhibited by ganciclovir, foscarnet, and cidofovir.[184–186] Most clinical experience has been with the treatment of HHV-6 encephalitis. Most reported cases used ganciclovir, foscarnet, or a combination of both with varying success.[156,172–176] Despite their in vitro activity against HHV-6, neither intravenous ganciclovir nor valganciclovir affected HHV-6 viral loads in a multicenter prospective clinical trial of CMV disease treatment.[171]

The β-herpes virus, HHV-7, is closely related to HHV-6 but its role in clinically relevant disease remains unclear. In children, HHV-7 has been associated with rare cases of exanthem subitum, febrile seizures, and encephalitis.[187] A few cases of encephalitis and myelitis have been attributed to HHV-7 among hematopoetic stem cell transplant recipients,.[188,189] In comparison with HHV-6, however, little data exist supporting organ-specific infections with HHV-7 in transplant recipients. Like HHV-6, HHV-7 has been proposed to act as an immunomodulatory virus, potentially lowering the barrier to other opportunistic infections, including CMV.[190–192] A recent prospective multicenter cohort examined the effect of HHV-7 viremia in patients with diagnosed CMV disease and found no correlation with duration of CMV disease or CMV disease outcomes.[171]

HHV-8

HHV-8 also known as Kaposi sarcoma–associated herpes virus, is responsible for the malignant entities of Kaposi sarcoma (KS) and primary effusion lymphoma (PEL), as well as some forms of multicentric Castleman disease (MCD).[193–195] HHV-8 belongs to the γ-herpes virus family along with EBV and infects CD-19 positive B cells in its latent form.[196] Unlike the other herpes viruses discussed earlier, the seroprevalence to HHV-8 is highly variable, depending on geography and behavioral risk factors.[197–200] Of 13,984 Americans sampled in the National Health and Nutrition Survey, 1.5% were found to be seropositive for HHV-8.[201] The highest rate of HHV-8 seropositivity in the United States was found in men who have sex with men, with a prevalence rate estimated to be 8.2%.[201] Worldwide prevalence varies dramatically, with some areas of sub-Saharan Africa estimated to have 30% to 50% seropositivity.[199,202]

Transmission of HHV-8 is believed to occur through sexual activity and possibly through saliva.[197,199,201] In endemic regions both means of transmission probably occur.[196,199] Elsewhere, such as in North America, sexual activity is believed to be the primary mode of transmission.[201] Transmission of HHV-8 has also been documented through solid-organ and hematopoetic stem cell transplantation.[203–205]

Manifestations of HHV-8 disease in transplant recipients are variable. In the Middle East, where seroprevalence for HHV-8 reaches 25%, KS is the most common malignancy following renal transplant.[198] The incidence is lower in North America. Prior series describing KS following solid-organ transplant reported onset of disease ranging from 2 to 23 months after transplant.[205–207] Lesions may present as focal nodules on the skin, within organs (including allografts), or as disseminated disease with lymph node, bone marrow, and splenic infiltration.[203,204,207,208] The diagnosis of KS is made by pathologic examination of affected tissues.

As with EBV-associated PTLD, reduction in immunosuppression is the first-line therapy for KS and is often curative.[202] Some investigators have suggested that using sirolimus instead of other calcineurin inhibitors may provide additional treatment effect by inhibition of vascular endothelial cell growth factor.[209,210] Chemotherapy and radiation may also be necessary in cases where reduction of immunosuppression is ineffective or not possible.[202,208] Antiviral medications have not been shown to be useful in the treatment of KS.[211,212]

Other rare manifestations of HHV-8 reported in transplant recipients include MCD and PEL.[213–217] MCD is an aggressive lymphoproliferative disorder characterized by fever, diffuse lymphadenopathy, wasting, and hepatosplenomegally.[218] HHV-8 is not always found in MCD, but is common, with virus detected in 75% of MCD lesions in 1 series.[219] The diagnosis of MCD is made by tissue biopsy. Other causes of diffuse lymphadenopathy, such as disseminated mycobacterial and fungal infections, should be ruled out. The reported outcomes of MCD in transplant recipients are poor, with rapidly fatal disease or allograft failure in several reports.[214,215,220,221] Treatments with immunomodulatory agents, chemotherapy, and antivirals have all been used with variable results.[218,222]

PEL, also known as body cavity lymphoma, typically presents with a refractory exudative effusion in 1 of several potential spaces within the body. Lymphomatous cells fill the affected cavity, with tumor foci often studding the serous membranes.[223] The most frequent location is the pleural space, however pericardial, peritoneal, and intracranial cases are also reported.[223] Diagnosis is made by pathologic evaluation of effusion cells. HHV-8 PCR of the effusion may also be helpful in making a diagnosis. Other causes of exudative effusions should be ruled out, including infectious entities such as tuberculosis and empyema. Treatment experience of transplant-associated PEL is limited. Reduction in immunosuppression may be useful, as with KS and MCD.[202] Antivirals have not been shown to offer much benefit and chemotherapy remains the treatment of choice in most cases.[222,223]

SUMMARY

The herpes viruses are responsible for a wide range of diseases in patients following transplant. The development of effective antiviral prophylaxis against HSV and VZV has substantially reduced the morbidity and mortality associated with these infections. Nonetheless, primary disease and reactivation of HSV and VZV can cause significant harm if not treated promptly. The role of EBV as a major cause of PTLD continues to pose a significant challenge. Current therapies focus on reduction of immunosuppression, chemotherapy, and rituximab therapy. There are few data to support antiviral therapy for EBV-associated PTLD, however ganciclovir may have a prophylactic effect, either by indirect or direct means. HHV-6 and -7 may have several indirect effects on transplant patients, including increased risk of infections and rejection episodes. These effects may be related to the viruses' effect on immune cell function. The evidence for HHV-6 as a cause of posttransplant encephalitis is growing. Treatment with ganciclovir and/or foscarnet may be beneficial. The role of HHV-8 in posttransplant KS is well established. Reduction in immune suppression is the mainstay of therapy; in some cases alteration of immunosuppression to include sirolimus may be effective. Other manifestations of HHV-8 infection, including PEL and MCD may require chemotherapy in conjunction with reduction in immunosuppression. Antivirals have not been shown to be beneficial in the treatment of KS or PEL.

REFERENCES

1. Balfour HH Jr, Chace BA, Stapleton JT, et al. A randomized, placebo-controlled trial of oral acyclovir for the prevention of cytomegalovirus disease in recipients of renal allografts. N Engl J Med 1989;320(21):1381–7.
2. Snydman DR. Epidemiology of infections after solid-organ transplantation. Clin Infect Dis 2001;33(Suppl 1):S5–8.
3. Montoya J, Giraldo L, Efron B, et al. Infectious complications among 620 consecutive heart transplant patients at Stanford University Medical Center. Clin Infect Dis 2001;33:629–40.
4. Singh N, Dummer JS, Kusne S, et al. Infections with cytomegalovirus and other herpesviruses in 121 liver transplant recipients: transmission by donated organ and the effect of OKT3 antibodies. J Infect Dis 1988;158(1):124–31.
5. Dummer JS, Armstrong J, Somers J, et al. Transmission of infection with herpes simplex virus by renal transplantation. J Infect Dis 1987;155(2):202–6.
6. Koneru B, Tzakis AG, DePuydt LE, et al. Transmission of fatal herpes simplex infection through renal transplantation. Transplantation 1988;45(3):653–6.
7. Malkin J. Epidemiology of genital herpes simplex virus infection in developed countries. Herpes 2004;11(Suppl 1):24.
8. Malkin J, Morand P, Malvy D. Seroprevalence of HSV-1 and HSV-2 in the general French population. Sex Transm Dis 2002;78:201–3.
9. Vyse A, Gay N, Slomka M. The burden of infection with HSV-1 and HSV-2 in England and Wales: implications for the changing epidemiology of genital herpes. Sex Transm Dis 2000;76:183–7.
10. Xu F, Sternberg MR, Kottiri BJ, et al. Trends in herpes simplex virus type 1 and type 2 seroprevalence in the United States. JAMA 2006;296(8):964–73.

11. Gane E, Saliba F, Valdecasas GJ, et al. Randomised trial of efficacy and safety of oral ganciclovir in the prevention of cytomegalovirus disease in liver-transplant recipients. The Oral Ganciclovir International Transplantation Study Group [corrected]. Lancet 1997;350(9093):1729–33.
12. Lowance D, Neumayer HH, Legendre CM, et al. Valacyclovir for the prevention of cytomegalovirus disease after renal transplantation. International Valacyclovir Cytomegalovirus Prophylaxis Transplantation Study Group. N Engl J Med 1999; 340(19):1462–70.
13. Meyers JD, Flournoy N, Thomas ED. Infection with herpes simplex virus and cell-mediated immunity after marrow transplant. J Infect Dis 1980;142(3): 338–46.
14. Meyers JD, Wade JC, Mitchell CD, et al. Multicenter collaborative trial of intravenous acyclovir for treatment of mucocutaneous herpes simplex virus infection in the immunocompromised host. Am J Med 1982;73(1A):229–35.
15. Saral R, Burns WH, Laskin OL, et al. Acyclovir prophylaxis of herpes-simplex-virus infections. N Engl J Med 1981;305(2):63–7.
16. Seale L, Jones CJ, Kathpalia S, et al. Prevention of herpesvirus infections in renal allograft recipients by low-dose oral acyclovir. JAMA 1985;254(24): 3435–8.
17. Kusne S, Schwartz M, Breinig MK, et al. Herpes simplex virus hepatitis after solid organ transplantation in adults. J Infect Dis 1991;163(5):1001–7.
18. Pettersson E, Hovi T, Ahonen J, et al. Prophylactic oral acyclovir after renal transplantation. Transplantation 1985;39(3):279–81.
19. Naraqi S, Jackson GG, Jonasson O, et al. Prospective study of prevalence, incidence, and source of herpesvirus infections in patients with renal allografts. J Infect Dis 1977;136(4):531–40.
20. Corey L. Herpes simplex virus. In: Mandell G, Bennett J, Dolin R, editors. 6th edition, Principles and practice of infectious diseases, vol. 2. Philadelphia (PA): Elsevier; 2005. p. 1762–80.
21. Hann IM, Prentice HG, Blacklock HA, et al. Acyclovir prophylaxis against herpes virus infections in severely immunocompromised patients: randomised double blind trial. Br Med J (Clin Res Ed) 1983;287(6389):384–8.
22. Buss DH, Scharyj M. Herpesvirus infection of the esophagus and other visceral organs in adults. Incidence and clinical significance. Am J Med 1979;66(3):457–62.
23. Cunha BA, Eisenstein LE, Dillard T, et al. Herpes simplex virus (HSV) pneumonia in a heart transplant: diagnosis and therapy. Heart Lung 2007;36(1):72–8.
24. Herout V, Vortel V, Vondrackova A. Herpes simplex involvement of the lower respiratory tract. Am J Clin Pathol 1966;46(4):411–9.
25. Morgan HR, Finland M. Isolation of herpes virus from a case of atypical pneumonia and erythema multiforme exudativum with studies of four additional cases. Am J Med Sci 1949;217(1):92–5.
26. Nash G. Necrotizing tracheobronchitis and bronchopneumonia consistent with herpetic infection. Hum Pathol 1972;3(2):283–91.
27. Nash G, Foley FD. Herpetic infection of the middle and lower respiratory tract. Am J Clin Pathol 1970;54(6):857–63.
28. Ramsey PG, Fife KH, Hackman RC, et al. Herpes simplex virus pneumonia: clinical, virologic, and pathologic features in 20 patients. Ann Intern Med 1982; 97(6):813–20.
29. Bruynseels P, Jorens PG, Demey HE, et al. Herpes simplex virus in the respiratory tract of critical care patients: a prospective study. Lancet 2003;362(9395): 1536–41.

30. Camps K, Jorens PG, Demey HE, et al. Clinical significance of herpes simplex virus in the lower respiratory tract of critically ill patients. Eur J Clin Microbiol Infect Dis 2002;21(10):758–9.
31. Klainer AS, Oud L, Randazzo J, et al. Herpes simplex virus involvement of the lower respiratory tract following surgery. Chest 1994;106(Suppl 1):8S–14S [discussion: 34S–5S].
32. Liebau P, Kuse E, Winkler M, et al. Management of herpes simplex virus type 1 pneumonia following liver transplantation. Infection 1996;24(2):130–5.
33. Tuxen DV, Wilson JW, Cade JF. Prevention of lower respiratory herpes simplex virus infection with acyclovir in patients with the adult respiratory distress syndrome. Am Rev Respir Dis 1987;136(2):402–5.
34. Schuller D, Spessert C, Fraser VJ, et al. Herpes simplex virus from respiratory tract secretions: epidemiology, clinical characteristics, and outcome in immunocompromised and nonimmunocompromised hosts. Am J Med 1993;94(1):29–33.
35. Campsen J, Hendrickson R, Bak T, et al. Herpes simplex in a liver transplant recipient. Liver Transpl 2006;12(7):1171–3.
36. Basse G, Mengelle C, Kamar N, et al. Disseminated herpes simplex type-2 (HSV-2) infection after solid-organ transplantation. Infection 2008;36(1):62–4.
37. Duckro AN, Sha BE, Jakate S, et al. Herpes simplex virus hepatitis: expanding the spectrum of disease. Transpl Infect Dis 2006;8(3):171–6.
38. Kaufman B, Gandhi SA, Louie E, et al. Herpes simplex virus hepatitis: case report and review. Clin Infect Dis 1997;24(3):334–8.
39. Taylor RJ, Saul SH, Dowling JN, et al. Primary disseminated herpes simplex infection with fulminant hepatitis following renal transplantation. Arch Intern Med 1981;141(11):1519–21.
40. Bissig KD, Zimmermann A, Bernasch D, et al. Herpes simplex virus hepatitis 4 years after liver transplantation. J Gastroenterol 2003;38(10):1005–8.
41. Adler M, Goldman M, Liesnard C, et al. Diffuse herpes simplex virus colitis in a kidney transplant recipient successfully treated with acyclovir. Transplantation 1987;43(6):919–21.
42. Delis S, Kato T, Ruiz P, et al. Herpes simplex colitis in a child with combined liver and small bowel transplant. Pediatr Transplant 2001;5(5):374–7.
43. el-Serag HB, Zwas FR, Cirillo NW, et al. Fulminant herpes colitis in a patient with Crohn's disease. J Clin Gastroenterol 1996;22(3):220–3.
44. Fishbein PG, Tuthill R, Kressel H, et al. Herpes simplex esophagitis: a cause of upper-gastrointestinal bleeding. Dig Dis Sci 1979;24(7):540–4.
45. Howiler W, Goldberg HI. Gastroesophageal involvement in herpes simplex. Gastroenterology 1976;70(5 Pt 1):775–8.
46. Mosimann F, Cuenoud PF, Steinhauslin F, et al. Herpes simplex esophagitis after renal transplantation. Transpl Int 1994;7(2):79–82.
47. Naik HR, Chandrasekar PH. Herpes simplex virus (HSV) colitis in a bone marrow transplant recipient. Bone Marrow Transplant 1996;17(2):285–6.
48. Watts SJ, Alexander LC, Fawcett K, et al. Herpes simplex esophagitis in a renal transplant patient treated with cyclosporine A: a case report. Am J Gastroenterol 1986;81(3):185–8.
49. Gomez E, Melon S, Aguado S, et al. Herpes simplex virus encephalitis in a renal transplant patient: diagnosis by polymerase chain reaction detection of HSV DNA. Am J Kidney Dis 1997;30(3):423–7.
50. Raschilas F, Wolff M, Delatour F, et al. Outcome of and prognostic factors for herpes simplex encephalitis in adult patients: results of a multicenter study. Clin Infect Dis 2002;35(3):254–60.

51. Lakeman FD, Whitley RJ. Diagnosis of herpes simplex encephalitis: application of polymerase chain reaction to cerebrospinal fluid from brain-biopsied patients and correlation with disease. National Institute of Allergy and Infectious Diseases Collaborative Antiviral Study Group. J Infect Dis 1995;171(4):857–63.
52. Whitley RJ, Alford CA, Hirsch MS, et al. Vidarabine versus acyclovir therapy in herpes simplex encephalitis. N Engl J Med 1986;314(3):144–9.
53. Shepp DH, Dandliker PS, Flournoy N, et al. Once-daily intravenous acyclovir for prophylaxis of herpes simplex virus reactivation after marrow transplantation. J Antimicrob Chemother 1985;16(3):389–95.
54. Chen Y, Scieux C, Garrait V, et al. Resistant herpes simplex virus type 1 infection: an emerging concern after allogeneic stem cell transplantation. Clin Infect Dis 2000;31(4):927–35.
55. Erard V, Wald A, Corey L, et al. Use of long-term suppressive acyclovir after hematopoietic stem-cell transplantation: impact on herpes simplex virus (HSV) disease and drug-resistant HSV disease. J Infect Dis 2007;196(2):266–70.
56. Morfin F, Thouvenot D. Herpes simplex virus resistance to antiviral drugs. J Clin Virol 2003;26(1):29–37.
57. Nugier F, Colin JN, Aymard M, et al. Occurrence and characterization of acyclovir-resistant herpes simplex virus isolates: report on a two-year sensitivity screening survey. J Med Virol 1992;36(1):1–12.
58. Herpes simplex virus (HSV)-1 and -2, and varicella zoster virus (VZV). Am J Transplant 2004;4(s10):69–71.
59. Alcaide ML, Abbo L, Pano JR, et al. Herpes zoster infection after liver transplantation in patients receiving induction therapy with alemtuzumab. Clin Transplant 2008;22(4):502–7.
60. Arness T, Pedersen R, Dierkhising R, et al. Varicella zoster virus-associated disease in adult kidney transplant recipients: incidence and risk-factor analysis. Transpl Infect Dis 2008;10(4):260–8.
61. Manuel O, Kumar D, Singer LG, et al. Incidence and clinical characteristics of herpes zoster after lung transplantation. J Heart Lung Transplant 2008;27(1):11–6.
62. Locksley RM, Flournoy N, Sullivan KM, et al. Infection with varicella-zoster virus after marrow transplantation. J Infect Dis 1985;152(6):1172–81.
63. Boeckh M, Kim HW, Flowers ME, et al. Long-term acyclovir for prevention of varicella zoster virus disease after allogeneic hematopoietic cell transplantation–a randomized double-blind placebo-controlled study. Blood 2006;107(5):1800–5.
64. Han CS, Miller W, Haake R, et al. Varicella zoster infection after bone marrow transplantation: incidence, risk factors and complications. Bone Marrow Transplant 1994;13(3):277–83.
65. Leung TF, Chik KW, Li CK, et al. Incidence, risk factors and outcome of varicella-zoster virus infection in children after haematopoietic stem cell transplantation. Bone Marrow Transplant 2000;25(2):167–72.
66. Koc Y, Miller KB, Schenkein DP, et al. Varicella zoster virus infections following allogeneic bone marrow transplantation: frequency, risk factors, and clinical outcome. Biol Blood Marrow Transplant 2000;6(1):44–9.
67. Gnann J. Herpes simplex and varicella zoster virus infection after hemopoietic stem cell or solid organ transplantation. Philadelphia: Lippincott, Williams and Wilkins; 2003.
68. Fuks L, Shitrit D, Fox BD, et al. Herpes zoster after lung transplantation: incidence, timing, and outcome. Ann Thorac Surg 2009;87(2):423–6.

69. Gourishankar S, McDermid JC, Jhangri GS, et al. Herpes zoster infection following solid organ transplantation: incidence, risk factors and outcomes in the current immunosuppressive era. Am J Transplant 2004;4(1):108–15.
70. Herrero JI, Quiroga J, Sangro B, et al. Herpes zoster after liver transplantation: incidence, risk factors, and complications. Liver Transpl 2004;10(9):1140–3.
71. Lauzurica R, Bayes B, Frias C, et al. Disseminated varicella infection in adult renal allograft recipients: role of mycophenolate mofetil. Transplant Proc 2003; 35(5):1758–9.
72. Weinberg A, Horslen SP, Kaufman SS, et al. Safety and immunogenicity of varicella-zoster virus vaccine in pediatric liver and intestine transplant recipients. Am J Transplant 2006;6(3):565–8.
73. Khan S, Erlichman J, Rand EB. Live virus immunization after orthotopic liver transplantation. Pediatr Transplant 2006;10(1):78–82.
74. Kraft JN, Shaw JC. Varicella infection caused by Oka strain vaccine in a heart transplant recipient. Arch Dermatol 2006;142(7):943–5.
75. Levitsky J, Te HS, Faust TW, et al. Varicella infection following varicella vaccination in a liver transplant recipient. Am J Transplant 2002;2(9):880–2.
76. Sauerbrei A, Prager J, Hengst U, et al. Varicella vaccination in children after bone marrow transplantation. Bone Marrow Transplant 1997;20(5):381–3.
77. Merck. Varivax varicella virus vaccine live [PDF file]. Available at: http://www.merck.com/product/usa/pi_circulars/v/varivax/varivax_pi.pdf. 2009. Accessed August 8, 2009.
78. Hata A, Asanuma H, Rinki M, et al. Use of an inactivated varicella vaccine in recipients of hematopoietic-cell transplants. N Engl J Med 2002;347(1):26–34.
79. Feldhoff CM, Balfour HH Jr, Simmons RL, et al. Varicella in children with renal transplants. J Pediatr 1981;98(1):25–31.
80. McGregor RS, Zitelli BJ, Urbach AH, et al. Varicella in pediatric orthotopic liver transplant recipients. Pediatrics 1989;83(2):256–61.
81. Parnham AP, Flexman JP, Saker BM, et al. Primary varicella in adult renal transplant recipients: a report of three cases plus a review of the literature. Clin Transplant 1995;9(2):115–8.
82. Fall AJ, Aitchison JD, Krause A, et al. Donor organ transmission of varicella zoster due to cardiac transplantation. Transplantation 2000;70(1):211–3.
83. Hyland JM, Butterworth J. Severe acute visceral pain from varicella zoster virus. Anesth Analg 2003;97(4):1117–8.
84. Koskiniemi M, Piiparinen H, Rantalaiho T, et al. Acute central nervous system complications in varicella zoster virus infections. J Clin Virol 2002;25(3): 293–301.
85. Aberle SW, Puchhammer-Stockl E. Diagnosis of herpesvirus infections of the central nervous system. J Clin Virol 2002;25(Suppl 1):S79–85.
86. Puchhammer-Stockl E, Popow-Kraupp T, Heinz FX, et al. Detection of varicella-zoster virus DNA by polymerase chain reaction in the cerebrospinal fluid of patients suffering from neurological complications associated with chicken pox or herpes zoster. J Clin Microbiol 1991;29(7):1513–6.
87. Glaser CA, Honarmand S, Anderson LJ, et al. Beyond viruses: clinical profiles and etiologies associated with encephalitis. Clin Infect Dis 2006;43(12):1565–77.
88. Gilden D. Varicella zoster virus and central nervous system syndromes. Herpes 2004;11(Suppl 2):89A–94A.
89. Tyring S, Belanger R, Bezwoda W, et al. A randomized, double-blind trial of famciclovir versus acyclovir for the treatment of localized dermatomal herpes zoster in immunocompromised patients. Cancer Invest 2001;19(1):13–22.

90. American Academy of Pediatrics. Varicella zoster virus. 25th edition. Elk Grove (IL): American Academy of Pediatrics; 2000.
91. Marin M, Guris D, Chaves SS, et al. Prevention of varicella: recommendations of the Advisory Committee on Immunization Practices (ACIP). MMWR Recomm Rep 2007;56(RR-4):1–40.
92. A new product (VariZIG™) for postexposure prophylaxis of varicella available under an investigational new drug application expanded access protocol. MMWR Morb Mortal Wkly Rep 2006;55(8):209–10.
93. Epstein-Barr virus and lymphoproliferative disorders after transplantation. Am J Transplant 2004;4(Suppl 10):59–65.
94. Nalesnik MA. The diverse pathology of post-transplant lymphoproliferative disorders: the importance of a standardized approach. Transpl Infect Dis 2001;3(2):88–96.
95. Preiksaitis JK. New developments in the diagnosis and management of post-transplantation lymphoproliferative disorders in solid organ transplant recipients. Clin Infect Dis 2004;39(7):1016–23.
96. Karras A, Thervet E, Legendre C. Hemophagocytic syndrome in renal transplant recipients: report of 17 cases and review of literature. Transplantation 2004;77(2):238–43.
97. Lee ES, Locker J, Nalesnik M, et al. The association of Epstein-Barr virus with smooth-muscle tumors occurring after organ transplantation. N Engl J Med 1995;332(1):19–25.
98. Jenkins FJ, Rowe DT, Rinaldo CR Jr. Herpesvirus infections in organ transplant recipients. Clin Diagn Lab Immunol 2003;10(1):1–7.
99. Johannsen E, Schooley R, Kaye K. Epstein-Barr virus (infectious mononucleosis). In: Mandell G, Bennett J, Dolin R, editors, Principles and practice of infectious diseases, vol. 2. Philadelphia (PA): Elsevier; 2005. p. 1801–20.
100. Baskin HJ, Hedlund G. Neuroimaging of herpesvirus infections in children. Pediatr Radiol 2007;37(10):949–63.
101. Alfieri C, Tanner J, Carpentier L, et al. Epstein-Barr virus transmission from a blood donor to an organ transplant recipient with recovery of the same virus strain from the recipient's blood and oropharynx. Blood 1996;87(2):812–7.
102. Haque T, Thomas JA, Falk KI, et al. Transmission of donor Epstein-Barr virus (EBV) in transplanted organs causes lymphoproliferative disease in EBV-seronegative recipients. J Gen Virol 1996;77(Pt 6):1169–72.
103. Frizzera G, Hanto DW, Gajl-Peczalska KJ, et al. Polymorphic diffuse B-cell hyperplasias and lymphomas in renal transplant recipients. Cancer Res 1981;41(11 Pt 1):4262–79.
104. Hanto DW, Gajl-Peczalska KJ, Frizzera G, et al. Epstein-Barr virus (EBV) induced polyclonal and monoclonal B-cell lymphoproliferative diseases occurring after renal transplantation. Clinical, pathologic, and virologic findings and implications for therapy. Ann Surg 1983;198(3):356–69.
105. Yousem SA, Randhawa P, Locker J, et al. Posttransplant lymphoproliferative disorders in heart-lung transplant recipients: primary presentation in the allograft. Hum Pathol 1989;20(4):361–9.
106. Diaz-Guzman E, Farver C, Kanne JP, et al. A 65-year-old man with odynophagia and a lung mass. Chest 2009;135(3):876–9.
107. Khan MS, Ahmed S, Challacombe B, et al. Post-transplant lymphoproliferative disorder (PTLD) presenting as painful lymphocele 12 years after a cadaveric renal transplant. Int Urol Nephrol 2008;40(2):547–50.

108. Lee WK, Lau EW, Duddalwar VA, et al. Abdominal manifestations of extranodal lymphoma: spectrum of imaging findings. AJR Am J Roentgenol 2008;191(1): 198–206.
109. Kunitomi A, Arima N, Ishikawa T. Epstein-Barr virus-associated post-transplant lymphoproliferative disorders presented as interstitial pneumonia; successful recovery with rituximab. Haematologica 2007;92(4):e49–52.
110. Ellis D, Jaffe R, Green M, et al. Epstein-Barr virus-related disorders in children undergoing renal transplantation with tacrolimus-based immunosuppression. Transplantation 1999;68(7):997–1003.
111. Ho M, Miller G, Atchison RW, et al. Epstein-Barr virus infections and DNA hybridization studies in posttransplantation lymphoma and lymphoproliferative lesions: the role of primary infection. J Infect Dis 1985;152(5):876–86.
112. Swinnen LJ, Costanzo-Nordin MR, Fisher SG, et al. Increased incidence of lymphoproliferative disorder after immunosuppression with the monoclonal antibody OKT3 in cardiac-transplant recipients. N Engl J Med 1990;323(25):1723–8.
113. Walker RC, Marshall WF, Strickler JG, et al. Pretransplantation assessment of the risk of lymphoproliferative disorder. Clin Infect Dis 1995;20(5):1346–53.
114. Keay S, Oldach D, Wiland A, et al. Posttransplantation lymphoproliferative disorder associated with OKT3 and decreased antiviral prophylaxis in pancreas transplant recipients. Clin Infect Dis 1998;26(3):596–600.
115. Cox KL, Lawrence-Miyasaki LS, Garcia-Kennedy R, et al. An increased incidence of Epstein-Barr virus infection and lymphoproliferative disorder in young children on FK506 after liver transplantation. Transplantation 1995;59(4):524–9.
116. Manez R, Breinig MC, Linden P, et al. Posttransplant lymphoproliferative disease in primary Epstein-Barr virus infection after liver transplantation: the role of cytomegalovirus disease. J Infect Dis 1997;176(6):1462–7.
117. Weinstock DM, Ambrossi GG, Brennan C, et al. Preemptive diagnosis and treatment of Epstein-Barr virus-associated post transplant lymphoproliferative disorder after hematopoietic stem cell transplant: an approach in development. Bone Marrow Transplant 2006;37(6):539–46.
118. Preiksaitis JK, Keay S. Diagnosis and management of posttransplant lymphoproliferative disorder in solid-organ transplant recipients. Clin Infect Dis 2001; 33(Suppl 1):S38–46.
119. Tsai DE, Douglas L, Andreadis C, et al. EBV PCR in the diagnosis and monitoring of posttransplant lymphoproliferative disorder: results of a two-arm prospective trial. Am J Transplant 2008;8(5):1016–24.
120. Wheless SA, Gulley ML, Raab-Traub N, et al. Post-transplantation lymphoproliferative disease: Epstein-Barr virus DNA levels, HLA-A3, and survival. Am J Respir Crit Care Med 2008;178(10):1060–5.
121. Harris NL. Posttransplant lymphoproliferative disorders (PTLD). In: Jaffe E, Harris N, Stein H, et al, editors. Pathology and genetics: tumours of haematopoietic and lymphoid tissues. WHO classification of tumours. Lyon (France): IARC Press; 2001. p. 264–9.
122. Harris NL, Ferry JA, Swerdlow SH. Posttransplant lymphoproliferative disorders: summary of Society for Hematopathology Workshop. Semin Diagn Pathol 1997; 14(1):8–14.
123. Starzl TE, Nalesnik MA, Porter KA, et al. Reversibility of lymphomas and lymphoproliferative lesions developing under cyclosporin-steroid therapy. Lancet 1984; 1(8377):583–7.
124. Tsai DE, Hardy CL, Tomaszewski JE, et al. Reduction in immunosuppression as initial therapy for posttransplant lymphoproliferative disorder: analysis of

prognostic variables and long-term follow-up of 42 adult patients. Transplantation 2001;71(8):1076–88.
125. Hanto DW, Frizzera G, Gajl-Peczalska KJ, et al. Epstein-Barr virus-induced B-cell lymphoma after renal transplantation: acyclovir therapy and transition from polyclonal to monoclonal B-cell proliferation. N Engl J Med 1982;306(15):913–8.
126. Andersson J, Skoldenberg B, Ernberg I, et al. Acyclovir treatment in primary Epstein-Barr virus infection. A double-blind placebo-controlled study. Scand J Infect Dis Suppl 1985;47:107–15.
127. Paya CV, Fung JJ, Nalesnik MA, et al. Epstein-Barr virus-induced posttransplant lymphoproliferative disorders. ASTS/ASTP EBV-PTLD Task Force and The Mayo Clinic Organized International Consensus Development Meeting. Transplantation 1999;68(10):1517–25.
128. Yao QY, Ogan P, Rowe M, et al. Epstein-Barr virus-infected B cells persist in the circulation of acyclovir-treated virus carriers. Int J Cancer 1989;43(1):67–71.
129. Choquet S, Leblond V, Herbrecht R, et al. Efficacy and safety of rituximab in B-cell post-transplantation lymphoproliferative disorders: results of a prospective multicenter phase 2 study. Blood 2006;107(8):3053–7.
130. Norin S, Kimby E, Ericzon BG, et al. Posttransplant lymphoma–a single-center experience of 500 liver transplantations. Med Oncol 2004;21(3):273–84.
131. Trappe RU, Choquet S, Reinke P, et al. Salvage therapy for relapsed posttransplant lymphoproliferative disorders (PTLD) with a second progression of PTLD after upfront chemotherapy: the role of single-agent rituximab. Transplantation 2007;84(12):1708–12.
132. Oertel SH, Verschuuren E, Reinke P, et al. Effect of anti-CD 20 antibody rituximab in patients with post-transplant lymphoproliferative disorder (PTLD). Am J Transplant 2005;5(12):2901–6.
133. Rooney CM, Smith CA, Ng CYC, et al. Infusion of cytotoxic T cells for the prevention and treatment of Epstein-Barr virus-induced lymphoma in allogeneic transplant recipients. Blood 1998;92(5):1549–55.
134. Gustafsson A, Levitsky V, Zou J-Z, et al. Epstein-Barr virus (EBV) load in bone marrow transplant recipients at risk to develop posttransplant lymphoproliferative disease: prophylactic infusion of EBV-specific cytotoxic T cells. Blood 2000;95(3):807–14.
135. Savoldo B, Goss JA, Hammer MM, et al. Treatment of solid organ transplant recipients with autologous Epstein Barr virus-specific cytotoxic T lymphocytes (CTLs). Blood 2006;108(9):2942–9.
136. Haque T, Taylor C, Wilkie GM, et al. Complete regression of posttransplant lymphoproliferative disease using partially HLA-matched Epstein Barr virus-specific cytotoxic T cells. Transplantation 2001;72(8):1399–402.
137. Haque T, Wilkie GM, Jones MM, et al. Allogeneic cytotoxic T-cell therapy for EBV-positive posttransplantation lymphoproliferative disease: results of a phase 2 multicenter clinical trial. Blood 2007;110(4):1123–31.
138. Haque T, Wilkie GM, Taylor C, et al. Treatment of Epstein-Barr-virus-positive post-transplantation lymphoproliferative disease with partly HLA-matched allogeneic cytotoxic T cells. Lancet 2002;360(9331):436–42.
139. Comoli P, Labirio M, Basso S, et al. Infusion of autologous Epstein-Barr virus (EBV)-specific cytotoxic T cells for prevention of EBV-related lymphoproliferative disorder in solid organ transplant recipients with evidence of active virus replication. Blood 2002;99(7):2592–8.
140. Khanna R, Bell S, Sherritt M, et al. Activation and adoptive transfer of Epstein–Barr virus-specific cytotoxic T cells in solid organ transplant patients with

posttransplant lymphoproliferative disease. Proc Natl Acad Sci U S A 1999; 96(18):10391–6.
141. Choquet S, Trappe R, Leblond V, et al. CHOP-21 for the treatment of post-transplant lymphoproliferative disorders (PTLD) following solid organ transplantation. Haematologica 2007;92(2):273–4.
142. Elstrom RL, Andreadis C, Aqui NA, et al. Treatment of PTLD with rituximab or chemotherapy. Am J Transplant 2006;6(3):569–76.
143. Garrett TJ, Chadburn A, Barr ML, et al. Posttransplantation lymphoproliferative disorders treated with cyclophosphamide-doxorubicin-vincristine-prednisone chemotherapy. Cancer 1993;72(9):2782–5.
144. Mamzer-Bruneel MF, Lome C, Morelon E, et al. Durable remission after aggressive chemotherapy for very late post-kidney transplant lymphoproliferation: a report of 16 cases observed in a single center. J Clin Oncol 2000;18(21):3622–32.
145. Everly MJ, Bloom RD, Tsai DE, et al. Posttransplant lymphoproliferative disorder. Ann Pharmacother 2007;41(11):1850–8.
146. Karras A, Thervet E, Le Meur Y, et al. Successful renal retransplantation after post-transplant lymphoproliferative disease. Am J Transplant 2004;4(11): 1904–9.
147. Darenkov IA, Marcarelli MA, Basadonna GP, et al. Reduced incidence of Epstein-Barr virus-associated posttransplant lymphoproliferative disorder using preemptive antiviral therapy. Transplantation 1997;64(6):848–52.
148. Davis CL, Harrison KL, McVicar JP, et al. Antiviral prophylaxis and the Epstein Barr virus-related post-transplant lymphoproliferative disorder. Clin Transplant 1995;9(1):53–9.
149. Funch DP, Walker AM, Schneider G, et al. Ganciclovir and acyclovir reduce the risk of post-transplant lymphoproliferative disorder in renal transplant recipients. Am J Transplant 2005;5(12):2894–900.
150. Green M, Kaufmann M, Wilson J, et al. Comparison of intravenous ganciclovir followed by oral acyclovir with intravenous ganciclovir alone for prevention of cytomegalovirus and Epstein-Barr virus disease after liver transplantation in children. Clin Infect Dis 1997;25(6):1344–9.
151. Bakker NA, Verschuuren EA, Erasmus ME, et al. Epstein-Barr virus-DNA load monitoring late after lung transplantation: a surrogate marker of the degree of immunosuppression and a safe guide to reduce immunosuppression. Transplantation 2007;83(4):433–8.
152. Salahuddin SZ, Ablashi DV, Markham PD, et al. Isolation of a new virus, HBLV, in patients with lymphoproliferative disorders. Science 1986;234(4776):596–601.
153. Gentile G. Post-transplant HHV-6 diseases. Herpes 2000;7(1):24–7.
154. Leach CT, Sumaya CV, Brown NA. Human herpesvirus-6: clinical implications of a recently discovered, ubiquitous agent. J Pediatr 1992;121(2):173–81.
155. Brown NA, Sumaya CV, Liu CR, et al. Fall in human herpesvirus 6 seropositivity with age. Lancet 1988;2(8607):396.
156. Lau YL, Peiris M, Chan GC, et al. Primary human herpes virus 6 infection transmitted from donor to recipient through bone marrow infusion. Bone Marrow Transplant 1998;21(10):1063–6.
157. Cervera C, Marcos MA, Linares L, et al. A prospective survey of human herpesvirus-6 primary infection in solid organ transplant recipients. Transplantation 2006;82(7):979–82.
158. Zerr DM, Corey L, Kim HW, et al. Clinical outcomes of human herpesvirus 6 reactivation after hematopoietic stem cell transplantation. Clin Infect Dis 2005; 40(7):932–40.

159. de Pagter PJ, Schuurman R, Meijer E, et al. Human herpesvirus type 6 reactivation after haematopoietic stem cell transplantation. J Clin Virol 2008;43(4):361–6.
160. de Pagter PJ, Schuurman R, Visscher H, et al. Human herpes virus 6 plasma DNA positivity after hematopoietic stem cell transplantation in children: an important risk factor for clinical outcome. Biol Blood Marrow Transplant 2008;14(7):831–9.
161. Wang LR, Dong LJ, Zhang MJ, et al. The impact of human herpesvirus 6B reactivation on early complications following allogeneic hematopoietic stem cell transplantation. Biol Blood Marrow Transplant 2006;12(10):1031–7.
162. Yamane A, Mori T, Suzuki S, et al. Risk factors for developing human herpesvirus 6 (HHV-6) reactivation after allogeneic hematopoietic stem cell transplantation and its association with central nervous system disorders. Biol Blood Marrow Transplant 2007;13(1):100–6.
163. DesJardin JA, Gibbons L, Cho E, et al. Human herpesvirus 6 reactivation is associated with cytomegalovirus infection and syndromes in kidney transplant recipients at risk for primary cytomegalovirus infection. J Infect Dis 1998;178(6):1783–6.
164. Dockrell DH, Prada J, Jones MF, et al. Seroconversion to human herpesvirus 6 following liver transplantation is a marker of cytomegalovirus disease. J Infect Dis 1997;176(5):1135–40.
165. Lehto JT, Halme M, Tukiainen P, et al. Human herpesvirus-6 and -7 after lung and heart-lung transplantation. J Heart Lung Transplant 2007;26(1):41–7.
166. Ratnamohan VM, Chapman J, Howse H, et al. Cytomegalovirus and human herpesvirus 6 both cause viral disease after renal transplantation. Transplantation 1998;66(7):877–82.
167. Yoshikawa T, Suga S, Asano Y, et al. A prospective study of human herpesvirus-6 infection in renal transplantation. Transplantation 1992;54(5):879–83.
168. Humar A, Malkan G, Moussa G, et al. Human herpesvirus-6 is associated with cytomegalovirus reactivation in liver transplant recipients. J Infect Dis 2000;181(4):1450–3.
169. Herbein G, Strasswimmer J, Altieri M, et al. Longitudinal study of human herpesvirus 6 infection in organ transplant recipients. Clin Infect Dis 1996;22(1):171–3.
170. Razonable RR, Paya CV. The impact of human herpesvirus-6 and -7 infection on the outcome of liver transplantation. Liver Transpl 2002;8(8):651–8.
171. Humar A, Asberg A, Kumar D, et al. An assessment of herpesvirus co-infections in patients with CMV disease: correlation with clinical and virologic outcomes. Am J Transplant 2009;9(2):374–81.
172. Singh N, Paterson DL. Encephalitis caused by human herpesvirus-6 in transplant recipients: relevance of a novel neurotropic virus. Transplantation 2000;69(12):2474–9.
173. Bollen AE, Wartan AN, Krikke AP, et al. Amnestic syndrome after lung transplantation by human herpes virus-6 encephalitis. J Neurol 2001;248(7):619–20.
174. Mookerjee BP, Vogelsang G. Human herpes virus-6 encephalitis after bone marrow transplantation: successful treatment with ganciclovir. Bone Marrow Transplant 1997;20(10):905–6.
175. Mori T, Mihara A, Yamazaki R, et al. Myelitis associated with human herpes virus 6 (HHV-6) after allogeneic cord blood transplantation. Scand J Infect Dis 2007;39(3):276–8.
176. Seeley WW, Marty FM, Holmes TM, et al. Post-transplant acute limbic encephalitis: clinical features and relationship to HHV6. Neurology 2007;69(2):156–65.

177. Vu T, Carrum G, Hutton G, et al. Human herpesvirus-6 encephalitis following allogeneic hematopoietic stem cell transplantation. Bone Marrow Transplant 2007;39(11):705–9.
178. Fotheringham J, Akhyani N, Vortmeyer A, et al. Detection of active human herpesvirus-6 infection in the brain: correlation with polymerase chain reaction detection in cerebrospinal fluid. J Infect Dis 2007;195(3):450–4.
179. Luppi M, Barozzi P, Maiorana A, et al. Human herpesvirus 6 infection in normal human brain tissue. J Infect Dis 1994;169(4):943–4.
180. Caserta MT, McDermott M, Dewhurst S, et al. Human herpesvirus 6 (HHV6) DNA persistence and reactivation in healthy children. J Pediatr 2004; 145(4):478–84.
181. Singh N, Carrigan DR, Gayowski T, et al. Variant B human herpesvirus-6 associated febrile dermatosis with thrombocytopenia and encephalopathy in a liver transplant recipient. Transplantation 1995;60(11):1355–7.
182. Revest M, Camus C, D'Halluin PN, et al. Fatal human herpes virus 6 primary infection after liver transplantation. Transplantation 2007;83(10):1404–5.
183. Randhawa PS, Jenkins FJ, Nalesnik MA, et al. Herpesvirus 6 variant A infection after heart transplantation with giant cell transformation in bile ductular and gastroduodenal epithelium. Am J Surg Pathol 1997;21(7):847–53.
184. Burns WH, Sandford GR. Susceptibility of human herpesvirus 6 to antivirals in vitro. J Infect Dis 1990;162(3):634–7.
185. Agut H, Aubin JT, Huraux JM. Homogeneous susceptibility of distinct human herpesvirus 6 strains to antivirals in vitro. J Infect Dis 1991;163(6):1382–3.
186. Reymen D, Naesens L, Balzarini J, et al. Antiviral activity of selected acyclic nucleoside analogues against human herpesvirus 6. Antiviral Res 1995;28(4): 343–57.
187. Ward KN. Human herpesviruses-6 and -7 infections. Curr Opin Infect Dis 2005; 18(3):247–52.
188. Ward KN, White RP, Mackinnon S, et al. Human herpesvirus-7 infection of the CNS with acute myelitis in an adult bone marrow recipient. Bone Marrow Transplant 2002;30(12):983–5.
189. Yoshikawa T, Yoshida J, Hamaguchi M, et al. Human herpesvirus 7-associated meningitis and optic neuritis in a patient after allogeneic stem cell transplantation. J Med Virol 2003;70(3):440–3.
190. Kidd IM, Clark DA, Sabin CA, et al. Prospective study of human betaherpesviruses after renal transplantation: association of human herpesvirus 7 and cytomegalovirus co-infection with cytomegalovirus disease and increased rejection. Transplantation 2000;69(11):2400–4.
191. Osman HK, Peiris JS, Taylor CE, et al. "Cytomegalovirus disease" in renal allograft recipients: is human herpesvirus 7 a co-factor for disease progression? J Med Virol 1996;48(4):295–301.
192. Tong CY, Bakran A, Williams H, et al. Association of human herpesvirus 7 with cytomegalovirus disease in renal transplant recipients. Transplantation 2000; 70(1):213–6.
193. Moore PS, Chang Y. Detection of herpesvirus-like DNA sequences in Kaposi's sarcoma in patients with and without HIV infection. N Engl J Med 1995; 332(18):1181–5.
194. Cesarman E, Chang Y, Moore PS, et al. Kaposi's sarcoma-associated herpesvirus-like DNA sequences in AIDS-related body-cavity-based lymphomas. N Engl J Med 1995;332(18):1186–91.
195. Antman K, Chang Y. Kaposi's sarcoma. N Engl J Med 2000;342(14):1027–38.

196. Moore PS. The emergence of Kaposi's sarcoma-associated herpesvirus (human herpesvirus 8). N Engl J Med 2000;343(19):1411–3.
197. Melbye M, Cook PM, Hjalgrim H, et al. Risk factors for Kaposi's-sarcoma-associated herpesvirus (KSHV/HHV-8) seropositivity in a cohort of homosexual men, 1981–1996. Int J Cancer 1998;77(4):543–8.
198. Ahmadpoor P, Ilkhanizadeh B, Sharifzadeh P, et al. Seroprevalence of human herpes virus-8 in renal transplant recipients: a single center study from Iran. Transplant Proc 2007;39(4):1000–2.
199. Butler LM, Dorsey G, Hladik W, et al. Kaposi sarcoma-associated herpesvirus (KSHV) seroprevalence in population-based samples of African children: evidence for at least 2 patterns of KSHV transmission. J Infect Dis 2009; 200(3):430–8.
200. Fu B, Sun F, Li B, et al. Seroprevalence of Kaposi's sarcoma-associated herpesvirus and risk factors in Xinjiang, China. J Med Virol 2009;81(8):1422–31.
201. Engels EA, Atkinson JO, Graubard BI, et al. Risk factors for human herpesvirus 8 infection among adults in the United States and evidence for sexual transmission. J Infect Dis 2007;196(2):199–207.
202. Human herpesvirus-8 (HHV-8, KSHV). Am J Transplant 2004;4(s10):67–9.
203. Dudderidge TJ, Khalifa M, Jeffery R, et al. Donor-derived human herpes virus 8-related Kaposi's sarcoma in renal allograft ureter. Transpl Infect Dis 2008;10(3): 221–6.
204. Luppi M, Barozzi P, Schulz TF, et al. Bone marrow failure associated with human herpesvirus 8 infection after transplantation. N Engl J Med 2000;343(19): 1378–85.
205. Parravicini C, Olsen SJ, Capra M, et al. Risk of Kaposi's sarcoma-associated herpes virus transmission from donor allografts among Italian posttransplant Kaposi's sarcoma patients. Blood 1997;90(7):2826–9.
206. Bergallo M, Costa C, Margio S, et al. Human herpes virus 8 infection in kidney transplant patients from an area of northwestern Italy (Piemonte region). Nephrol Dial Transplant 2007;22(6):1757–61.
207. Boeckle E, Boesmueller C, Wiesmayr S, et al. Kaposi sarcoma in solid organ transplant recipients: a single center report. Transplant Proc 2005;37(4): 1905–9.
208. Verucchi G, Calza L, Trevisani F, et al. Human herpesvirus-8-related Kaposi's sarcoma after liver transplantation successfully treated with cidofovir and liposomal daunorubicin. Transpl Infect Dis 2005;7(1):34–7.
209. Stallone G, Schena A, Infante B, et al. Sirolimus for Kaposi's sarcoma in renal-transplant recipients. N Engl J Med 2005;352(13):1317–23.
210. Lebbe C, Euvrard S, Barrou B, et al. Sirolimus conversion for patients with post-transplant Kaposi's sarcoma. Am J Transplant 2006;6(9):2164–8.
211. Robles R, Lugo D, Gee L, et al. Effect of antiviral drugs used to treat cytomegalovirus end-organ disease on subsequent course of previously diagnosed Kaposi's sarcoma in patients with AIDS. J Acquir Immune Defic Syndr Hum Retrovirol 1999;20(1):34–8.
212. Little RF, Merced-Galindez F, Staskus K, et al. A pilot study of cidofovir in patients with Kaposi sarcoma. J Infect Dis 2003;187(1):149–53.
213. Jones D, Ballestas ME, Kaye KM, et al. Primary-effusion lymphoma and Kaposi's sarcoma in a cardiac-transplant recipient. N Engl J Med 1998;339(7):444–9.
214. Al Otaibi T, Al Sagheir A, Ludwin D, et al. Post renal transplant Castleman's disease resolved after graft nephrectomy: a case report. Transplant Proc 2007;39(4):1276–7.

215. Cagirgan S, Cirit M, Ok E, et al. Castleman's disease in a renal allograft recipient. Nephron 1997;76(3):352–3.
216. Dotti G, Fiocchi R, Motta T, et al. Primary effusion lymphoma after heart transplantation: a new entity associated with human herpesvirus-8. Leukemia 1999; 13(5):664–70.
217. Melo NC, Sales MM, Santana AN, et al. Pleural primary effusion lymphoma in a renal transplant recipient. Am J Transplant 2008;8(4):906–7.
218. Stebbing J, Pantanowitz L, Dayyani F, et al. HIV-associated multicentric Castleman's disease. Am J Hematol 2008;83(6):498–503.
219. Soulier J, Grollet L, Oksenhendler E, et al. Kaposi's sarcoma-associated herpesvirus-like DNA sequences in multicentric Castleman's disease. Blood 1995; 86(4):1276–80.
220. Mandel C, Silberstein M, Hennessy O. Case report: fatal pulmonary Kaposi's sarcoma and Castleman's disease in a renal transplant recipient. Br J Radiol 1993;66(783):264–5.
221. Theate I, Michaux L, Squifflet JP, et al. Human herpesvirus 8 and Epstein-Barr virus-related monotypic large B-cell lymphoproliferative disorder coexisting with mixed variant of Castleman's disease in a lymph node of a renal transplant recipient. Clin Transplant 2003;17(5):451–4.
222. Casper C. Defining a role for antiviral drugs in the treatment of persons with HHV-8 infection. Herpes 2006;13(2):42–7.
223. Gaidano G, Carbone A. Primary effusion lymphoma: a liquid phase lymphoma of fluid-filled body cavities. Adv Cancer Res 2001;80:115–46.

Respiratory Viral Infections in Transplant and Oncology Patients

Deepali Kumar, MD, MSc, FRCPC*, Atul Humar, MD, MSc, FRCPC

KEYWORDS

• Hematopoietic stem cell transplant • Solid organ transplant
• Influenza • Cancer

Respiratory viral infections (RVI) are a significant cause of morbidity and mortality in the immunocompromised host. In the last two decades, there has been significant advancement in the epidemiology and laboratory diagnosis of RVI with discoveries of new pathogens, such as bocavirus, KI and WU polyomaviruses, and novel coronaviruses (CoV). In addition, the clinical consequences of many respiratory viruses in the immunocompetent and immunocompromised host continue to be studied. Many therapeutics have also now become available, although their efficacy in transplant recipients remains uncertain. This section describes the current knowledge of RVI as it relates to solid organ transplant (SOT), hematopoietic stem cell transplant (HSCT), and oncology settings.

EPIDEMIOLOGY, TRANSMISSION, PATHOGENESIS

Respiratory viruses that are commonly recognized in the human host including the transplant recipient are influenza A and B, parainfluenza 1 to 4, respiratory syncytial virus (RSV), and adenovirus (AdV). Other viruses including CoV, enteroviruses, rhinovirus, and human metapneumovirus (hMPV) have gained importance in the past decade. In addition, bocavirus, parvovirus 4 and 5, polyomaviruses, and mimivirus have also been described, although there is limited literature in the transplant setting for these viruses. The prevalence of respiratory viruses in a given season depends on exposure, virulence of the virus, the types of circulating viruses, and detection methods used. Most respiratory viruses are transmitted by direct contact or aerosolized droplets.[1] Incubation periods range from 1 to 10 days, although those for newly described viruses (bocavirus, parvovirus 4 and 5, and mimivirus) are unknown.

Department of Medicine, Transplant Infectious Diseases, University of Alberta, 6-030 Katz-Rexall Center for Health Research, Edmonton, Alberta T6G 2E1, Canada
* Corresponding author.
E-mail address: Deepali.Kumar@ualberta.ca

Infect Dis Clin N Am 24 (2010) 395–412
doi:10.1016/j.idc.2010.01.007 id.theclinics.com
0891-5520/10/$ – see front matter © 2010 Elsevier Inc. All rights reserved.

The incidence of RVI following HSCT has ranged from 3.5% to 29%.[2–5] Older studies are more likely to underestimate the incidence, however, because the RVI detection methodologies used were generally less sensitive and limited to fewer viruses.

The outcome of RVIs in HSCT recipients depends on several factors including whether the transplant was myeloablative versus nonmyeloablative, the presence of lymphopenia, and intensity of immunosuppression. In one series from a large cancer center, 343 RVIs in patients with hematologic malignancy and HSCT were identified over a 2-year period.[6] Progression to lower respiratory infection occurred in 35% of patients and did not depend on the type of infecting virus. Risk factors for progression included an underlying diagnosis of leukemia, age greater than 65 years, and severe neutropenia or lymphopenia. Lymphopenia as a risk factor in allogeneic and autologous HSCT has also been identified in other studies.[3,4] Lower tract infection is more common in those receiving myeloablative conditioning than in nonmyeloablative transplants.[7] Aside from direct morbidity and mortality, RVI may also be a risk factor for the development of invasive aspergillosis in allogeneic HSCT[8]; whether this represents an overall immunosuppressed state needs further study.

The incidence of RVI in SOT recipients is 7.7% to 64%.[9–13] Lung transplant recipients seem to have a greater frequency of RVI than other SOT recipients, likely because of the direct communication of the allograft with the environment and the poor immune response in the allograft. The risk of progression to lower tract disease is not well defined; however, it is likely dependent on time posttransplant and intensity of immunosuppression and the type of transplant. Because of poor immune responses in the allograft, lung transplant recipients likely have a greater risk of lower tract disease.

CLINICAL PRESENTATION AND COMPLICATIONS

There is significant overlap in the symptoms of respiratory viruses and it is difficult to distinguish clinically which respiratory virus is causing symptoms in a given patient. Common symptoms of upper respiratory tract illness include malaise, sore throat, coryza, cough, and fever. The presence of dyspnea may signal lower respiratory tract infection (LRTI) by the virus or bacterial superinfection. Chest radiograph may show diffuse interstitial infiltrates but can also show airspace disease. The most common chest CT finding is ground-glass attenuation; centrilobular nodules 3 to 10 mm in size including a tree-in-bud appearance can also be seen. Airspace consolidation can be present in up to one third of patients on CT chest scan.[14] A "crazy-paving" pattern has been described on high-resolution chest CT scan, which consists of interlobular and intralobular septal thickening superimposed on an area of ground-glass opacification. Although not specific for RVI, one study found that 70% of patients with this pattern had viral pneumonitis.[15] Progression from upper tract to lower tract infection can occur, although the incidence is quite variable. This is likely caused by the varying immunosuppressives, timing of infection from transplant, and other underlying diseases. Asymptomatic shedding of respiratory viruses has been shown to occur in both solid organ and HSCT recipients.[16] Transplant recipients have been postulated to be "superspreaders" of virus given the high viral loads of respiratory viruses found in respiratory secretions.[17] In addition, prolonged shedding of respiratory viruses is often noted. Transplant recipients may serve as sentinals for a given infection in the community, because they may be the first to become infected with an emerging virus signaling the beginning of an outbreak.

LABORATORY DIAGNOSIS

Traditionally, the laboratory diagnosis of respiratory viruses has been difficult and limited to relatively few viruses. In the past, acute and convalescent sera have been used to diagnose viral infections. In the transplant or oncology patient, however, humoral responses to viral infections are often not detectable or significantly delayed. Virus isolation in cell lines has also been used. Tube culture results are generally available in 8 to 10 days and lead to a delayed diagnosis. Direct fluorescent antibody (DFA) testing using a nasopharyngeal aspirate or swab is available in most clinical laboratories and provides a rapid result in 3 to 5 hours. This test is commonly limited, however, to influenza A and B; parainfluenza 1, 2, and 3; RSV; and AdV. It is also limited in its sensitivity of detection. With the recognition of other viruses, such as CoV (including severe acute respiratory syndrome [SARS]–associated CoV), hMPV, and rhinovirus as significant pathogens leading to disease, nucleic acid amplification testing (NAT) has taken a leading role in the diagnosis of RVIs. Multiplex polymerase chain reaction (PCR), microbead detection, or DNA microarrays have the capability of searching for several viruses in one test. Molecular detection of several respiratory viruses simultaneously using NAT-based assays is now being used in several clinical laboratories.[18] The detection and study of some viruses, such as human bocavirus, is dependent on NAT. In general, NAT testing is more sensitive than other methods.[19] One issue with such sensitive methods is the detection of asymptomatic viral infection. One study in HSCT recipients tested 688 nasal wash specimens from 131 patients in the first 100 days posttransplant by conventional DFA and PCR.[2] PCR significantly increased the yield of viruses; however, those viruses only detected by PCR had lower viral loads, many of which represented asymptomatic infections. Coinfection with two or more respiratory viruses may also be detected using such sensitive methods; in this case, it may be difficult to determine toward which virus treatment should be directed.

Influenza

Influenza is a negative sense, single-stranded RNA virus of the Orthomyxoviridae family. Influenza viruses undergo antigenic changes at a high frequency. Smaller antigenic changes are termed "antigenic drift" and produce minor variations in surface glycoproteins, such as substitutions in antibody-binding sites that can result in reinfection. Larger antigenic shifts can occur because of reassortment of genes, however, when two influenza viruses simultaneously infect one host. Antigenic shift can also occur as a result of direct mutation that allows for cross-species infection.

Complications of influenza infection seem to be common in HSCT and SOT populations. There seems to be a relatively high rate of progression to viral pneumonia in some reports, especially in lung transplant recipients and HSCT recipients.[20,21] In one study of organ transplant recipients over a 10-year period, the rate of influenza infection ranged from 2.8 cases per 1000 person years (liver transplant) to 41.8 cases per 1000 person years (lung transplant).[21,22] Complications including secondary bacterial pneumonia (17%) and extrapulmonary complications, such as myocarditis and myositis, were observed. This is in contrast to a report by Ljungman and colleagues[22] on 12 influenza cases in renal transplant recipients. Only one patient developed viral pneumonia and one had bronchitis. The remaining 10 patients recovered without complications. Severe disease has been commonly reported in HSCT recipients with attributable mortality rates as high as 43%.[20] A large review of 62 HSCT recipients with influenza showed that pneumonia developed in those who were infected sooner posttransplant and had lymphopenia.[23] In patients not treated with antivirals, 18% progressed to pneumonia. Shedding was longer in those on steroid doses of greater than 1 mg/kg/d and it was suggested that oseltamivir may decrease this shedding. More recently, in a review of 19 patients with influenza, none with upper respiratory tract infection (URTI) progressed to LRTI and there was no mortality, although most patients were treated with oseltamivir. Shedding was present for a median of 12 days and correlated inversely with the presence of lymphopenia.[24] Lymphopenia (absolute lymphocyte count ≤200 cells/mL) was a specific risk factor identified for progression to influenza pneumonia.[6] Influenza A and B infection following autologous HSCT have also been associated with mortality.[4] In pediatric cancer patients, influenza was also an important cause of morbidity.[25]

The diagnosis of influenza can be made using several methods: serology, virus culture, DFA, and PCR. A nasopharyngeal swab or lower respiratory sampling can be used.

Therapy of influenza A or B with neuraminidase inhibitors (oseltamivir or zanamivir) is the mainstay of management (**Table 1**). In immunosuppressed hosts, oseltamivir can be started at any time during the course of the illness at an oral dose of 75 mg twice daily for five days. A dose of 150 mg twice daily has also been suggested by some experts, as has extending the therapeutic course for

Table 1
Suggested therapy for RVIs in transplant and oncology patients

Respiratory Virus	Diagnosis	Isolation Precautions[1]	Suggested Management
Influenza	DFA, NAT, serology, culture	Droplet Airborne for pandemic strains	Oseltamivir, 75–150 mg po bid × 5–10 d Zanamivir, 2 puffs bid × 5 d Amantadine, 100 mg bid Rimantadine, 100 mg bid
RSV	DFA, NAT	Droplet and contact	Ribavirin IVIg or RSV-Ig Palivizumab
Parainfluenza	DFA, NAT	Droplet	Ribavirin (aerosolized, po, IV)
Adenovirus	DFA, NAT	Droplet	Cidofovir, 3 mg/kg IV once weekly Ribavirin? IVIG
Coronavirus	NAT	Droplet Airborne for SARS-CoV	Supportive care Ribavirin (for SARS-CoV)
Human metapneumovirus	NAT	Droplet	Ribavirin? Supportive care
Rhinovirus	NAT	Droplet	Supportive care
Parvovirus B19	NAT, serology	Droplet	IVIG
Bocavirus	NAT	Droplet	Supportive care
WU/KI viruses	NAT	Droplet	Supportive care

Not all diagnostic tests are available in all clinical laboratories. Some diagnostic tests are primarily used for research purposes.

Doses of antivirals are standard doses for adults with normal creatinine clearance.

Abbreviations: DFA, direct fluorescent antibody; IVIG, intravenous immunoglobin; NAT, nucleic acid amplification testing; RSV, respiratory syncytial virus; SARS-CoV, severe acute respiratory syndrome associated coronavirus.

patients who remain symptomatic after 5 days. Zanamivir is a sialic acid analog that is available as an inhaled preparation and has been shown to be effective against influenza A in the general population when started within 48 hours of symptom onset.[26–28] Zanamivir has also been used successfully in HSCT recipients with influenza A or B.[29] The recommended dose of zanamivir is 10 mg (or two puffs) twice daily for 5 days. In the study by Johny and colleagues,[29] zanamivir was used until viral excretion ceased. Concerns have also been raised regarding the pulmonary bioavailability of zanamivir in immunocompromised patients.[30] Future clinical trials in this area and in the use of combination antivirals for the transplant population are needed. Resistance to oseltamivir has developed in a large proportion of influenza A–H1N1 viruses and some influenza A–H5N1 and influenza B viruses.[31] Conversely, H3N2 viruses have a high rate of resistance to zanamivir but remain susceptible to oseltamivir. The M2 inhibitor class (amantadine and rimantadine) can also be used in transplant recipients with influenza A but their use is limited because of side effects and antiviral resistance.[32] Ribavirin also has in vitro activity against influenza and could potentially be used in combination with other antivirals.[33,34] In addition, novel compounds, such as peramivir and combination antiviral therapies are also being studied in clinical trials.

The most commonly used trivalent inactivated subunit vaccine is revised annually and contains two influenza A and one influenza B strains. The vaccine is recommended for all transplant recipients, transplant candidates, their household contacts, and health care workers in contact with immunocompromised patients.[35–37] The immunogenicity of the vaccine is variable depending on the population studied. In HSCT recipients, vaccine responses are absent before 6 months posttransplant and it is recommended to wait until 6 months to administer the vaccine.[36] Similarly, in SOT recipients, vaccine can be administered any time after 3 to 6 months posttransplant. There are no data to support acute or chronic rejection as a consequence of vaccination in this population. The intranasal preparation is a live attenuated vaccine and is not recommended for the immunocompromised population.

Pandemic influenza is of particular concern in transplant and oncology centers. The current pandemic of swine origin H1N1 virus likely arose from cross-species adaptation of the virus from swine-to-human and successful human-to-human transmission. At the time of this writing, more than 168,000 persons were reported infected and more than 1150 deaths worldwide. Risk factors for severe disease include infants less than 1 year, underlying lung disease, diabetes, and pregnancy. Immunosuppressed patients are also at risk for severe disease, although there are no specific data on transplant or oncology patients; however, as greater knowledge becomes available, risk factors for severe disease or death will be more clearly defined. The impact on transplant programs in part depends on the virulence of the virus and the amount of resources required to manage critically ill patients.

Parainfluenza

Parainfluenza viruses (PIV) comprise a group of four serotypes (1–4) of single-stranded RNA paramyxoviruses. PIV occurs year-round and can cause a number of clinical syndromes including croup and bronchiolitis, the common cold, and pneumonia. In transplant recipients, the spectrum of PIV ranges from asymptomatic to respiratory failure and death. In a large retrospective review of HSCT patients in the 1990s, those with upper respiratory infection survived but those with pneumonia had a universal mortality despite ribavirin therapy.[38] Asymptomatic parainfluenza infection has been detected in a surveillance study of HSCT patients and could be a possible mode of transmission in outbreaks.[5,39] PIV-3 in particular has caused nosocomial outbreaks on HSCT units as a result of person-to-person transmission.[39–44] Mortality rates up to 33% are seen in outbreak situations.[42,44] Other syndromes in transplantation associated with PIV include Guillain-Barré syndrome, acute disseminated encephalomyelitis, and parotitis.[45–47] In lung transplant recipients, the incidence of PIV has been estimated to be 5.3% of patients.[48] LRTI can occur in 10% to 66%. Bronchiolitis obliterans syndrome (BOS) can be a long-term consequence of this infection. Radiologic features can include peribronchial small nodules of less than 5 mm diameter on CT chest.[49] Intravenous and oral ribavirin have been used for therapy of infection in transplant recipients with conflicting results.[50–54]

Respiratory Syncytial Virus

RSV is possibly the most important cause of morbidity and mortality of all respiratory viruses affecting the transplant recipient. RSV causes severe lower respiratory tract disease in transplant patients. In one study risk factors for the progression of RSV were lack of RSV-directed antiviral therapy and age.[6] In pediatric studies, both lymphopenia and age less than 2 years have also been shown to be an important risk factors for progression.[55] RSV-related mortality in children treated for acute myeloid leukemia was 10%.[56] Diagnosis of RSV can be performed using standard DFA technique, culture, or NAT. The xTAG RVP assay has been reported to have a sensitivity of 100% for RSV detection with specificity ranging from 97% to 99%.[57] The primary therapy that has been most studied is aerosolized ribavirin given 2 g three times a day or 6 g over 18 hours. The logistical and cost issues with aerosol therapy limit its use in many centers. A negative pressure room must be used. The drug is teratogenic to those in close contact. A small randomized trial of aerosolized ribavirin versus standard care for upper respiratory RSV infection in HSCT recipients showed a decrease in viral load in the ribavirin arm but no difference in the progression to pneumonia.[58] Oral ribavirin has been suggested as an alternative. In a study of five lung transplant recipients, oral ribavirin and pulse solumedrol (10–15 mg/kg/d for 3 days) were given for RSV LRTI and was well-tolerated and seemed to be effective.[59] In a case series of 18 lung transplant recipients with RSV given intravenous ribavirin with corticosteroids, no mortality was seen although hemolytic anemia occurred.[60] Palivizumab is a monoclonal antibody specific for RSV. It has also been used in conjunction with antivirals in the treatment of RSV pneumonia.[61] A survey of pediatric SOT centers in the United States showed that 49% of centers used RSV prophylaxis, most of whom used palivizumab in infants up to 24 months.[62] Another humanized monoclonal antibody (motavizumab) is under investigation. In addition, an RNAi molecule (ALN-RSV01) that silences the nucleocapsid gene of the RSV genome is also in clinical trials. No vaccine is available, although clinical trials are ongoing.

Human Metapneumovirus

hMPV is a negative-sense nonsegmented RNA paramyxovirus closely related in structure to RSV. It is increasingly recognized as a cause of upper and lower respiratory infection during winter months. The incidence in HSCT patients is 2.7% to 7.2%.[5,63–65] Retrospectively, hMPV was found to be a cause of infection in 3% of HSCT patients diagnosed with idiopathic pneumonia.[63] It is unknown how often hMPV upper tract infection progresses to lower tract infection; however, fatal cases of progressive respiratory failure early posttransplantation have been described.[63,66] Persistent asymptomatic hMPV has also been recognized in HSCT recipients.[67] In lung transplantation, most hMPV infections seem to be symptomatic and can lead to graft dysfunction.[68,69] The diagnosis of hMPV is based on nucleic acid detection. Supportive care is the mainstay of treatment. A reduction of immunosuppression may be of benefit. Ribavirin has shown activity in vitro and in animal models.[70–72] As well, there are reports of successful treatment of human cases with ribavirin with or without concomitant immune globulin.[73–75] Candidate vaccines for hMPV are being investigated in animal models.[76,77]

CoV Including SARS CoV

CoV have also emerged as important causes of upper and lower tract RVI in transplantation. The incidence of human CoV (hCoV) in transplant recipients has likely been underestimated because of the limitations of diagnostic testing. With the increasing use of NAT, however, the strains of hCoV described in transplant recipients now include OC43, 229E, NL63, SARS, and HKU1. A prospective study identified hCoV in 5.4% of bronchoalveolar lavage fluid specimens; transplantation (lung or liver) was the most common underlying medical condition occurring in almost half the patients.[78] In prospective studies of lung transplant recipients, coronavirus comprised 16.7% to 24% of specimens positive for respiratory viruses and lead to significant short- and long-term declines in forced expiratory pressure in 1 second.[11,79] Severe cases have also been described early post-HSCT.[80] Diagnosis of CoV is based on nucleic acid detection but culture using human hepatoma cell line (HUH7) and serology can also be used. There is no specific therapy for CoV infection.

In 2003, an outbreak of severe respiratory illness was described in China, Hong Kong, and Canada that eventually affected persons in several countries worldwide.[81–83] This was predominantly a health care–associated outbreak and significant mortality was seen in previously healthy persons. The etiologic agent was identified to be a CoV termed "severe acute respiratory syndrome–associated CoV" (SARS-CoV).[84] Common symptoms were fever, myalgias, and cough followed by dyspnea. Laboratory markers included lymphopenia, thrombocytopenia, and an elevated lactate dehydrogenase.[85] A characteristic viral pneumonitis was seen on chest radiograph. Several patients were given intravenous or oral ribavirin with corticosteroids often with adverse effects, such as hemolytic anemia (61%–76%) and hypocalcemia (58%).[85–87] A liver transplant recipient who acquired SARS following an outpatient hospital visit had a fatal outcome; he infected a significant number of health care workers.[88] In addition, tissue levels of SARS-CoV in a lung transplant recipient were several log-fold greater than in immunocompetent patients.[89] These observations in transplant recipients led to the term "super-shedders" of virus.[17] Although the spread of SARS-CoV was eventually controlled by effective infection control measures, the exercise in identification and management of an emerging virus provides important lessons for the future. Transplant patients are sentinals for emerging infections because of their immunosuppressed state and contact with the health care system. In addition, they generally have higher levels of virus in secretions. With widespread infections in the community, there is also a theoretical risk of transmission of a respiratory virus from a donor to a recipient, especially during lung transplantation but also theoretically from other organs and tissues.[88] Emerging viruses are also important for both HSCT and SOT programs and can lead to a complete halt of transplant activity, especially if resources need to be diverted for medical management of the general population.[17] Individual programs must review strategies for care of their transplant patients during respiratory virus outbreaks.

Adenovirus

AdV are nonenveloped DNA viruses with at least 52 known serotypes that are categorized into serogroups A to G. AdV are capable of causing a variety of illness in immunocompetent and immunocompromised hosts.[90] This includes URTI and LRTI, conjunctivitis, keratoconjunctivitis and pharyngoconjunctival fever, enteritis, hepatitis, encephalitis, and disseminated disease. In HSCT recipients, an incidence of 5% to 47% has been reported. In SOT recipients, an incidence of 5.8% to 10% has been noted.[91–93] Variations in incidence depend on the type of diagnostic technique and type of transplant studied and age, with incidence being generally higher in the pediatric population.[94] Most likely, AdV in this population is acquired from the community but other possibilities are donor-derived infection or reactivation disease. Diagnosis can be made by indirect methods, such as serology, or methods that directly demonstrate the presence of virus, such as NAT and culture. DFA is not as sensitive a test for AdV as NAT.[95] In situ hybridization, immunohistochemistry, or PCR of fixed tissue can also identify adenovirus. Monitoring for AdV, similar to cytomegalovirus, may permit early detection in certain high-risk settings. Monitoring for AdV in peripheral blood seemed to predict disease in a cohort of allo-HSCT recipients[96] but was not beneficial in SOT recipients. In a surveillance study using blood PCR for AdV, it was found that self-limited adenoviremia can occur in 7% of SOT patients with 58% being asymptomatic.[91] Although AdV disease may manifest with these clinical syndromes in transplant patients, several cases of AdV-related hemorrhagic cystitis have also been described in HSCT and kidney transplant recipients. Hofland and colleagues[97] reviewed 37 cases of AdV hemorrhagic cystitis in kidney transplant patients. All cases occurred within the first year posttransplant and most presented with fever, dysuria, and hematuria. Graft dysfunction was present in most patients and viral changes or acute rejection may be seen in kidney biopsies. AdV species B predominates with serotypes 7, 11, 34, and 35 causing most disease. There is no specific therapy for AdV; acyclovir and ganciclovir generally do not have activity because AdV does not encode a thymidine kinase; vidarabine has in vitro activity against AdV and has also been used to treat AdV hemorrhagic cystitis[98]; however, clinical studies have focused on cidofovir and ribavirin. There are reports of successful treatment of disseminated disease with cidofovir.[99–101] Intravenous immunoglobulin (IVIg) has also been used in conjunction with antivirals[99]; however, IVIg may not contain sufficient quantity of antibody against all serotypes. Adoptive transfer of T cells has also been used with documented AdV-specific T-cell response in recipients.[102,103] Donor lymphocyte infusion has also been attempted. Overall AdV-related mortality was 19% in allogeneic stem cell transplant recipients despite antivirals[104] and especially high in those who received T-cell depleted grafts. Mortality rates are quite high (up to 75%) for adenoviral pneumonia or hepatitis. Lower, although significant, mortality rates (29%) for hemorrhagic cystitis or colitis are also seen.[105] Immune reconstitution plays an important role in the clearance of AdV; decreasing doses of immunosuppressive medication is important.

Rhinovirus

With the advancement of molecular diagnostic techniques for the detection of a broad-range of respiratory viruses, rhinovirus is likely the most frequently detected virus. Rhinovirus is a member of the Picornaviridae family and is well accepted as a major cause of URTI. LRTI can also occur especially in immunocompromised hosts. In one review of 15 patients with underlying hematologic malignancy and rhinovirus infection, lower respiratory tract involvement was present in 13% of cases at the onset of infection and progression to LRTI was seen in a further 13%.[106] Fatal cases in HSCT patients attributed to rhinovirus have also been described.[107] Persistent chronic infection with rhinovirus has also been described in lung transplant recipients and may lead to graft dysfunction.[108] Up to 20% of lung transplant recipients may have repeated detection of rhinovirus. In addition, the likelihood of rhinoviral persistence increases if it is acquired soon after transplant.[109] Detection in asymptomatic patients, however, is common. A low-level viral load of rhinovirus was found in bronchoalveolar lavage specimens from many asymptomatic patients.[109] Pleconaril, a specific inhibitor of picornaviruses, seemed effective in clinical trials of immunocompetent persons with rhinovirus infection but is no longer available.[110] There is no specific therapy for rhinovirus and the management of a patient in whom rhinovirus is isolated is unclear. No intervention is likely necessary in the asymptomatic patient. If upper respiratory infection is present, many experts suggest decreasing exogenous immunosuppression if possible. For lower tract infection, immunosuppression should be reduced. There is no evidence that adjunct therapies, such as IVIg, corticosteroid therapy, or antibacterial prophylaxis, have a role to play in such infections.

Parvovirus B19

Parvovirus is a single-stranded DNA virus of the genus *Erythrovirus*. Although most infections are nonspecific flulike illnesses, specific clinical syndromes have been described. In children, parvovirus can cause a facial rash resembling "slapped cheeks"; adults with parvovirus can have a polyarthropathy syndrome. The virus can also lead to transient aplastic crisis in those with chronic hemolytic anemia and hydrops fetalis leading to intrauterine fetal death in pregnant women. Onset of parvovirus-associated syndromes can occur at any time posttransplant and has been described as early as 2 weeks. Acquisition of the virus is likely caused by inhalation of infected aerosols as in the immunocompetent host but also transmission from the donor is a possibility. It is also possible that parvovirus reactivates, although little is known about parvovirus latency or cellular reservoirs. Parvovirus B19 has been isolated from the lower respiratory tract of lung transplant recipients.[111] There are also reports of pneumonitis in transplant recipients.[112,113] Infection in transplant recipients is unlike that of immunocompetent patients in that viral replication can persist for prolonged periods of time.[114] Parvovirus has well-established association with hematologic abnormalities including pure red cell aplasia and acute or chronic anemia in transplant recipients. Because anemia is such a common problem in transplant recipients, it is important to search for parvovirus in cases of unexplained or recalcitrant anemia. Other cell lineages may also be affected and lead to leucopenia and thrombocytopenia. Serologic studies have limited use because they can be confounded by transfusion or immunoglobulin therapy. In addition, transplant recipients may not mount an antibody response. Instead, direct detection of virus by qualitative or quantitative DNA PCR is the most useful method. There is no specific antiviral therapy for parvovirus infection, although various management options have been suggested. These consist of a decrease in immunosuppression or IVIg. Various dose regimens of IVIg have been used and range from 0.4 to 1 g/kg for 4 to 10 days.

Bocavirus

Human bocavirus is a recently described member of the Parvoviridae family that also includes parvovirus B19 and parvovirus 4.[115] The first description of bocavirus was in 2005 by Allander and colleagues[116] in respiratory secretions of children. There have since been several studies worldwide in which seroprevalence has ranged from 1.5% to 19%. The virus has predominantly been found in children and many studies show its association with clinical upper and lower respiratory tract disease. It is found more frequently in symptomatic rather than asymptomatic individuals but has also been found as a copathogen with other respiratory viruses. Disseminated disease with bocavirus has been reported in a child with pulmonary infiltrates after HSCT where the virus was detected in respiratory, blood, and stool specimens.[117] Whether bocavirus is pathogenic in adults is not well-established and descriptions in adults are rare.[118] Miyakis and colleagues[119] did not find bocavirus in bronchoalveolar lavage specimens from adult lung transplant recipients and symptomatic nontransplant controls. The detection of human bocavirus DNA is primarily based on PCR methodology using primers specific for viral genes NP1, NS1, and VP1/2 and remains a research tool. Serologic testing using antibody specific to human bocavirus' viral capsid proteins has also been described.[120,121] There are no readily available tests for bocavirus in the clinical setting, although these could potentially be added to existing multiplex platforms in the future. As with many of the respiratory viruses, there is no specific therapy for bocavirus.

KI and WU Polyomaviruses

KI and WU are recently described polyomaviruses that have also been associated with upper and lower respiratory tract disease. WU was first described in respiratory specimens from Australia and subsequently from respiratory specimens worldwide; most patients have been children, although a few adults are also among the cohorts.[122–127] The association of WU and KI viruses with disease has been debated in the literature especially given that coinfection with another respiratory virus is found in 70% to 80% of patients.[122,127] There is limited literature for these viruses in the transplant setting. In a study of 200 hospitalized patients with respiratory illness, KI was significantly more frequent in HSCT recipients (17.8% vs 5.1%; $P = .01$).[126] Another study used real-time PCR for polyomavirus detection in immunocompetent and immunocompromised patients.[128] KI virus was found in three immunocompromised patients, although two had coinfections making it difficult to interpret the extent to which the virus was pathogenic. PCR is generally the exclusive method for detection of these viruses. Further study will determine their significance in the immunocompromised host.

CLINICAL SIGNIFICANCE OF RVI IN LUNG TRANSPLANT RECIPIENTS

Community-acquired RVI occurring after lung transplantation has been associated with acute rejection and BOS. Several retrospective and prospective studies have shown this association.[11,79,129,130] One prospective study followed 50 lung transplant recipients with RVIs and compared them with 50 controls.[79] Those with RVIs had a greater incidence of acute rejection, BOS, and death. The risk of BOS was 25% in RVI-positive versus 9% in RVI-negative patients.[11] In most studies, no individual virus has been more associated with progression to BOS; however, a more recent study found that a significant percentage of lung transplant recipients with paramyxovirus infection progressed to BOS but not with rhinovirus or CoV.[11] In addition, when hMPV was compared with RSV infections in lung transplant recipients, 63% and 72% of patients, respectively, developed graft dysfunction; however, progression to BOS was seen in only those infected with RSV.[69] How viruses trigger rejection or the progression to BOS is unclear but the mechanism is likely a cytokine-mediated inflammatory cascade that recruits T cells to the allograft further resulting in intraluminal proliferation of fibroblasts.[131] The therapy of RVI post–lung transplant is variable. Most experts agree that if available, specific antiviral therapy should be given for symptomatic infections regardless of the duration of symptoms. In most circumstances, a decrease in immunosuppression is recommended for many posttransplant viral infections, including respiratory viruses. Many experts also use high-dose steroids (5–10 mg/kg/d for 3 consecutive days), however, in the presence or absence of specific antiviral therapy, to prevent acute rejection and progression to BOS.[59,60] Whether specific antiviral therapy reduces the risk of progression to BOS-OB is controversial.[51,132]

INFECTION CONTROL MEASURES

General infection control measures for respiratory viruses include droplet precautions, which involves placing the patient in a single room. Persons entering the room should wear a gown, gloves, mask, and eye protection. In most situations, a surgical mask is appropriate; however, for more contagious viruses, a fit-tested N95 mask is required. When performing procedures, a face shield should be worn. Negative pressure isolation is also suggested for more virulent viruses. During an outbreak on a transplant unit, the following measures may reduce transmission and increase patient safety: temporarily discontinuing new transplants, discharging patients who are admitted for investigation or elective procedures, daily screening of staff for symptoms of respiratory illness, sending ill staff home promptly, and minimizing outpatient appointments and procedures for transplant patients. In an outbreak on a transplant ward, inpatients should be offered chemoprophylaxis if available. For example, during an influenza outbreak at a large HSCT center, oseltamivir prophylaxis, 75 mg daily, was shown to be safe and well-tolerated.[133]

SUMMARY

RVI continue to gain importance in transplant and oncology. New molecular techniques allow for rapid identification and identification of a greater number of viruses. The significance of newly found viruses in immunosuppressed patients continues to evolve. Treatment of RVI is limited and some infections, such as RSV, have a high mortality rate despite standard antiviral therapy. Prevention of infection with infection control measures and immunization against pathogens for which vaccines are available is important. Further research to improve diagnostics and therapeutic options in this population is needed.

REFERENCES

1. Siegel JD, Rhinehart E, Jackson M, et al. 2007 Guideline for isolation precautions: preventing transmission of infectious agents in health care settings. Am J Infect Control 2007;35:S65.
2. Kuypers J, Campbell AP, Cent A, et al. Comparison of conventional and molecular detection of respiratory viruses in hematopoietic cell transplant recipients. Transpl Infect Dis 2009;11(4):298–303.
3. Ljungman P, Ward KN, Crooks BN, et al. Respiratory virus infections after stem cell transplantation: a prospective study from the Infectious Diseases Working Party of the European Group for Blood and Marrow Transplantation. Bone Marrow Transplant 2001;28:479.
4. Martino R, Porras RP, Rabella N, et al. Prospective study of the incidence, clinical features, and outcome of symptomatic upper and lower respiratory tract infections by respiratory viruses in adult recipients of hematopoietic stem cell transplants for hematologic malignancies. Biol Blood Marrow Transplant 2005; 11:781.
5. Peck AJ, Englund JA, Kuypers J, et al. Respiratory virus infection among hematopoietic cell transplant recipients: evidence for asymptomatic parainfluenza virus infection. Blood 2007;110:1681.

6. Chemaly RF, Ghosh S, Bodey GP, et al. Respiratory viral infections in adults with hematologic malignancies and human stem cell transplantation recipients: a retrospective study at a major cancer center. Medicine (Baltimore) 2006;85:278.
7. Schiffer JT, Kirby K, Sandmaier B, et al. Timing and severity of community acquired respiratory virus infections after myeloablative versus non-myeloablative hematopoietic stem cell transplantation. Haematologica 2009;94:1101.
8. Martino R, Pinana JL, Parody R, et al. Lower respiratory tract respiratory virus infections increase the risk of invasive aspergillosis after a reduced-intensity allogeneic hematopoietic SCT. Bone Marrow Transplant 2009;44(11):749–56.
9. Bonatti H, Pruett TL, Brandacher G, et al. Pneumonia in solid organ recipients: spectrum of pathogens in 217 episodes. Transplant Proc 2009;41:371.
10. Garbino J, Soccal PM, Aubert JD, et al. Respiratory viruses in bronchoalveolar lavage: a hospital-based cohort study in adults. Thorax 2009;64:399.
11. Gottlieb J, Schulz TF, Welte T, et al. Community-acquired respiratory viral infections in lung transplant recipients: a single season cohort study. Transplantation 2009;87:1530.
12. Lopez-Medrano F, Aguado JM, Lizasoain M, et al. Clinical implications of respiratory virus infections in solid organ transplant recipients: a prospective study. Transplantation 2007;84:851.
13. Milstone AP, Brumble LM, Barnes J, et al. A single-season prospective study of respiratory viral infections in lung transplant recipients. Eur Respir J 2006;28:131.
14. Franquet T, Rodriguez S, Martino R, et al. Thin-section CT findings in hematopoietic stem cell transplantation recipients with respiratory virus pneumonia. AJR Am J Roentgenol 2006;187:1085.
15. Marchiori E, Escuissato DL, Gasparetto TD, et al. Crazy-paving patterns on high-resolution CT scans in patients with pulmonary complications after hematopoietic stem cell transplantation. Korean J Radiol 2009;10:21.
16. van Kraaij MG, van Elden LJ, van Loon AM, et al. Frequent detection of respiratory viruses in adult recipients of stem cell transplants with the use of real-time polymerase chain reaction, compared with viral culture. Clin Infect Dis 2005;40:662.
17. Kumar D, Humar A. Pandemic influenza and its implications for transplantation. Am J Transplant 2006;6:1512.
18. Mahony JB. Detection of respiratory viruses by molecular methods. Clin Microbiol Rev 2008;21:716.
19. Fox JD. Nucleic acid amplification tests for detection of respiratory viruses. J Clin Virol 2007;40(Suppl 1):S15.
20. Ison MG, Hayden FG. Viral infections in immunocompromised patients: what's new with respiratory viruses? Curr Opin Infect Dis 2002;15:355.
21. Vilchez RA, McCurry K, Dauber J, et al. Influenza virus infection in adult solid organ transplant recipients. Am J Transplant 2002;2:287.
22. Ljungman P, Andersson J, Aschan J, et al. Influenza A in immunocompromised patients. Clin Infect Dis 1993;17:244.
23. Nichols WG, Guthrie KA, Corey L, et al. Influenza infections after hematopoietic stem cell transplantation: risk factors, mortality, and the effect of antiviral therapy. Clin Infect Dis 2004;39:1300.
24. Khanna N, Steffen I, Studt JD, et al. Outcome of influenza infections in outpatients after allogeneic hematopoietic stem cell transplantation. Transpl Infect Dis 2009;11:100.

25. Tasian SK, Park JR, Martin ET, et al. Influenza-associated morbidity in children with cancer. Pediatr Blood Cancer 2008;50:983.
26. Randomised trial of efficacy and safety of inhaled zanamivir in treatment of influenza A and B virus infections. The MIST (Management of Influenza in the Southern Hemisphere Trialists) Study Group. Lancet 1998;352:1877.
27. Hayden FG, Osterhaus AD, Treanor JJ, et al. Efficacy and safety of the neuraminidase inhibitor zanamivir in the treatment of influenzavirus infections. GG167 Influenza Study Group. N Engl J Med 1997;337:874.
28. Makela MJ, Pauksens K, Rostila T, et al. Clinical efficacy and safety of the orally inhaled neuraminidase inhibitor zanamivir in the treatment of influenza: a randomized, double-blind, placebo-controlled European study. J Infect 2000;40:42.
29. Johny AA, Clark A, Price N, et al. The use of zanamivir to treat influenza A and B infection after allogeneic stem cell transplantation. Bone Marrow Transplant 2002;29:113.
30. Medeiros R, Rameix-Welti MA, Lorin V, et al. Failure of zanamivir therapy for pneumonia in a bone-marrow transplant recipient infected by a zanamivir-sensitive influenza A (H1N1) virus. Antivir Ther 2007;12:571.
31. Sheu TG, Deyde VM, Okomo-Adhiambo M, et al. Surveillance for neuraminidase inhibitor resistance among human influenza A and B viruses circulating worldwide from 2004 to 2008. Antimicrob Agents Chemother 2008;52:3284.
32. Monto AS. Antivirals and influenza: frequency of resistance. Pediatr Infect Dis J 2008;27:S110.
33. Ilyushina NA, Hay A, Yilmaz N, et al. Oseltamivir-ribavirin combination therapy for highly pathogenic H5N1 influenza virus infection in mice. Antimicrob Agents Chemother 2008;52:3889.
34. Smee DF, Hurst BL, Wong MH, et al. Effects of double combinations of amantadine, oseltamivir, and ribavirin on influenza A (H5N1) virus infections in cell culture and in mice. Antimicrob Agents Chemother 2009;53:2120.
35. Guidelines for vaccination of solid organ transplant candidates and recipients. Am J Transplant 2004;4(Suppl 10):160.
36. Ljungman P, Avetisyan G. Influenza vaccination in hematopoietic SCT recipients. Bone Marrow Transplant 2008;42:637.
37. Ljungman P, Engelhard D, de la Camara R, et al. Vaccination of stem cell transplant recipients: recommendations of the Infectious Diseases Working Party of the EBMT. Bone Marrow Transplant 2005;35:737.
38. Elizaga J, Olavarria E, Apperley J, et al. Parainfluenza virus 3 infection after stem cell transplant: relevance to outcome of rapid diagnosis and ribavirin treatment. Clin Infect Dis 2001;32:413.
39. Nichols WG, Erdman DD, Han A, et al. Prolonged outbreak of human parainfluenza virus 3 infection in a stem cell transplant outpatient department: insights from molecular epidemiologic analysis. Biol Blood Marrow Transplant 2004;10:58.
40. Cortez KJ, Erdman DD, Peret TC, et al. Outbreak of human parainfluenza virus 3 infections in a hematopoietic stem cell transplant population. J Infect Dis 2001;184:1093.
41. Hohenthal U, Nikoskelainen J, Vainionpaa R, et al. Parainfluenza virus type 3 infections in a hematology unit. Bone Marrow Transplant 2001;27:295.
42. Jalal H, Bibby DF, Bennett J, et al. Molecular investigations of an outbreak of parainfluenza virus type 3 and respiratory syncytial virus infections in a hematology unit. J Clin Microbiol 2007;45:1690.

43. Piralla A, Percivalle E, Di Cesare-Merlone A, et al. Multicluster nosocomial outbreak of parainfluenza virus type 3 infection in a pediatric oncohematology unit: a phylogenetic study. Haematologica 2009;94:833.
44. Zambon M, Bull T, Sadler CJ, et al. Molecular epidemiology of two consecutive outbreaks of parainfluenza 3 in a bone marrow transplant unit. J Clin Microbiol 1998;36:2289.
45. Au WY, Lie AK, Cheung RT, et al. Acute disseminated encephalomyelitis after para-influenza infection post bone marrow transplantation. Leuk Lymphoma 2002;43:455.
46. Lange T, Franke G, Niederwieser D. Parotitis associated with a parainfluenza virus type 3 infection during aplasia after unrelated allogeneic stem cell transplantation. Leuk Lymphoma 2006;47:1714.
47. Rodriguez V, Kuehnle I, Heslop HE, et al. Guillain-Barre syndrome after allogeneic hematopoietic stem cell transplantation. Bone Marrow Transplant 2002;29:515.
48. Vilchez RA, Dauber J, McCurry K, et al. Parainfluenza virus infection in adult lung transplant recipients: an emergent clinical syndrome with implications on allograft function. Am J Transplant 2003;3:116.
49. Ferguson PE, Sorrell TC, Bradstock KF, et al. Parainfluenza virus type 3 pneumonia in bone marrow transplant recipients: multiple small nodules in high-resolution lung computed tomography scans provide a radiological clue to diagnosis. Clin Infect Dis 2009. [Epub ahead of print].
50. Chakrabarti S, Collingham KE, Holder K, et al. Pre-emptive oral ribavirin therapy of paramyxovirus infections after haematopoietic stem cell transplantation: a pilot study. Bone Marrow Transplant 2001;28:759.
51. McCurdy LH, Milstone A, Dummer S. Clinical features and outcomes of paramyxoviral infection in lung transplant recipients treated with ribavirin. J Heart Lung Transplant 2003;22:745.
52. Nichols WG, Gooley T, Boeckh M. Community-acquired respiratory syncytial virus and parainfluenza virus infections after hematopoietic stem cell transplantation: the Fred Hutchinson Cancer Research Center experience. Biol Blood Marrow Transplant 2001;7(Suppl):11S.
53. Shima T, Yoshimoto G, Nonami A, et al. Successful treatment of parainfluenza virus 3 pneumonia with oral ribavirin and methylprednisolone in a bone marrow transplant recipient. Int J Hematol 2008;88:336.
54. Wright JJ, O'Driscoll G. Treatment of parainfluenza virus 3 pneumonia in a cardiac transplant recipient with intravenous ribavirin and methylprednisolone. J Heart Lung Transplant 2005;24:343.
55. El Saleeby CM, Somes GW, DeVincenzo JP, et al. Risk factors for severe respiratory syncytial virus disease in children with cancer: the importance of lymphopenia and young age. Pediatrics 2008;121:235.
56. Sung L, Alonzo TA, Gerbing RB, et al. Respiratory syncytial virus infections in children with acute myeloid leukemia: a report from the Children's Oncology Group. Pediatr Blood Cancer 2008;51:784.
57. Mahony J, Chong S, Merante F, et al. Development of a respiratory virus panel test for detection of twenty human respiratory viruses by use of multiplex PCR and a fluid microbead-based assay. J Clin Microbiol 2007;45:2965.
58. Boeckh M, Englund J, Li Y, et al. Randomized controlled multicenter trial of aerosolized ribavirin for respiratory syncytial virus upper respiratory tract infection in hematopoietic cell transplant recipients. Clin Infect Dis 2007; 44:245.

59. Pelaez A, Lyon GM, Force SD, et al. Efficacy of oral ribavirin in lung transplant patients with respiratory syncytial virus lower respiratory tract infection. J Heart Lung Transplant 2009;28:67.
60. Glanville AR, Scott AI, Morton JM, et al. Intravenous ribavirin is a safe and cost-effective treatment for respiratory syncytial virus infection after lung transplantation. J Heart Lung Transplant 2005;24:2114.
61. Chavez-Bueno S, Mejias A, Merryman RA, et al. Intravenous palivizumab and ribavirin combination for respiratory syncytial virus disease in high-risk pediatric patients. Pediatr Infect Dis J 2007;26:1089.
62. Michaels MG, Fonseca-Aten M, Green M, et al. Respiratory syncytial virus prophylaxis: a survey of pediatric solid organ transplant centers. Pediatr Transplant 2009;13:451.
63. Englund JA, Boeckh M, Kuypers J, et al. Brief communication: fatal human metapneumovirus infection in stem-cell transplant recipients. Ann Intern Med 2006;144:344.
64. Kamboj M, Gerbin M, Huang CK, et al. Clinical characterization of human metapneumovirus infection among patients with cancer. J Infect 2008;57:464.
65. Oliveira R, Machado A, Tateno A, et al. Frequency of human metapneumovirus infection in hematopoietic SCT recipients during 3 consecutive years. Bone Marrow Transplant 2008;42:265.
66. Evashuk KM, Forgie SE, Gilmour S, et al. Respiratory failure associated with human metapneumovirus infection in an infant posthepatic transplant. Am J Transplant 2008;8:1567.
67. Debiaggi M, Canducci F, Sampaolo M, et al. Persistent symptomless human metapneumovirus infection in hematopoietic stem cell transplant recipients. J Infect Dis 2006;194:474.
68. Gerna G, Vitulo P, Rovida F, et al. Impact of human metapneumovirus and human cytomegalovirus versus other respiratory viruses on the lower respiratory tract infections of lung transplant recipients. J Med Virol 2006;78:408.
69. Hopkins P, McNeil K, Kermeen F, et al. Human metapneumovirus in lung transplant recipients and comparison to respiratory syncytial virus. Am J Respir Crit Care Med 2008;178:876.
70. Hamelin ME, Prince GA, Boivin G. Effect of ribavirin and glucocorticoid treatment in a mouse model of human metapneumovirus infection. Antimicrob Agents Chemother 2006;50:774.
71. Wyde PR, Chetty SN, Jewell AM, et al. Comparison of the inhibition of human metapneumovirus and respiratory syncytial virus by ribavirin and immune serum globulin in vitro. Antiviral Res 2003;60:51.
72. Wyde PR, Moylett EH, Chetty SN, et al. Comparison of the inhibition of human metapneumovirus and respiratory syncytial virus by NMSO3 in tissue culture assays. Antiviral Res 2004;63:51.
73. Bonney D, Razali H, Turner A, et al. Successful treatment of human metapneumovirus pneumonia using combination therapy with intravenous ribavirin and immune globulin. Br J Haematol 2009;145:667.
74. Raza K, Ismailjee SB, Crespo M, et al. Successful outcome of human metapneumovirus (hMPV) pneumonia in a lung transplant recipient treated with intravenous ribavirin. J Heart Lung Transplant 2007;26:862.
75. Safdar A. Immune modulatory activity of ribavirin for serious human metapneumovirus disease: early I.V. therapy may improve outcomes in immunosuppressed SCT recipients. Bone Marrow Transplant 2008;41:707.

76. Herfst S, Fouchier RA. Vaccination approaches to combat human metapneumovirus lower respiratory tract infections. J Clin Virol 2008;41:49.
77. Herfst S, Schrauwen EJ, de Graaf M, et al. Immunogenicity and efficacy of two candidate human metapneumovirus vaccines in cynomolgus macaques. Vaccine 2008;26:4224.
78. Garbino J, Crespo S, Aubert JD, et al. A prospective hospital-based study of the clinical impact of non-severe acute respiratory syndrome (Non-SARS)-related human coronavirus infection. Clin Infect Dis 2006;43:1009.
79. Kumar D, Erdman D, Keshavjee S, et al. Clinical impact of community-acquired respiratory viruses on bronchiolitis obliterans after lung transplant. Am J Transplant 2005;5:2031.
80. Pene F, Merlat A, Vabret A, et al. Coronavirus 229E-related pneumonia in immunocompromised patients. Clin Infect Dis 2003;37:929.
81. Drosten C, Gunther S, Preiser W, et al. Identification of a novel coronavirus in patients with severe acute respiratory syndrome. N Engl J Med 1967;348:2003.
82. Ksiazek TG, Erdman D, Goldsmith CS, et al. A novel coronavirus associated with severe acute respiratory syndrome. N Engl J Med 2003;348:1953.
83. Rota PA, Oberste MS, Monroe SS, et al. Characterization of a novel coronavirus associated with severe acute respiratory syndrome. Science 2003;300:1394.
84. Adachi D, Johnson G, Draker R, et al. Comprehensive detection and identification of human coronaviruses, including the SARS-associated coronavirus, with a single RT-PCR assay. J Virol Methods 2004;122:29.
85. Booth CM, Matukas LM, Tomlinson GA, et al. Clinical features and short-term outcomes of 144 patients with SARS in the greater Toronto area. JAMA 2003;289:2801.
86. Chiou HE, Liu CL, Buttrey MJ, et al. Adverse effects of ribavirin and outcome in severe acute respiratory syndrome: experience in two medical centers. Chest 2005;128:263.
87. Knowles SR, Phillips EJ, Dresser L, et al. Common adverse events associated with the use of ribavirin for severe acute respiratory syndrome in Canada. Clin Infect Dis 2003;37:1139.
88. Kumar D, Tellier R, Draker R, et al. Severe Acute Respiratory Syndrome (SARS) in a liver transplant recipient and guidelines for donor SARS screening. Am J Transplant 2003;3:977.
89. Farcas GA, Poutanen SM, Mazzulli T, et al. Fatal severe acute respiratory syndrome is associated with multiorgan involvement by coronavirus. J Infect Dis 2005;191:193.
90. Echavarria M. Adenoviruses in immunocompromised hosts. Clin Microbiol Rev 2008;21:704.
91. Humar A, Kumar D, Mazzulli T, et al. A surveillance study of adenovirus infection in adult solid organ transplant recipients. Am J Transplant 2005;5:2555.
92. McGrath D, Falagas ME, Freeman R, et al. Adenovirus infection in adult orthotopic liver transplant recipients: incidence and clinical significance. J Infect Dis 1998;177:459.
93. Michaels MG, Green M, Wald ER, et al. Adenovirus infection in pediatric liver transplant recipients. J Infect Dis 1992;165:170.
94. Ljungman P. Treatment of adenovirus infections in the immunocompromised host. Eur J Clin Microbiol Infect Dis 2004;23:583.
95. Fox JD. Respiratory virus surveillance and outbreak investigation. J Clin Virol 2007;40(Suppl 1):S24.

96. Lion T, Baumgartinger R, Watzinger F, et al. Molecular monitoring of adenovirus in peripheral blood after allogeneic bone marrow transplantation permits early diagnosis of disseminated disease. Blood 2003;102:1114.
97. Hofland CA, Eron LJ, Washecka RM. Hemorrhagic adenovirus cystitis after renal transplantation. Transplant Proc 2004;36:3025.
98. Bordigoni P, Carret AS, Venard V, et al. Treatment of adenovirus infections in patients undergoing allogeneic hematopoietic stem cell transplantation. Clin Infect Dis 2001;32:1290.
99. Doan ML, Mallory GB, Kaplan SL, et al. Treatment of adenovirus pneumonia with cidofovir in pediatric lung transplant recipients. J Heart Lung Transplant 2007;26:883.
100. Refaat M, McNamara D, Teuteberg J, et al. Successful cidofovir treatment in an adult heart transplant recipient with severe adenovirus pneumonia. J Heart Lung Transplant 2008;27:699.
101. Ribaud P, Scieux C, Freymuth F, et al. Successful treatment of adenovirus disease with intravenous cidofovir in an unrelated stem-cell transplant recipient. Clin Infect Dis 1999;28:690.
102. Feuchtinger T, Matthes-Martin S, Richard C, et al. Safe adoptive transfer of virus-specific T-cell immunity for the treatment of systemic adenovirus infection after allogeneic stem cell transplantation. Br J Haematol 2006;134:64.
103. Leen AM, Christin A, Myers GD, et al. Cytotoxic T lymphocyte therapy with donor T cells prevents and treats adenovirus and Epstein-Barr virus infections after haploidentical and matched unrelated stem cell transplant. Blood 2009;114(19):4283–92.
104. Neofytos D, Ojha A, Mookerjee B, et al. Treatment of adenovirus disease in stem cell transplant recipients with cidofovir. Biol Blood Marrow Transplant 2007;13:74.
105. Symeonidis N, Jakubowski A, Pierre-Louis S, et al. Invasive adenoviral infections in T-cell-depleted allogeneic hematopoietic stem cell transplantation: high mortality in the era of cidofovir. Transpl Infect Dis 2007;9:108.
106. Parody R, Rabella N, Martino R, et al. Upper and lower respiratory tract infections by human enterovirus and rhinovirus in adult patients with hematological malignancies. Am J Hematol 2007;82:807.
107. Gutman JA, Peck AJ, Kuypers J, et al. Rhinovirus as a cause of fatal lower respiratory tract infection in adult stem cell transplantation patients: a report of two cases. Bone Marrow Transplant 2007;40:809.
108. Kaiser L, Aubert JD, Pache JC, et al. Chronic rhinoviral infection in lung transplant recipients. Am J Respir Crit Care Med 2006;174:1392.
109. Gerna G, Piralla A, Rovida F, et al. Correlation of rhinovirus load in the respiratory tract and clinical symptoms in hospitalized immunocompetent and immunocompromised patients. J Med Virol 2009;81:1498.
110. Hayden FG, Herrington DT, Coats TL, et al. Efficacy and safety of oral pleconaril for treatment of colds due to picornaviruses in adults: results of 2 double-blind, randomized, placebo-controlled trials. Clin Infect Dis 2003;36:1523.
111. Costa C, Terlizzi ME, Solidoro P, et al. Detection of parvovirus B19 in the lower respiratory tract. J Clin Virol 2009;46(2):150–3.
112. Beske F, Modrow S, Sorensen J, et al. Parvovirus B19 pneumonia in a child undergoing allogeneic hematopoietic stem cell transplantation. Bone Marrow Transplant 2007;40:89.
113. Janner D, Bork J, Baum M, et al. Severe pneumonia after heart transplantation as a result of human parvovirus B19. J Heart Lung Transplant 1994;13:336.

114. Waldman M, Kopp JB. Parvovirus-B19-associated complications in renal transplant recipients. Nat Clin Pract Nephrol 2007;3:540.
115. Allander T. Human bocavirus. J Clin Virol 2008;41:29.
116. Allander T, Tammi MT, Eriksson M, et al. Cloning of a human parvovirus by molecular screening of respiratory tract samples. Proc Natl Acad Sci U S A 2005;102:12891.
117. Schenk T, Strahm B, Kontny U, et al. Disseminated bocavirus infection after stem cell transplant. Emerg Infect Dis 2007;13:1425.
118. Kupfer B, Vehreschild J, Cornely O, et al. Severe pneumonia and human bocavirus in adult. Emerg Infect Dis 2006;12:1614.
119. Miyakis S, van Hal SJ, Barratt J, et al. Absence of human Bocavirus in bronchoalveolar lavage fluid of lung transplant patients. J Clin Virol 2009;44:179.
120. Kantola K, Hedman L, Allander T, et al. Serodiagnosis of human bocavirus infection. Clin Infect Dis 2008;46:540.
121. Lindner J, Karalar L, Schimanski S, et al. Clinical and epidemiological aspects of human bocavirus infection. J Clin Virol 2008;43:391.
122. Bialasiewicz S, Whiley DM, Lambert SB, et al. Presence of the newly discovered human polyomaviruses KI and WU in Australian patients with acute respiratory tract infection. J Clin Virol 2008;41:63.
123. Bialasiewicz S, Whiley DM, Lambert SB, et al. A newly reported human polyomavirus, KI virus, is present in the respiratory tract of Australian children. J Clin Virol 2007;40:15.
124. Gaynor AM, Nissen MD, Whiley DM, et al. Identification of a novel polyomavirus from patients with acute respiratory tract infections. PLoS Pathog 2007;3:e64.
125. Le BM, Demertzis LM, Wu G, et al. Clinical and epidemiologic characterization of WU polyomavirus infection, St. Louis, Missouri. Emerg Infect Dis 2007;13:1936.
126. Mourez T, Bergeron A, Ribaud P, et al. Polyomaviruses KI and WU in immunocompromised patients with respiratory disease. Emerg Infect Dis 2009;15:107.
127. Norja P, Ubillos I, Templeton K, et al. No evidence for an association between infections with WU and KI polyomaviruses and respiratory disease. J Clin Virol 2007;40:307.
128. Bialasiewicz S, Whiley DM, Lambert SB, et al. Detection of BK, JC, WU, or KI polyomaviruses in faecal, urine, blood, cerebrospinal fluid and respiratory samples. J Clin Virol 2009;45:249.
129. Billings JL, Hertz MI, Savik K, et al. Respiratory viruses and chronic rejection in lung transplant recipients. J Heart Lung Transplant 2002;21:559.
130. Khalifah AP, Hachem RR, Chakinala MM, et al. Respiratory viral infections are a distinct risk for bronchiolitis obliterans syndrome and death. Am J Respir Crit Care Med 2004;170:181.
131. Husain S, Singh N. Bronchiolitis obliterans and lung transplantation: evidence for an infectious etiology. Semin Respir Infect 2002;17:310.
132. Ison MG, Sharma A, Shepard JA, et al. Outcome of influenza infection managed with oseltamivir in lung transplant recipients. J Heart Lung Transplant 2008;27:282.
133. Vu D, Peck AJ, Nichols WG, et al. Safety and tolerability of oseltamivir prophylaxis in hematopoietic stem cell transplant recipients: a retrospective case-control study. Clin Infect Dis 2007;45:187.

Antiviral Drug Resistance: Mechanisms and Clinical Implications

Lynne Strasfeld, MD*, Sunwen Chou, MD

KEYWORDS

- Drug resistance • Transplant • Cytomegalovirus
- Herpes simplex virus • Varicella zoster virus
- Hepatitis B virus

In the setting of intensive immunosuppression for the management of rejection in solid organ transplant (SOT) recipients, or graft-versus-host disease (GVHD) in hematopoietic stem cell transplant (HSCT) recipients, antiviral therapy is commonly used and drug-resistant viruses are increasingly encountered. Prolonged antiviral drug exposure and ongoing viral replication due to immunosuppression are key factors in the development of antiviral drug resistance, which may manifest as persistent or increasing viremia or disease despite therapy. Consequences of drug resistance range from toxicity inherent in use of second-line antivirals, to severe disease and even death from progressive viral infection when no effective alternative treatments are available. In this article, the authors review the mechanisms, implications, and management of resistance to antiviral drugs used to treat several viral infections that play a significant role in the clinical course of transplant recipients and oncology patients: cytomegalovirus (CMV), herpes simplex virus (HSV), varicella zoster virus (VZV), and hepatitis B virus (HBV).

HERPESVIRUSES

Antiviral Agents and Mechanism of Action

All of the currently licensed drugs for systemic treatment of herpesvirus infections share the same target, viral DNA polymerase. The most commonly used drugs are the nucleoside analogues acyclovir and ganciclovir. Acyclovir, its more bioavailable prodrug valacyclovir, and famciclovir (the prodrug of penciclovir) are used for HSV

Dr Chou was supported by NIH grant AI39938.
Division of Infectious Diseases, Oregon Health & Science University, 3181 SW Sam Jackson Park Road, mail code L457, Portland, OR 97239, USA
* Corresponding author.
E-mail address: strasfel@ohsu.edu

Infect Dis Clin N Am 24 (2010) 413–437
doi:10.1016/j.idc.2010.01.001
id.theclinics.com
0891-5520/10/$ – see front matter © 2010 Elsevier Inc. All rights reserved.

and VZV infections but have weak anti-CMV activity. Ganciclovir and its valine ester prodrug valganciclovir have in vitro activity against HSV, VZV, and CMV, and are Food and Drug Administration (FDA)-approved for CMV infection, for which antiviral potency outweighs the increased toxicity as compared with acyclovir.

Acyclovir is monophosphorylated by thymidine kinase (TK) expressed by HSV (UL23) or VZV (ORF36) and then converted by cellular kinases to the active form, acyclovir triphosphate. Acyclovir triphosphate inhibits HSV and VZV replication by competitive inhibition of viral DNA polymerase and by chain termination of viral DNA strands.[1,2] Selectivity is related to preferential activation of acyclovir by viral TK and to the greater sensitivity of viral compared with cellular DNA polymerase to acyclovir triphosphate. Penciclovir, the active metabolite of famciclovir, has a similar mechanism of activation and action. Ganciclovir is monophosphorylated by the CMV UL97 kinase, or HSV or VZV TK, with subsequent antiviral action analogous to acyclovir. Unlike acyclovir, ganciclovir is not an obligate chain terminator, but rather causes a slowing and subsequent cessation of viral DNA chain elongation.[3]

Foscarnet, a pyrophosphate analogue, and cidofovir, a nucleotide analogue, do not depend on prior activation by viral enzymes. Foscarnet binds selectively to viral DNA polymerase at the pyrophosphate-binding site, blocking cleavage of the pyrophosphate moiety from deoxynucleotide triphosphates, in turn halting DNA chain elongation. Cidofovir is phosphorylated by cellular enzymes, and once activated acts as a potent inhibitor of the viral DNA polymerase. Foscarnet and cidofovir are typically used as second- and third-line herpesvirus drugs, respectively, when there is either suspected or documented resistance to initial therapy or dose-limiting toxicities of first-line drugs.

Use of these antiviral drugs may be affected by dose-limiting toxicities. Although acyclovir is usually considered relatively nontoxic, high doses are associated with nephrotoxicity[4] and encephalopathy.[5,6] High-dose valacyclovir has been associated with thrombotic microangiopathy in immunocompromised hosts.[7] Ganciclovir and valganciclovir frequently cause myelosuppression, especially neutropenia.[8,9] Foscarnet is associated with significant nephrotoxicity and electrolyte abnormalities.[10,11] Cidofovir is associated with nephrotoxicity and neutropenia when administered intravenously,[12] and with application site irritation when administered topically.[13]

In Vitro Evaluation of Antiviral Susceptibility

In vitro drug susceptibility testing of herpesviruses is by phenotypic and/or genotypic assays. Phenotypic assays measure drug susceptibility by culturing a calibrated viral inoculum under serial drug dilutions, thereby arriving at the drug concentration required to inhibit viral growth by 50% or 90% from the level observed without drug, referred to as the IC_{50} or IC_{90}, respectively. The IC_{50} is the value usually reported because it is more reproducible than the IC_{90} value. The IC_{50} threshold for susceptible strains is assay dependent, with the cutoff for sensitivity typically set at 3 to 5 times the mean IC_{50} for susceptible strains. In the classic plaque reduction assay (PRA), viral growth is measured as the number of visible plaques formed in cell culture monolayers after a fixed incubation period. The PRA is poorly standardized as to what constitutes a viral plaque, is labor-intensive, and is affected by a variety of culture conditions such as the type, density, and growth phase of cells, the viral inoculum, and the drug concentration range. Efforts were made to standardize a PRA technique for CMV susceptibility testing,[14] though in practice a great deal of variability remains, and the assay is clinically impractical because of the slow growth of CMV and the increasing use of molecular diagnostic assays that do not yield a live isolate for phenotypic testing. On the other hand, phenotypic testing for the more rapidly growing HSV is a preferred approach to resistance testing for this virus. To improve assay efficiency and reduce subjectivity, plaque counting can be replaced by viral quantitation methods that depend on assay of viral antigen or nucleic acid, or a reporter gene that is activated by viral infection. A reporter-based yield reduction system has been used for rapid phenotypic testing of HSV clinical isolates and laboratory strains.[15]

Genotypic assays depend on knowledge of the viral mutations causing resistance to specific antiviral drugs and the level of resistance and cross-resistance conferred by single and multiple mutations. These assays work best when a limited number of characteristic mutations are regularly encountered in connection with resistance to a specific drug, and are well supported by an accessible information database necessary for accurate interpretation. Genotypic tests have a faster turnaround time than phenotype assays and use a common technology of polymerase chain reaction (PCR) amplification of viral sequences followed by analysis for diagnostic mutations. A viral culture isolate is not needed, and viral DNA can be amplified directly from blood, fluid, or tissue specimens. Limitations of genotypic assays include difficulties with interpretation of viral sequence changes not found in the current information database, and the effective levels of resistance that result from combinations of mutations. There are also technical issues relating to DNA amplification and the sensitivity of detection of viral mutations when present as a minor subpopulation mixed with wild-type virus.

Genotype-phenotype correlations are confirmed by recombinant phenotyping, also known as marker transfer, whereby individual mutations suspected of causing drug resistance are transferred to baseline viral strains and their effect on drug susceptibility is established by phenotypic assays. A large volume of this work has been done for CMV because of the dominant role of genotypic resistance testing for this virus. Recombinant phenotyping has also been done to determine the significance of various TK and DNA polymerase gene mutations for HSV and VZV drug resistance,[16,17] but given the number and variety of TK resistance mutations, resistance testing of HSV and VZV isolates is more reliant on phenotypic approaches.

HERPES SIMPLEX VIRUS

Epidemiology of Antiviral Resistance

Acyclovir, valacyclovir, and famciclovir are drugs of choice for mucocutaneous HSV infections and for preventive treatment, while intravenous acyclovir is used for serious invasive disease such as encephalitis. The first clinical cases of acyclovir-resistant HSV were reported in 1982, shortly after initial use of systemically administered acyclovir.[18,19] Despite the subsequent widespread use of acyclovir, clinically evident drug resistance remains largely confined to the immunocompromised population, and the frequency of isolation of acyclovir-resistant HSV has remained stable over time.[20] Drug-resistant HSV disease is rare in immunocompetent hosts (<1% in various reports), and typically is cleared without adverse clinical outcome.[20–24] In immunocompromised hosts the prevalence ranges from 3.5% to 14%, with the most the most immunosuppressed subset having the highest risk for resistance.[20–25] Prolonged use of acyclovir is an important risk factor for resistant HSV, but drug-resistant HSV has been isolated in the absence of a known history of acyclovir exposure.[26]

Mechanisms of Resistance

Resistance of HSV to acyclovir is related to viral TK or DNA polymerase mutations.[27] As viral TK is not essential for HSV replication, more than 90% of acyclovir resistance in clinical isolates is associated with TK mutations.[28] TK mutations may result in either a loss of TK activity (TK deleted or deficient virus) or, less commonly, an alteration in TK substrate specificity (TK altered virus).[28] Mutations in the TK gene are often due to addition or deletion of nucleotides in homopolymer runs of guanines and cytosines, resulting in frameshifting and loss of TK function.[29,30] The specific TK mutations resulting from penciclovir exposure differ from those selected by acyclovir cross-resistance is expected with TK deficient mutants, though certain acyclovir-resistant TK altered mutants appear to retain in vitro sensitivity to penciclovir.[31] In addition, resistance to ganciclovir is presumed in the case of TK-deficient mutants.[32] Drug-resistant TK mutants retain susceptibility to drugs that are not dependent on virally mediated phosphorylation, including foscarnet and cidofovir, unless a viral DNA polymerase mutation is also present. Given the essential role of viral DNA polymerase in viral replication, mutations in this gene occur less frequently and have been observed to cluster in functional domains II and III. The cross-resistance patterns of these mutations vary and are evaluated by recombinant phenotyping.[3,33]

Clinical Implications and Management of Resistant Virus

The clinical implications of antiviral-resistant HSV are related to the direct effects of viral infection as well as the toxicities of second-line agents. Unchecked viral replication can lead to progressive and sometimes fatal invasive HSV disease.[32,34,35] Recurrent, chronic, and extensive mucocutaneous HSV ulcerations have been observed in immunocompromised individuals with drug-resistant virus.[36] Drug-resistant HSV has been associated with decreased neurovirulence in murine models when compared with wild-type virus,[37,38] with TK null mutants having the greatest reduction in virulence.[39] Though previously thought to lack the ability to establish and reactivate from latency, it is now appreciated that TK null mutants may be able to do so by way of reversion, due to ribosomal frameshifting or replication errors that create subpopulations of TK altered virus.[40,41] Human data for decreased pathogenicity of drug-resistant HSV are lacking.

In clinical practice, management of suspected or proven acyclovir-resistant HSV is generally with foscarnet, or less often with cidofovir. Management is often done empirically based on the frequency of TK mutations, but cross-resistance may result from DNA polymerase mutations, and emergence of both foscarnet and cidofovir resistance while on therapy has been reported.[36,42] Vidarabine, a purine analogue phosphorylated by cellular kinases with selectivity for HSV DNA polymerase, has in vitro activity against HSV,[43] but clinical experience has been disappointing for acyclovir-resistant HSV in the human immunodeficiency virus (HIV)-infected population.[44] Topical imiquimod, an immunomodulatory agent, or topical cidofovir have been used successfully to treat some cases of drug-resistant mucocutaneous HSV infection.[45,46] Topical treatments avoid the potential nephrotoxicity of systemically administered foscarnet or cidofovir. Management of drug-resistant HSV should include efforts to improve the immune status of the patient, when possible, by decreasing immunosuppressive therapy.

VARICELLA ZOSTER VIRUS

Epidemiology of Antiviral Resistance

The same antiviral drugs are used for VZV as for HSV. Given that acyclovir has less potent activity against VZV than HSV, intravenous administration, frequent and high oral doses, or the more bioavailable oral prodrugs (valacyclovir or famciclovir) are needed to ensure therapeutic antiviral blood levels.[47] Acyclovir-resistant VZV clinical isolates have been reported uncommonly and mostly in the HIV population[48–51] with a few cases in oncology and transplant recipients.[52,53] Unlike HSV, there are no large surveillance studies of antiviral drug-resistant VZV, and available information exists as case reports and series. Of note, there are 2 cases in the pediatric oncology literature of chronic disseminated varicella disease attributable to the VZV vaccine strain Oka with in vitro documentation of acyclovir resistance.[54,55]

Mechanisms of Resistance

Like HSV, VZV also expresses a TK, and VZV drug resistance is for the most part attributable to TK mutations,[3] which often result in a premature stop codon that makes the virus TK deficient appear to cluster at particular VZV TK gene loci.[3,53] Suggest that acyclovir-resistance mutations in gene those conferring resistance to foscarnet.[3] Not much is known of penciclovir-resistant clinical isolates. Although acyclovir and penciclovir may select in vitro for different patterns of cross-resistance to other antivirals, cross-resistance between the 2 drugs is expected.[56]

Clinical Implications and Management of Resistant Virus

Similar to HSV, the clinical implications of drug-resistant VZV relate to the direct effects of viral replication and to the toxicities of alternative antiviral agents. Cases of visceral dissemination and death due to progressive VZV infection unresponsive to antiviral treatment were reported in HIV-infected subjects.[51] A chronic verrucous form of VZV is associated with drug-resistant virus in immunocompromised hosts.[52,55,57,58] Some VZV DNA polymerase mutants selected under foscarnet in cell culture have a slow-growth phenotype,[59] perhaps suggesting attenuated virulence, although this has not been clinically validated.

Management of suspected or proven acyclovir-resistant VZV is generally with foscarnet, as described mostly in HIV-infected individuals[51,60] and some oncology patients.[52,54,55] Emergence of foscarnet resistance was detected in a few patients being treated with the drug for acyclovir-resistant VZV,[60,61] and attributed to a viral DNA polymerase mutation.[61] Although the literature on cidofovir treatment for drug-resistant VZV is very limited,[62] cidofovir is expected to retain activity against acyclovir-resistant TK mutants.[63] Vidarabine shows in vitro activity against VZV DNA polymerase mutants,[64] though clinical experience is limited.[65] Susceptibility testing of VZV isolates should be performed when drug resistance is suspected on clinical grounds, and any immunosuppressive therapy should be minimized.

CYTOMEGALOVIRUS

Epidemiology of Antiviral Resistance

CMV is a well-recognized opportunistic pathogen in those with AIDS, in SOT and HSCT recipients, and occasionally in nontransplant oncology patients, particularly following major T-cell suppressive regimens.[66] Ganciclovir and valganciclovir are currently the principal drugs used for prevention and treatment of CMV infection, and are widely used in transplant populations. Shortly following the introduction of ganciclovir in the late 1980s, cases of ganciclovir resistance in immunocompromised hosts began to appear in the literature.[67] Much of our knowledge about CMV drug resistance comes from studies of CMV retinitis in the AIDS population in the 1990s.[68,69] More recently, studies have highlighted the problem in the SOT population.[70–78] The overall incidence of ganciclovir resistance among SOT recipients is 0% to 13%, and varies according to the type of organ transplant, the immunosuppressive regimen and antiviral prophylaxis used, and the specific criteria for determining resistance.[79] CMV seronegative recipients of organs from seropositive donors (D+/R− subset), those with prolonged ganciclovir exposure and potent immunosuppression, and lung transplant recipients are at higher risk for developing antiviral drug resistance. In the HSCT setting, the development of ganciclovir resistance is reported to be uncommon and generally limited to case reports and small case series,[80–85] with the exception of the pediatric population for which there have been reports of rapid emergence of resistance[86–88]; this may relate to less ganciclovir exposure in the HSCT population, where a preemptive as opposed to a prophylactic approach to CMV disease prevention is favored. Emergence of resistance to foscarnet and cidofovir has also been reported in the SOT and HSCT population.[76,80,81,86,89–91]

Mechanism of Resistance

The literature on CMV drug resistance mutations is extensive,[92–99] especially for ganciclovir. More than 90% of resistant CMV isolates obtained following ganciclovir exposure contain one or more characteristic mutations in the viral UL97 kinase gene,[98] which apparently decrease the phosphorylation of ganciclovir without impairing the important functions of this kinase in viral replication.[98,100,101] Unlike the case with HSV TK mutations, CMV UL97 drug resistance mutations cluster tightly at codons 460, 520, and 590-607 (**Fig. 1**). Mutations M460V/I, H520Q, C592G, A594V, L595S, and C603W are among the most frequently encountered in ganciclovir-resistant isolates.[98] These mutations individually confer moderate ganciclovir resistance, with an IC_{50} ratio of 5 to 10, except for C592G, which confers low-level ganciclovir resistance with an IC_{50} ratio of about 2.5.[98] These IC_{50} ratios are based on recombinant phenotyping data,[99] which are also available for many other less common UL97 mutations. The accumulated genotype-phenotype correlations are the basis for the CMV genotypic resistance testing that is available in various commercial and academic laboratories.

CMV UL54 DNA polymerase mutations can confer resistance to any or all of the current anti-CMV drugs Many ganciclovir resistance mutations are located in the exonuclease domains (**Fig. 2**) and typically confer cross-resistance to cidofovir.[92,94] Mutations in and between catalytic regions II (eg, codons 700 and 715), III (eg, codons 802 and 809), VI (eg, codon 781), and at some nonconserved loci (eg, codon 756) confer foscarnet resistance, as well as low-grade ganciclovir or cidofovir cross-resistance in the case of mutations at region III.[3,92,95] Uncommonly, single UL54 mutations can confer simultaneous resistance to ganciclovir, cidofovir, and foscarnet.[89,94,97] The serial emergence of multiple mutations in patients on prolonged CMV antiviral therapy

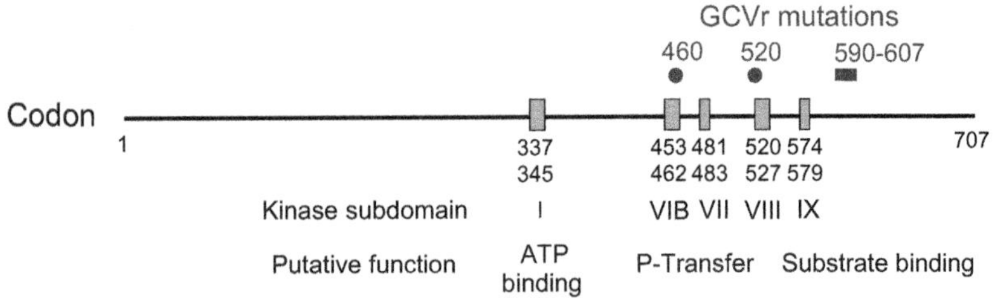

Fig. 1. Map of CMV UL97 gene functional domains and resistance mutations. Ganciclovir resistance (GCVr) mutations are clustered at codons 460, 520, and 590-607. In the latter region mutations A594V, L595S, C592G, and C603W are some of the most common, but a variety of point and in-frame deletion mutations are known to confer varying degrees of GCV resistance. Not all sequence changes at codons 590 to 607 confer ganciclovir resistance. ATP, adenosine triphosphate.

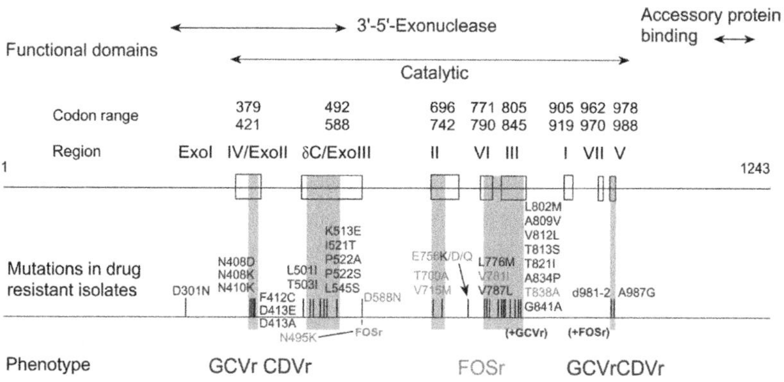

Fig. 2. Map of CMV DNA polymerase functional domains, resistance mutations, and associated phenotypes. All listed mutations have been found in clinical isolates and validated by recombinant phenotyping. Shaded regions indicate where resistance mutations are clustered, with associated phenotypes indicated below. GCVr, ganciclovir resistance; CDVr, cidofovir resistance; FOSr, foscarnet resistance. (*Updated from* Chou S, Lurain NS, Thompson KD, et al. Viral DNA polymerase mutations associated with drug resistance in human cytomegalovirus. J Infect Dis 2003;188:32–9; with permission.)

is well documented.[93,102] A UL97 mutation conferring ganciclovir typically appears first, followed by the addition of one or more UL54 polymerase mutations after prolonged therapy. The eventual phenotype of these isolates is often high-level resistance to ganciclovir, with additional resistance to foscarnet and/or cidofovir.

Clinical Implications and Management of Resistant Virus

As with untreated CMV infection, the clinical consequences of infection with drug-resistant CMV range from asymptomatic to severe. While asymptomatic infection with drug-resistant virus has been noted, especially in clinical antiviral trials for disease prevention,[103] and persistent viremia without overt disease also occurs, has been reported more commonly in connection with,[75,77,80,83,84] probably because the host factors that predispose to serious CMV disease are the same as those that favor the emergence of drug resistance. There is insufficient evidence to assess the relative clinical virulence of wild-type and drug-resistant CMV strains, even though several drug-resistant CMV DNA polymerase mutants have been reported to have a slow-growth phenotype in vitro.[3,80,86,96]

CMV drug resistance should be suspected in the setting of high or rising viral load and/or progressive CMV disease despite appropriate induction doses of antiviral therapy for at least 2 weeks, and with a history of cumulative antiviral drug exposure of at least 6 weeks, except in some pediatric settings as noted earlier. When resistance is suspected, laboratory testing for resistance should be pursued and immunosuppressive therapy should be minimized. There are no controlled studies to guide the treatment of drug-resistant CMV infection. The degree of drug resistance, the antiviral drug(s) and dose used, the competence of host immune response, and the site and extent of CMV disease all play a role in determining outcome.

In the absence of immediate, life- or sight-threatening CMV disease, selection of antiviral therapy should be guided by genotypic analysis of UL97 and UL54 genes. The degree of phenotypic resistance known to be associated with a particular gene mutation(s) has significant implications for choice of therapy. Low-grade ganciclovir resistance in the case of non–life- or sight-threatening disease can potentially be addressed with higher-dose intravenous ganciclovir.[78,79,104,105] High-grade ganciclovir resistance with a major UL97 resistance mutation and suspected resistance in the case of life- or sight-threatening disease is best managed with foscarnet. Use of foscarnet is often complicated by nephrotoxicity, and long-term use is rarely tolerated. Cidofovir is another option for ganciclovir-resistant CMV, providing there is not a polymerase mutation conferring cross-resistance to ganciclovir and cidofovir. Significant nephrotoxicity has been associated with cidofovir use in HSCT recipients[106]; however, the experience in SOT recipients is limited. Combination therapy with ganciclovir and foscarnet has been recommended for treatment of drug-resistant CMV infection, based on limited in vitro data[107] and a small case series advocating reduced-dose ganciclovir and escalating-dose foscarnet.[108] Despite the lack of controlled studies, combination treatment is a common practice in cases of documented multidrug resistance or cases of life- or sight-threatening disease unresponsive to monotherapy.

Given the significant limitations of the currently available therapies for drug-resistant CMV infection, alternative agents, both investigational compounds and drugs currently licensed for other indications, have been studied. Maribavir, a benzimidazole riboside, is a potent inhibitor of the CMV UL97 kinase, an enzyme important in various aspects of CMV replication. Because maribavir inhibits UL97-mediated ganciclovir phosphorylation, it antagonizes the antiviral action of ganciclovir, but may have an additive anti-CMV effect when combined with foscarnet or cidofovir.[109] No cross-resistance has been observed between maribavir and other current anti-CMV drugs.[110] Maribavir-resistant laboratory CMV strains have been isolated in vitro[111,112] and have been found to contain mutations in the UL97 and/or UL27 genes, which confer high- and low-grade resistance, respectively.[111–113] Maribavir was successfully tested in phase 1 and 2 trials, which suggested low toxicity and in vivo antiviral activity.[114] However, two phase 3 trials as a CMV prophylactic agent in HSCT and liver transplant recipients did not meet expectations of antiviral efficacy at the dosing regimens chosen. Higher doses of maribavir could still be useful in treating drug-resistant CMV, although clinical experience to date is limited to several transplant recipients, some of whom may have benefited, albeit maribavir-resistant virus was isolated in one case.[115]

Other experimental anti-CMV therapies are considerably less clinically developed than maribavir. Inhibitors of viral DNA cleavage and processing include tomeglovir (BAY-384766), and a benzimidazole D-riboside, GW-275175X, both of which underwent preliminary clinical studies to demonstrate tolerability, but neither of which has proceeded to more advanced clinical trials.[116] In vitro resistance to tomeglovir maps to the CMV UL89, UL56, and UL104 genes,[117] supporting the novel mechanism of action and expected lack of cross-resistance to current drugs. A lipid ester oral prodrug of cidofovir (hexadecyloxypropyl-CDV, or CMX001) has been shown to have in vitro and in vivo activity against CMV, with excellent oral bioavailability and minimal nephrotoxicity in preclinical studies.[118–120] CMX001 may offer a better alternative to the intravenous cidofovir formulation currently available. Cyclopropavir, a purine nucleoside analogue, has been shown to have potent in vitro and in vivo activity against CMV[121,122] but has not undergone clinical trials. While cyclopropavir appears to have a mechanism of action similar to ganciclovir, one study reported that some ganciclovir-resistant isolates exhibited only slightly reduced susceptibility to cyclopropavir[122]; more data are needed on the extent of cross-resistance between the 2 drugs.

Several drugs licensed for other indications and with no defined viral target appear to have anti-CMV activity, although clinical experience is limited to case reports, small case series, and retrospective cohort studies, with no controlled treatment data available. Their role in the treatment of drug-resistant CMV is unclear at this time but would likely be adjunctive to other antivirals. Several retrospective studies in SOT recipients,[123–129] as well as a few studies in HSCT recipients,[130,131] have demonstrated a lower incidence of CMV infection in patients who have received immunosuppressive regimens that included a target of rapamycin inhibitor, either sirolimus or everolimus. Leflunomide, an immunosuppressive drug with an indication for the treatment of rheumatoid arthritis, has been demonstrated to inhibit CMV replication in vitro and in a rat model.[132] Clinical data on the use of leflunomide for treatment of CMV infection in transplant recipients is mixed. When used as adjunctive therapy, a few successes have been reported in the treatment of drug-resistant CMV[81,133]; however, leflunomide is associated with significant hematologic and hepatic toxicity, and treatment failures have been reported as well.[134] Lastly, the antimalarial drug artesunate has been shown to have inhibitory activity against CMV in vitro and in vivo.[135,136] Artesunate appears to have additive effects with ganciclovir, foscarnet, and cidofovir.[135] There is one report of successful use in an HSCT recipient with foscarnet- and ganciclovir-resistant CMV infection.[137]

HEPATITIS B VIRUS

Antiviral Agents and Mechanism of Action

There are currently 7 FDA-approved agents for the treatment of hepatitis B. Three are nucleoside analogues (lamivudine, entecavir, and telbivudine) and 2 are nucleotide analogues (adefovir and tenofovir). Alpha-interferon, approved in 1992 for this indication, and more recently pegylated interferon, remains an important treatment option. Lastly, passive immunization with hepatitis B immune globulin (HBIG) liver transplantation, in combination with a nucleoside or nucleotide analogue for the prevention of HBV recurrence.[138,139]

All of the nucleoside and nucleotide analogues selectively target HBV DNA polymerase, which includes reverse transcriptase activity. Drugs in this class are phosphorylated by cellular enzymes to active form and then incorporated into growing DNA, resulting in premature chain termination, amongst other inhibitory functions related to viral replication. Drug-related side effects are generally minimal with this class, adefovir is associated with nephrotoxicity in up to 12% of liver transplant recipients,[140,141] and caution is advised in patients receiving concomitant nephrotoxins. Although these antiviral compounds are effective to varying degrees in providing long-term suppression, they do not eradicate HBV, which persists in hepatocytes in the form of covalently closed circular DNA (cccDNA).[142] In vitro studies have demonstrated that antiviral therapy has little or no effect on cccDNA.[143] Therefore, treatment of chronic HBV infection is typically prolonged and issues of antiviral drug resistance become important.

Historically, sequential and combination therapy was used to treat chronic HBV infection, with changes made in response to the frequent emergence of antiviral drug resistance. More recently, because of higher potency and lower rates of resistance, entecavir and tenofovir have largely supplanted lamivudine and adefovir as preferred first-line agents for antiviral naïve individuals.[144] For the significant number of patients who have been successfully treated with lamivudine and adefovir, with undetectable serum HBV DNA, there is no recommendation to change therapy.

In Vitro Evaluation of Antiviral Susceptibility

Genotypic resistance testing involves the detection of characteristic HBV polymerase gene mutations, which can be performed at varying levels of sensitivity using broadly applicable methods, such as standard sequencing of PCR products, restriction fragment length polymorphism, reverse hybridization, and single genome sequencing.[145]

Dideoxy sequencing is insensitive at detecting minor subpopulations of mutant virus that comprise less than 20% of the circulating virus population. The more sensitive assays can detect HBV DNA mutants that represent 5% to 10% of the entire HBV quasispecies, potentially allowing for earlier identification of genotypic resistance. With the advent of newer sequencing technologies, such as "ultra-deep" pyrosequencing, mutants comprising less than 1% of the viral pool can be identified and characterized.[146] The clinical utility and value of these more sensitive techniques remains to be determined. Genotypic testing is standard clinical practice as it is rapid and practical, but subject to the usual limitation that it cannot interpret novel or previously uncharacterized mutations and cannot directly assess such properties as the replication fitness of drug-resistant mutants.

Standardized phenotypic testing for HBV drug susceptibility has been limited by the absence of a cell culture system that allows fully permissive infection. A human hepatoma cell line maintained with dimethyl sulfoxide and hydrocortisone to promote cell differentiation and phenotypic stability[147] has been developed as a means of comparing the relative antiviral susceptibility and growth fitness of HBV mutants.[148] Cell culture systems may involve transient transfection of HBV clones or construction of cell lines that permanently express drug-resistant mutants.[149] Alternatively, biochemical assays of expressed HBV polymerase have been used to assess inhibition by drug, independent of cell culture. Although current HBV recombinant phenotyping approaches may not accurately model viral replication in vivo, they are necessary for validating the interpretation of genotypic resistance testing data.

Epidemiology of Antiviral Resistance

Given the high viral replication rate and the error-prone nature of HBV reverse transcriptase, emergence of drug resistance is expected.[150] Drug resistance has been associated with a variety of patient and viral factors. Host factors that contribute to an increased risk for drug resistance include older age, high body mass index (weight in kilograms divided by height in meters squared), medication noncompliance, immunosuppression, high pretreatment HBV DNA levels, baseline hepatic enzyme elevations, and abundant replication space (large number of uninfected hepatocytes, as in a newly transplanted liver).[151–156] The viral mutation frequency, the magnitude and rate of virus replication, and the overall replication fitness of the mutant are critical viral determinants in risk for drug resistance.[157]

Apart from host and virus factors, the potency and genetic barrier to resistance of the antiviral drug is of critical importance in determining risk for drug resistance.[150] The genetic barrier reflects the number and type of mutations that must be accumulated in order for the virus to develop significant drug resistance while maintaining adequate growth. Lamivudine is an intermediate potency drug with a low genetic barrier to resistance, resulting in high resistance rates. Adefovir is a low potency drug with an intermediate genetic barrier to resistance, and therefore an intermediate rate of resistance. Telbivudine is a high-potency drug, though with a low genetic barrier to resistance, and so resistance rates are intermediate. Lastly, entecavir and tenofovir are considered high-potency antivirals, with a high genetic barrier to resistance, and therefore low rates of resistance. Among antiviral-naïve patients, drug resistance has been reported in up to 70% of patients treated with 5 years of lamivudine therapy, 29% after 5 years of adefovir, 20% after 2 years of telbivudine, and 1% after 5 years of entecavir.[152,158–162] Resistance rates are significantly higher in patients with prior exposure to lamivudine, with rates of up to 18% at 1 year following switch to adefovir monotherapy and 51% at 5 years following switch to entecavir.[150,163]

Mechanism of Resistance

The HBV polymerase gene is the target for nucleoside and nucleotide analogues. The enzyme has 4 functional domains (terminal protein, spacer, Pol/rt [polymerase/reverse transcriptase], and RNaseH), with 7 catalytic subdomains (A–G) in the Pol/rt region (**Fig. 3**).[150] Antiviral drug-resistant strains have signature mutations in the reverse transcriptase domains of the viral polymerase gene, with most substitutions occurring in domains B, C, and D. Resistance mutations alter the interaction between HBV polymerase and drug.[164] Molecular modeling studies of the interaction of wild-type and mutant HBV polymerase with natural thymidine triphosphate substrate and with anti-HBV agents highlight the important conformational changes in mutants that confer drug resistance.[165] While the interaction of each nucleoside or nucleotide analogue with HBV polymerase appears to be mechanistically unique with regard to binding affinity and shifting after ligand attachment, all drug-resistant mutants seem to exhibit either altered binding of substrate or downstream structural changes that interfere with the inhibitory effect of drug on viral polymerase. After emergence of primary resistance mutations, compensatory mutations that restore replication capacity may arise, as well as secondary resistance mutations that increase drug resistance when they accumulate on the same viral genome.

High-level lamivudine resistance is most often caused by mutations M204I/V, which are in the YMDD (tyrosine-methionine-aspartate-aspartate) motif in the C domain of the polymerase gene,[166] and infrequently by A181V/T mutations.[167] M204V is almost always accompanied by compensatory mutations L180M and/or V173L, resulting in restored fitness of the mutant.[166,168] The M204I mutation confers high-level cross-resistance to telbivudine, but M204I/V mutations do not appear to reduce susceptibility to adefovir and tenofovir.[162,169] The signature mutation associated with

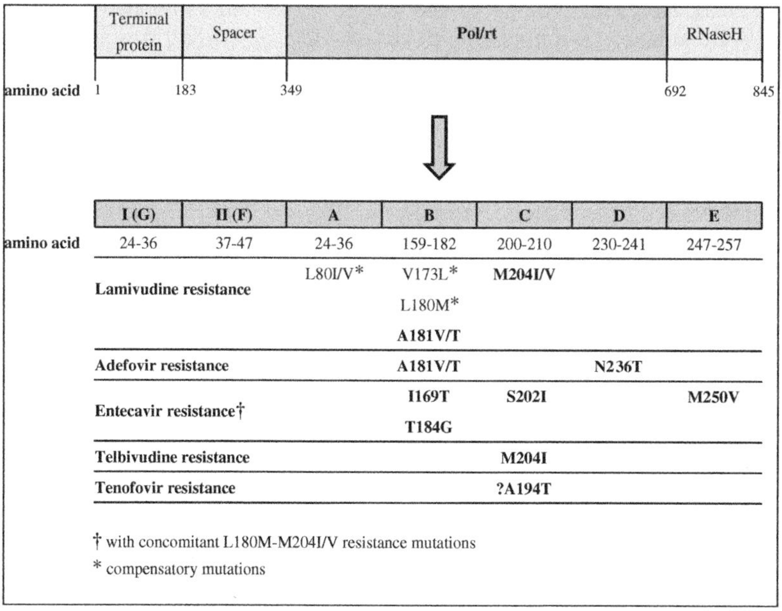

Fig. 3. Map of HBV polymerase gene functional domains (terminal protein, spacer, Pol/rt, RNaseH), catalytic subdomains (A–G), and resistance mutations. Pol/rt, polymerase/reverse transcriptase.

telbivudine resistance is M204I, either alone or in association with the secondary mutations L80I/V or L180M.[162]

N236T and A181V/T are adefovir-resistance mutations.[159,170] Although the resistance conferred by these mutations is less than that associated with M204I/V and lamivudine resistance, virological breakthrough is seen.[169–171] The N236T mutation reduces viral replicative capacity in vitro and confers cross-resistance to tenofovir but not to lamivudine or telbivudine.[172]

Resistance to entecavir appears to occur though a 2-hit mechanism, whereby classic lamivudine-resistant mutants (L180M, M204I/V) are selected in patients on lamivudine or, less frequently, in patients on primary therapy with entecavir.[173] During continued entecavir treatment, additional mutations at I169T and M250V or T184G and S202I are selected, conferring resistance to entecavir.[174–176]

Resistance to tenofovir currently appears to be unusual,[177] although more experience with this drug for treatment of chronic HBV is needed. There is a report of virologic breakthrough on tenofovir in 2 HBV/HIV coinfected patients with prior lamivudine exposure (L180M-M204V mutations) and an A194T mutation.[178] However, A194T was not shown to confer resistance to tenofovir in vitro,[179] suggesting that it may instead be a viral sequence polymorphism or a lamivudine compensatory mutation.[180]

Clinical Implications and Management of Resistant Virus

With the availability of safe and effective oral HBV antiviral agents in the late 1990s and the switch from HBIG monotherapy to combination therapy (HBIG plus antivirals) in HBV-infected liver transplant recipients, HBV recurrence rates have decreased significantly.[181–183] Antiviral drug resistance remains an important factor in HBV reinfection after liver transplantation. Clinical consequences of the emergence of drug-resistant HBV range from asymptomatic viremia to serum transaminase flares, worsening liver histology, hepatic decompensation and, occasionally, death.[152,171,184] Drug resistance is associated with virologic breakthrough,[185] defined as an increase in serum HBV DNA by at least 1.0 $\log_{10}$ (10-fold) above nadir, or the reappearance of serum HBV DNA with previously undetectable HBV DNA on 2 or more occasions at least 1 month apart while on treatment and after initial response is achieved in a medication-compliant patient.[145] Ultimately biochemical breakthrough, defined by elevation of hepatic transaminase values (hepatitis flare), occurs.

Genotypic resistance testing is important because not all virologic breakthrough is attributable to drug resistance. As many as 30% to 50% of viral breakthroughs observed in clinical trials are due to medication noncompliance,[145] a figure likely to be higher in clinical practice. When virologic breakthrough is associated with the emergence of resistance mutation(s), the inferred cross-resistance phenotype is used to develop a timely plan of action, such as a change to another drug or combination therapy.[186]

Management of lamivudine-resistant virus has involved the addition of adefovir, a strategy that has been shown to result in high rates of virologic suppression and a lower emergence rate of adefovir resistance than sequential monotherapy.[186,187] Tenofovir, a potent antiviral drug with excellent activity against lamivudine-resistant virus, appears to be superior to adefovir monotherapy for treatment of lamivudine-resistant virus[188]; comparison of tenofovir with combination adefovir-lamivudine in this setting, however, has not yet been reported in large-scale clinical studies. Entecavir is not a good option for lamivudine-resistant virus given the observed emergence of resistance.[176,189] Telbivudine resistance is associated with the M204I mutation, and although there are in vitro data demonstrating telbivudine activity against the lamivudine-resistant mutant,[190] clinical data are not available at this time. Telbuvidine should not be relied on for treatment of lamivudine-resistant virus, and management of telbivudine resistance should be similar to management of lamivudine resistance. Management of adefovir-resistant virus is dependent on the type of mutation(s) and the antiviral drug history of the patient. Lamivudine has proved to be effective in suppressing adefovir-resistant HBV with the N236 T mutation,[170,191] and it is presumed that telbivudine would also be effective based on in vitro data.[190] The durability of response in patients with previous lamivudine resistance, however, is unclear, with a report of reemergence of lamivudine resistance after reintroduction of drug.[192] There are in vitro data to suggest that entecavir may be a reasonable choice for N236T mutants,[193] with the caveat that the benefit may be short-lived in patients with prior lamivudine resistance. For patients with the N236T mutation, options include switching to or adding entecavir, adding lamivudine (or telbivudine), or switching to tenofovir. The activity of lamivudine (and likely telbivudine) against the A181 V adefovir-resistant mutants is decreased compared with wild-type HBV.[167] Whereas the A181T mutant has been shown in vitro to have decreased susceptibility to tenofovir,[167] in the clinical setting entecavir and tenofovir have been effective in suppressing replication of adefovir-resistant mutants.[194,195] In the case of an A181T mutation, management options include switching to or adding entecavir, or switching to tenofovir; lamivudine should not be used in this scenario given the risk of cross-resistance.[167]

There are no large-scale clinical studies yet available to guide the treatment of entecavir-resistant HBV. From in vitro data and case reports it appears that adefovir and tenofovir are effective for entecavir-resistant HBV.[176,196,197] Based for the most part on expert opinion, a recommended approach for entecavir-resistant virus is to add tenofovir or adefovir.[145,150,194] Data on management of tenofovir-resistant HBV are not yet available, given the low rate of resistance observed with early use of this drug.

Emtricitabine, a potent nucleoside analogue that is currently FDA-approved for the treatment of HIV, is currently in late phase clinical trial for management of chronic HBV.[198] At the target treatment dose of 200 mg daily, resistance to emtricitabine was observed in 9% of treatment-naïve patients at 1 year and rose to 20% after 2 years.[198] Emtricitabine resistance is conferred by the M204I/V mutation with or without the accompanying L180M and V173L mutations, therefore implying cross-resistance to lamivudine and telbivudine.

THE FUTURE

As antiviral therapy becomes widely used in immunosuppressed patient populations, concerns about drug resistance will require a better understanding of the relevant virus-, host-, and drug-related factors. Knowledge of genetic mechanisms and associated viral mutations has allowed for development of genotypic techniques for the timely diagnosis of resistance. The accuracy of this testing will be improved by recombinant phenotyping data that validate the drug resistance properties associated with the many viral sequence changes detected in clinical specimens. An accessible and authoritative database of drug resistance mutations needs to be available for each virus to guide therapeutic decisions. More comprehensive information on the epidemiologic, host, and drug exposure factors that favor the emergence of resistant virus can be used to develop better strategies for prevention, early detection, and appropriate treatment change. Ideally, controlled trials are needed to compare sequential and combination use of alternative therapies, optimize dosing schedules, and evaluate adjunctive therapies that seek to improve host conditions for antiviral drug efficacy. There is an ongoing need for less toxic but potent new antiviral drugs that preferably target different aspects of viral replication to reduce the risk of cross-resistance.

REFERENCES

1. Elion GB, Furman PA, Fyfe JA, et al. The selectivity of action of an antiherpetic agent, 9-(2-hydroxyethoxymethyl) guanine. Proc Natl Acad Sci USA 1977;74(12):5716–20.
2. Elion GB. Acyclovir: discovery, mechanism of action, and selectivity. J Med Virol 1993;41(Suppl 1):2–6.
3. Gilbert C, Bestman-Smith J, Boivin G. Resistance of herpesviruses to antiviral drugs: clinical impacts and molecular mechanisms. Drug Resist Updat 2002;5(2):88–114.
4. Wagstaff AJ, Faulds D, Goa KL. Aciclovir. A reappraisal of its antiviral activity, pharmacokinetic properties and therapeutic efficacy. Drugs 1994;47(1):153–205.
5. Haefeli WE, Schoenenberger RA, Weiss P, et al. Acyclovir-induced neurotoxicity: concentration-side effect relationship in acyclovir overdose. Am J Med 1993;94(2):212–5.
6. Lowance D, Neumayer HH, Legendre CM, et al. Valacyclovir for the prevention of cytomegalovirus disease after renal transplantation. International Valacyclovir Cytomegalovirus Prophylaxis Transplantation Study Group. N Engl J Med 1999;340(19):1462–70.
7. Ormrod D, Scott LJ, Perry CM. Valaciclovir: a review of its long term utility in the management of genital herpes simplex virus and cytomegalovirus infections. Drugs 2000;59(4):839–63.
8. Kalil AC, Freifeld AG, Lyden ER, et al. Valganciclovir for cytomegalovirus prevention in solid organ transplant patients: an evidence-based reassessment of safety and efficacy. PLoS One 2009;4(5):e5512.
9. Crumpacker CS. Ganciclovir. N Engl J Med 1996;335(10):721–9.
10. Wagstaff AJ, Bryson HM. Foscarnet. A reappraisal of its antiviral activity, pharmacokinetic properties and therapeutic use in immunocompromised patients with viral infections. Drugs 1994;48(2):199–226.
11. Deray G, Martinez F, Katlama C, et al. Foscarnet nephrotoxicity: mechanism, incidence and prevention. Am J Nephrol 1989;9(4):316–21.
12. Safrin S, Cherrington J, Jaffe HS. Clinical uses of cidofovir. Rev Med Virol 1997;7(3):145–56.
13. Lalezari J, Schacker T, Feinberg J, et al. A randomized, double-blind, placebo-controlled trial of cidofovir gel for the treatment of acyclovir-unresponsive mucocutaneous herpes simplex virus infection in patients with AIDS. J Infect Dis 1997;176(4):892–8.
14. Landry ML, Stanat S, Biron K, et al. A standardized plaque reduction assay for determination of drug susceptibilities of cytomegalovirus clinical isolates. Antimicrob Agents Chemother 2000;44(3):688–92.
15. Wang YC, Kao CL, Liu WT, et al. A cell line that secretes inducibly a reporter protein for monitoring herpes simplex virus infection and drug susceptibility. J Med Virol 2002;68(4):599–605.
16. Frobert E, Ooka T, Cortay JC, et al. Herpes simplex virus thymidine kinase mutations associated with resistance to acyclovir: a site-directed mutagenesis study. Antimicrob Agents Chemother 2005;49(3):1055–9.
17. Suzutani T, Saijo M, Nagamine M, et al. Rapid phenotypic characterization method for herpes simplex virus and varicella-zoster virus thymidine kinases to screen for acyclovir-resistant viral infection. J Clin Microbiol 2000;38(5):1839–44.

18. Burns WH, Saral R, Santos GW, et al. Isolation and characterisation of resistant Herpes simplex virus after acyclovir therapy. Lancet 1982;1(8269):421–3.
19. Sibrack CD, Gutman LT, Wilfert CM, et al. Pathogenicity of acyclovir-resistant herpes simplex virus type 1 from an immunodeficient child. J Infect Dis 1982; 146(5):673–82.
20. Stranska R, Schuurman R, Nienhuis E, et al. Survey of acyclovir-resistant herpes simplex virus in The Netherlands: prevalence and characterization. J Clin Virol 2005;32(1):7–18.
21. Nugier F, Colin JN, Aymard M, et al. Occurrence and characterization of acyclovir-resistant herpes simplex virus isolates: report on a two-year sensitivity screening survey. J Med Virol 1992;36(1):1–12.
22. Englund JA, Zimmerman ME, Swierkosz EM, et al. Herpes simplex virus resistant to acyclovir. A study in a tertiary care center. Ann Intern Med 1990; 112(6):416–22.
23. Christophers J, Clayton J, Craske J, et al. Survey of resistance of herpes simplex virus to acyclovir in northwest England. Antimicrob Agents Chemother 1998; 42(4):868–72.
24. Danve-Szatanek C, Aymard M, Thouvenot D, et al. Surveillance network for herpes simplex virus resistance to antiviral drugs: 3-year follow-up. J Clin Microbiol 2004;42(1):242–9.
25. Chakrabarti S, Pillay D, Ratcliffe D, et al. Resistance to antiviral drugs in herpes simplex virus infections among allogeneic stem cell transplant recipients: risk factors and prognostic significance. J Infect Dis 2000;181(6):2055–8.
26. Malvy D, Treilhaud M, Bouee S, et al. A retrospective, case-control study of acyclovir resistance in herpes simplex virus. Clin Infect Dis 2005;41(3): 320–6.
27. Coen DM, Schaffer PA. Two distinct loci confer resistance to acycloguanosine in herpes simplex virus type 1. Proc Natl Acad Sci U S A 1980;77(4):2265–9.
28. Morfin F, Thouvenot D. Herpes simplex virus resistance to antiviral drugs. J Clin Virol 2003;26(1):29–37.
29. Morfin F, Souillet G, Bilger K, et al. Genetic characterization of thymidine kinase from acyclovir-resistant and -susceptible herpes simplex virus type 1 isolated from bone marrow transplant recipients. J Infect Dis 2000;182(1):290–3.
30. Gaudreau A, Hill E, Balfour HH Jr, et al. Phenotypic and genotypic characterization of acyclovir-resistant herpes simplex viruses from immunocompromised patients. J Infect Dis 1998;178(2):297–303.
31. Bacon TH, Levin MJ, Leary JJ, et al. Herpes simplex virus resistance to acyclovir and penciclovir after two decades of antiviral therapy. Clin Microbiol Rev 2003; 16(1):114–28.
32. Ljungman P, Ellis MN, Hackman RC, et al. Acyclovir-resistant herpes simplex virus causing pneumonia after marrow transplantation. J Infect Dis 1990; 162(1):244–8.
33. Bestman-Smith J, Boivin G. Drug resistance patterns of recombinant herpes simplex virus DNA polymerase mutants generated with a set of overlapping cosmids and plasmids. J Virol 2003;77(14):7820–9.
34. Longerich T, Eisenbach C, Penzel R, et al. Recurrent herpes simplex virus hepatitis after liver retransplantation despite acyclovir therapy. Liver Transpl 2005; 11(10):1289–94.
35. Frangoul H, Wills M, Crossno C, et al. Acyclovir-resistant herpes simplex virus pneumonia post-unrelated stem cell transplantation: a word of caution. Pediatr Transplant 2007;11(8):942–4.

36. Chen Y, Scieux C, Garrait V, et al. Resistant herpes simplex virus type 1 infection: an emerging concern after allogeneic stem cell transplantation. Clin Infect Dis 2000;31(4):927–35.
37. Coen DM, Kosz-Vnenchak M, Jacobson JG, et al. Thymidine kinase-negative herpes simplex virus mutants establish latency in mouse trigeminal ganglia but do not reactivate. Proc Natl Acad Sci U S A 1989;86(12):4736–40.
38. Andrei G, Fiten P, Froeyen M, et al. DNA polymerase mutations in drug-resistant herpes simplex virus mutants determine in vivo neurovirulence and drug-enzyme interactions. Antivir Ther 2007;12(5):719–32.
39. Coen DM. Acyclovir-resistant, pathogenic herpesviruses. Trends Microbiol 1994;2(12):481–5.
40. Griffiths A, Chen SH, Horsburgh BC, et al. Translational compensation of a frameshift mutation affecting herpes simplex virus thymidine kinase is sufficient to permit reactivation from latency. J Virol 2003;77(8):4703–9.
41. Griffiths A, Link MA, Furness CL, et al. Low-level expression and reversion both contribute to reactivation of herpes simplex virus drug-resistant mutants with mutations on homopolymeric sequences in thymidine kinase. J Virol 2006; 80(13):6568–74.
42. Wyles DL, Patel A, Madinger N, et al. Development of herpes simplex virus disease in patients who are receiving cidofovir. Clin Infect Dis 2005;41(5): 676–80.
43. De Clercq E. The antiviral spectrum of (E)-5-(2-bromovinyl)-2′-deoxyuridine. J Antimicrob Chemother 1984;14(Suppl A):85–95.
44. Safrin S, Crumpacker C, Chatis P, et al. A controlled trial comparing foscarnet with vidarabine for acyclovir-resistant mucocutaneous herpes simplex in the acquired immunodeficiency syndrome. The AIDS Clinical Trials Group. N Engl J Med 1991;325(8):551–5.
45. Martinez V, Molina JM, Scieux C, et al. Topical imiquimod for recurrent acyclovir-resistant HSV infection. Am J Med 2006;119(5):e9–11.
46. Sims CR, Thompson K, Chemaly RF, et al. Oral topical cidofovir: novel route of drug delivery in a severely immunosuppressed patient with refractory multidrug-resistant herpes simplex virus infection. Transpl Infect Dis 2007;9(3):256–9.
47. Biron KK, Elion GB. In vitro susceptibility of varicella-zoster virus to acyclovir. Antimicrob Agents Chemother 1980;18(3):443–7.
48. Boivin G, Edelman CK, Pedneault L, et al. Phenotypic and genotypic characterization of acyclovir-resistant varicella-zoster viruses isolated from persons with AIDS. J Infect Dis 1994;170(1):68–75.
49. Jacobson MA, Berger TG, Fikrig S, et al. Acyclovir-resistant varicella zoster virus infection after chronic oral acyclovir therapy in patients with the acquired immunodeficiency syndrome (AIDS). Ann Intern Med 1990;112(3):187–91.
50. Saint-Leger E, Caumes E, Breton G, et al. Clinical and virologic characterization of acyclovir-resistant varicella-zoster viruses isolated from 11 patients with acquired immunodeficiency syndrome. Clin Infect Dis 2001;33(12):2061–7.
51. Breton G, Fillet AM, Katlama C, et al. Acyclovir-resistant herpes zoster in human immunodeficiency virus-infected patients: results of foscarnet therapy. Clin Infect Dis 1998;27(6):1525–7.
52. Crassard N, Souillet AL, Morfin F, et al. Acyclovir-resistant varicella infection with atypical lesions in a non-HIV leukemic infant. Acta Paediatr 2000;89(12):1497–9.
53. Morfin F, Thouvenot D, De Turenne-Tessier M, et al. Phenotypic and genetic characterization of thymidine kinase from clinical strains of varicella-zoster virus resistant to acyclovir. Antimicrob Agents Chemother 1999;43(10):2412–6.

54. Levin MJ, Dahl KM, Weinberg A, et al. Development of resistance to acyclovir during chronic infection with the Oka vaccine strain of varicella-zoster virus, in an immunosuppressed child. J Infect Dis 2003;188(7):954–9.
55. Bryan CJ, Prichard MN, Daily S, et al. Acyclovir-resistant chronic verrucous vaccine strain varicella in a patient with neuroblastoma. Pediatr Infect Dis J 2008;27(10):946–8.
56. Andrei G, De Clercq E, Snoeck R. In vitro selection of drug-resistant varicella-zoster virus (VZV) mutants (OKA strain): differences between acyclovir and penciclovir? Antiviral Res 2004;61(3):181–7.
57. Pahwa S, Biron K, Lim W, et al. Continuous varicella-zoster infection associated with acyclovir resistance in a child with AIDS. JAMA 1988;260(19):2879–82.
58. Linnemann CC Jr, Biron KK, Hoppenjans WG, et al. Emergence of acyclovir-resistant varicella zoster virus in an AIDS patient on prolonged acyclovir therapy. AIDS 1990;4(6):577–9.
59. Visse B, Huraux JM, Fillet AM. Point mutations in the varicella-zoster virus DNA polymerase gene confers resistance to foscarnet and slow growth phenotype. J Med Virol 1999;59(1):84–90.
60. Safrin S, Berger TG, Gilson I, et al. Foscarnet therapy in five patients with AIDS and acyclovir-resistant varicella-zoster virus infection. Ann Intern Med 1991; 115(1):19–21.
61. Visse B, Dumont B, Huraux JM, et al. Single amino acid change in DNA polymerase is associated with foscarnet resistance in a varicella-zoster virus strain recovered from a patient with AIDS. J Infect Dis 1998;178(Suppl 1):S55–7.
62. Schliefer K, Gumbel HO, Rockstroh JK, et al. Management of progressive outer retinal necrosis with cidofovir in a human immunodeficiency virus-infected patient. Clin Infect Dis 1999;29(3):684–5.
63. Snoeck R, Andrei G, De Clercq E. Novel agents for the therapy of varicella-zoster virus infections. Expert Opin Investig Drugs 2000;9(8):1743–51.
64. Kamiyama T, Kurokawa M, Shiraki K. Characterization of the DNA polymerase gene of varicella-zoster viruses resistant to acyclovir. J Gen Virol 2001;82(Pt 11):2761–5.
65. Reusser P, Cordonnier C, Einsele H, et al. European survey of herpesvirus resistance to antiviral drugs in bone marrow transplant recipients. Infectious diseases working party of the European group for blood and marrow transplantation (EBMT). Bone Marrow Transplant 1996;17(5):813–7.
66. Laurenti L, Piccioni P, Cattani P, et al. Cytomegalovirus reactivation during alemtuzumab therapy for chronic lymphocytic leukemia: incidence and treatment with oral ganciclovir. Haematologica 2004;89(10):1248–52.
67. Erice A, Chou S, Biron KK, et al. Progressive disease due to ganciclovir-resistant cytomegalovirus in immunocompromised patients. N Engl J Med 1989;320(5): 289–93.
68. Jabs DA, Enger C, Dunn JP, et al. Cytomegalovirus retinitis and viral resistance: ganciclovir resistance. CMV Retinitis and Viral Resistance Study Group. J Infect Dis 1998;177(3):770–3.
69. Jabs DA, Enger C, Forman M, et al. Incidence of foscarnet resistance and cidofovir resistance in patients treated for cytomegalovirus retinitis. The Cytomegalovirus Retinitis and Viral Resistance Study Group. Antimicrob Agents Chemother 1998;42(9):2240–4.
70. Reddy AJ, Zaas AK, Hanson KE, et al. A single-center experience with ganciclovir-resistant cytomegalovirus in lung transplant recipients: treatment and outcome. J Heart Lung Transplant 2007;26(12):1286–92.

71. Li F, Kenyon KW, Kirby KA, et al. Incidence and clinical features of ganciclovir-resistant cytomegalovirus disease in heart transplant recipients. Clin Infect Dis 2007;45(4):439–47.
72. Limaye AP, Raghu G, Koelle DM, et al. High incidence of ganciclovir-resistant cytomegalovirus infection among lung transplant recipients receiving preemptive therapy. J Infect Dis 2002;185(1):20–7.
73. Limaye AP, Corey L, Koelle DM, et al. Emergence of ganciclovir-resistant cytomegalovirus disease among recipients of solid-organ transplants. Lancet 2000; 356(9230):645–9.
74. Bhorade SM, Lurain NS, Jordan A, et al. Emergence of ganciclovir-resistant cytomegalovirus in lung transplant recipients. J Heart Lung Transplant 2002; 21(12):1274–82.
75. Eid AJ, Arthurs SK, Deziel PJ, et al. Emergence of drug-resistant cytomegalovirus in the era of valganciclovir prophylaxis: therapeutic implications and outcomes. Clin Transplant 2008;22(2):162–70.
76. Lurain NS, Bhorade SM, Pursell KJ, et al. Analysis and characterization of antiviral drug-resistant cytomegalovirus isolates from solid organ transplant recipients. J Infect Dis 2002;186(6):760–8.
77. Isada CM, Yen-Lieberman B, Lurain NS, et al. Clinical characteristics of 13 solid organ transplant recipients with ganciclovir-resistant cytomegalovirus infection. Transpl Infect Dis 2002;4(4):189–94.
78. Kruger RM, Shannon WD, Arens MQ, et al. The impact of ganciclovir-resistant cytomegalovirus infection after lung transplantation. Transplantation 1999; 68(9):1272–9.
79. Limaye AP. Ganciclovir-resistant cytomegalovirus in organ transplant recipients. Clin Infect Dis 2002;35(7):866–72.
80. Marfori JE, Exner MM, Marousek GI, et al. Development of new cytomegalovirus UL97 and DNA polymerase mutations conferring drug resistance after valganciclovir therapy in allogeneic stem cell recipients. J Clin Virol 2007;38(2):120–5.
81. Avery RK, Bolwell BJ, Yen-Lieberman B, et al. Use of leflunomide in an allogeneic bone marrow transplant recipient with refractory cytomegalovirus infection. Bone Marrow Transplant 2004;34(12):1071–5.
82. Erice A, Borrell N, Li W, et al. Ganciclovir susceptibilities and analysis of UL97 region in cytomegalovirus (CMV) isolates from bone marrow recipients with CMV disease after antiviral prophylaxis. J Infect Dis 1998;178(2):531–4.
83. Hamprecht K, Eckle T, Prix L, et al. Ganciclovir-resistant cytomegalovirus disease after allogeneic stem cell transplantation: pitfalls of phenotypic diagnosis by in vitro selection of an UL97 mutant strain. J Infect Dis 2003;187(1): 139–43.
84. Julin JE, van Burik JH, Krivit W, et al. Ganciclovir-resistant cytomegalovirus encephalitis in a bone marrow transplant recipient. Transpl Infect Dis 2002; 4(4):201–6.
85. Seo SK, Regan A, Cihlar T, et al. Cytomegalovirus ventriculoencephalitis in a bone marrow transplant recipient receiving antiviral maintenance: clinical and molecular evidence of drug resistance. Clin Infect Dis 2001;33(9):e105–8.
86. Springer KL, Chou S, Li S, et al. How evolution of mutations conferring drug resistance affects viral dynamics and clinical outcomes of cytomegalovirus-infected hematopoietic cell transplant recipients. J Clin Microbiol 2005;43(1): 208–13.
87. Eckle T, Lang P, Prix L, et al. Rapid development of ganciclovir-resistant cytomegalovirus infection in children after allogeneic stem cell transplantation in

the early phase of immune cell recovery. Bone Marrow Transplant 2002;30(7): 433–9.
88. Prix L, Hamprecht K, Holzhuter B, et al. Comprehensive restriction analysis of the UL97 region allows early detection of ganciclovir-resistant human cytomegalovirus in an immunocompromised child. J Infect Dis 1999;180(2):491–5.
89. Scott GM, Weinberg A, Rawlinson WD, et al. Multidrug resistance conferred by novel DNA polymerase mutations in human cytomegalovirus isolates. Antimicrob Agents Chemother 2007;51(1):89–94.
90. Rodriguez J, Casper K, Smallwood G, et al. Resistance to combined ganciclovir and foscarnet therapy in a liver transplant recipient with possible dual-strain cytomegalovirus coinfection. Liver Transpl 2007;13(10):1396–400.
91. Oshima K, Kanda Y, Kako S, et al. Case report: persistent cytomegalovirus (CMV) infection after haploidentical hematopoietic stem cell transplantation using in vivo alemtuzumab: emergence of resistant CMV due to mutations in the UL97 and UL54 genes. J Med Virol 2008;80(10):1769–75.
92. Chou S, Lurain NS, Thompson KD, et al. Viral DNA polymerase mutations associated with drug resistance in human cytomegalovirus. J Infect Dis 2003;188(1): 32–9.
93. Chou S, Marousek G, Guentzel S, et al. Evolution of mutations conferring multidrug resistance during prophylaxis and therapy for cytomegalovirus disease. J Infect Dis 1997;176(3):786–9.
94. Chou S, Marousek G, Li S, et al. Contrasting drug resistance phenotypes resulting from cytomegalovirus DNA polymerase mutations at the same exonuclease locus. J Clin Virol 2008;43(1):107–9.
95. Chou S, Marousek G, Parenti DM, et al. Mutation in region III of the DNA polymerase gene conferring foscarnet resistance in cytomegalovirus isolates from 3 subjects receiving prolonged antiviral therapy. J Infect Dis 1998;178(2):526–30.
96. Chou S, Marousek GI, Van Wechel LC, et al. Growth and drug resistance phenotypes resulting from cytomegalovirus DNA polymerase region III mutations observed in clinical specimens. Antimicrob Agents Chemother 2007;51(11):4160–2.
97. Chou S, Miner RC, Drew WL. A deletion mutation in region V of the cytomegalovirus DNA polymerase sequence confers multidrug resistance. J Infect Dis 2000;182(6):1765–8.
98. Chou S, Waldemer RH, Senters AE, et al. Cytomegalovirus UL97 phosphotransferase mutations that affect susceptibility to ganciclovir. J Infect Dis 2002; 185(2):162–9.
99. Chou S, Van Wechel LC, Lichy HM, et al. Phenotyping of cytomegalovirus drug resistance mutations by using recombinant viruses incorporating a reporter gene. Antimicrob Agents Chemother 2005;49(7):2710–5.
100. Prichard MN, Gao N, Jairath S, et al. A recombinant human cytomegalovirus with a large deletion in UL97 has a severe replication deficiency. J Virol 1999; 73(7):5663–70.
101. Wolf DG, Courcelle CT, Prichard MN, et al. Distinct and separate roles for herpesvirus-conserved UL97 kinase in cytomegalovirus DNA synthesis and encapsidation. Proc Natl Acad Sci U S A 2001;98(4):1895–900.
102. Smith IL, Cherrington JM, Jiles RE, et al. High-level resistance of cytomegalovirus to ganciclovir is associated with alterations in both the UL97 and DNA polymerase genes. J Infect Dis 1997;176(1):69–77.
103. Boivin G, Goyette N, Gilbert C, et al. Clinical impact of ganciclovir-resistant cytomegalovirus infections in solid organ transplant patients. Transpl Infect Dis 2005;7(3–4):166–70.

104. Cytomegalovirus. Am J Transplant 2004;4(Suppl 10):51–8.
105. West P, Schmiedeskamp M, Neeley H, et al. Use of high-dose ganciclovir for a resistant cytomegalovirus infection due to UL97 mutation. Transpl Infect Dis 2008;10(2):129–32.
106. Ljungman P, Deliliers GL, Platzbecker U, et al. Cidofovir for cytomegalovirus infection and disease in allogeneic stem cell transplant recipients. The infectious diseases working party of the European group for blood and marrow transplantation. Blood 2001;97(2):388–92.
107. Drew WL. Is combination antiviral therapy for CMV superior to monotherapy? J Clin Virol 2006;35(4):485–8.
108. Mylonakis E, Kallas WM, Fishman JA. Combination antiviral therapy for ganciclovir-resistant cytomegalovirus infection in solid-organ transplant recipients. Clin Infect Dis 2002;34(10):1337–41.
109. Chou S, Marousek GI. Maribavir antagonizes the antiviral action of ganciclovir on human cytomegalovirus. Antimicrob Agents Chemother 2006;50(10):3470–2.
110. Drew WL, Miner RC, Marousek GI, et al. Maribavir sensitivity of cytomegalovirus isolates resistant to ganciclovir, cidofovir or foscarnet. J Clin Virol 2006;37(2):124–7.
111. Chou S, Wechel LC, Marousek GI. Cytomegalovirus UL97 kinase mutations that confer maribavir resistance. J Infect Dis 2007;196(1):91–4.
112. Chou S, Marousek GI, Senters AE, et al. Mutations in the human cytomegalovirus UL27 gene that confer resistance to maribavir. J Virol 2004;78(13): 7124–30.
113. Chou S, Marousek GI. Accelerated evolution of maribavir resistance in a cytomegalovirus exonuclease domain II mutant. J Virol 2008;82(1):246–53.
114. Winston DJ, Young JA, Pullarkat V, et al. Maribavir prophylaxis for prevention of cytomegalovirus infection in allogeneic stem cell transplant recipients: a multicenter, randomized, double-blind, placebo-controlled, dose-ranging study. Blood 2008;111(11):5403–10.
115. Avery RK, Marty FM, Strasfeld L, et al. Oral maribavir (MBV) for treatment of resistant or refractory cytomegalovirus (CMV) infection in transplant recipients [abstract]. In: Programs and abstracts of the 49th Interscience Conference on Antimicrobial Agents and Chemotherapy (ICAAC). San Francisco, September 12–15, 2009.
116. Lischka P, Zimmermann H. Antiviral strategies to combat cytomegalovirus infections in transplant recipients. Curr Opin Pharmacol 2008;8(5):541–8.
117. Buerger I, Reefschlaeger J, Bender W, et al. A novel nonnucleoside inhibitor specifically targets cytomegalovirus DNA maturation via the UL89 and UL56 gene products. J Virol 2001;75(19):9077–86.
118. Ciesla SL, Trahan J, Wan WB, et al. Esterification of cidofovir with alkoxyalkanols increases oral bioavailability and diminishes drug accumulation in kidney. Antiviral Res 2003;59(3):163–71.
119. Quenelle DC, Collins DJ, Pettway LR, et al. Effect of oral treatment with (S)-HPMPA, HDP-(S)-HPMPA or ODE-(S)-HPMPA on replication of murine cytomegalovirus (MCMV) or human cytomegalovirus (HCMV) in animal models. Antiviral Res 2008;79(2):133–5.
120. Quenelle DC, Collins DJ, Wan WB, et al. Oral treatment of cowpox and vaccinia virus infections in mice with ether lipid esters of cidofovir. Antimicrob Agents Chemother 2004;48(2):404–12.
121. Kern ER, Bidanset DJ, Hartline CB, et al. Oral activity of a methylenecyclopropane analog, cyclopropavir, in animal models for cytomegalovirus infections. Antimicrob Agents Chemother 2004;48(12):4745–53.

122. Kern ER, Kushner NL, Hartline CB, et al. In vitro activity and mechanism of action of methylenecyclopropane analogs of nucleosides against herpesvirus replication. Antimicrob Agents Chemother 2005;49(3):1039–45.
123. Webster AC, Lee VW, Chapman JR, et al. Target of rapamycin inhibitors (TOR-I; sirolimus and everolimus) for primary immunosuppression in kidney transplant recipients. Cochrane Database Syst Rev 2006;(2):CD004290.
124. Hill JA, Hummel M, Starling RC, et al. A lower incidence of cytomegalovirus infection in de novo heart transplant recipients randomized to everolimus. Transplantation 2007;84(11):1436–42.
125. Kobashigawa JA, Miller LW, Russell SD, et al. Tacrolimus with mycophenolate mofetil (MMF) or sirolimus vs. cyclosporine with MMF in cardiac transplant patients: 1-year report. Am J Transplant 2006;6(6):1377–86.
126. Buchler M, Caillard S, Barbier S, et al. Sirolimus versus cyclosporine in kidney recipients receiving thymoglobulin, mycophenolate mofetil and a 6-month course of steroids. Am J Transplant 2007;7(11):2522–31.
127. Haririan A, Morawski K, West MS, et al. Sirolimus exposure during the early post-transplant period reduces the risk of CMV infection relative to tacrolimus in renal allograft recipients. Clin Transplant 2007;21(4):466–71.
128. Demopoulos L, Polinsky M, Steele G, et al. Reduced risk of cytomegalovirus infection in solid organ transplant recipients treated with sirolimus: a pooled analysis of clinical trials. Transplant Proc 2008;40(5):1407–10.
129. San Juan R, Aguado JM, Lumbreras C, et al. Impact of current transplantation management on the development of cytomegalovirus disease after renal transplantation. Clin Infect Dis 2008;47(7):875–82.
130. Cutler C, Kim HT, Hochberg E, et al. Sirolimus and tacrolimus without methotrexate as graft-versus-host disease prophylaxis after matched related donor peripheral blood stem cell transplantation. Biol Blood Marrow Transplant 2004;10(5):328–36.
131. Marty FM, Bryar J, Browne SK, et al. Sirolimus-based graft-versus-host disease prophylaxis protects against cytomegalovirus reactivation after allogeneic hematopoietic stem cell transplantation: a cohort analysis. Blood 2007;110(2):490–500.
132. Waldman WJ, Knight DA, Blinder L, et al. Inhibition of cytomegalovirus in vitro and in vivo by the experimental immunosuppressive agent leflunomide. Intervirology 1999;42(5–6):412–8.
133. Levi ME, Mandava N, Chan LK, et al. Treatment of multidrug-resistant cytomegalovirus retinitis with systemically administered leflunomide. Transpl Infect Dis 2006;8(1):38–43.
134. Battiwalla M, Paplham P, Almyroudis NG, et al. Leflunomide failure to control recurrent cytomegalovirus infection in the setting of renal failure after allogeneic stem cell transplantation. Transpl Infect Dis 2007;9(1):28–32.
135. Kaptein SJ, Efferth T, Leis M, et al. The anti-malaria drug artesunate inhibits replication of cytomegalovirus in vitro and in vivo. Antiviral Res 2006;69(2):60–9.
136. Efferth T, Romero MR, Wolf DG, et al. The antiviral activities of artemisinin and artesunate. Clin Infect Dis 2008;47(6):804–11.
137. Shapira MY, Resnick IB, Chou S, et al. Artesunate as a potent antiviral agent in a patient with late drug-resistant cytomegalovirus infection after hematopoietic stem cell transplantation. Clin Infect Dis 2008;46(9):1455–7.
138. Tung BY, Kowdley KV. Hepatitis B and liver transplantation. Clin Infect Dis 2005;41(10):1461–6.

139. Marzano A, Salizzoni M, Debernardi-Venon W, et al. Prevention of hepatitis B virus recurrence after liver transplantation in cirrhotic patients treated with lamivudine and passive immunoprophylaxis. J Hepatol 2001;34(6): 903–10.
140. Schiff ER, Lai CL, Hadziyannis S, et al. Adefovir dipivoxil therapy for lamivudine-resistant hepatitis B in pre- and post-liver transplantation patients. Hepatology 2003;38(6):1419–27.
141. Schiff E, Lai CL, Hadziyannis S, et al. Adefovir dipivoxil for wait-listed and post-liver transplantation patients with lamivudine-resistant hepatitis B: final long-term results. Liver Transpl 2007;13(3):349–60.
142. Wong DK, Yuen MF, Yuan H, et al. Quantitation of covalently closed circular hepatitis B virus DNA in chronic hepatitis B patients. Hepatology 2004;40(3): 727–37.
143. Moraleda G, Saputelli J, Aldrich CE, et al. Lack of effect of antiviral therapy in nondividing hepatocyte cultures on the closed circular DNA of woodchuck hepatitis virus. J Virol 1997;71(12):9392–9.
144. Keeffe EB, Dieterich DT, Han SH, et al. A treatment algorithm for the management of chronic hepatitis B virus infection in the United States: 2008 update. Clin Gastroenterol Hepatol 2008;6(12):1315–41 [quiz: 286].
145. Lok AS. How to diagnose and treat hepatitis B virus antiviral drug resistance in the liver transplant setting. Liver Transpl 2008;14(Suppl 2):S8–14.
146. Margeridon-Thermet S, Shulman NS, Ahmed A, et al. Ultra-deep pyrosequencing of hepatitis B virus quasispecies from nucleoside and nucleotide reverse-transcriptase inhibitor (NRTI)-treated patients and NRTI-naïve patients. J Infect Dis 2009;199(9):1275–85.
147. Gripon P, Rumin S, Urban S, et al. Infection of a human hepatoma cell line by hepatitis B virus. Proc Natl Acad Sci U S A 2002;99(24):15655–60.
148. Villet S, Billioud G, Pichoud C, et al. In vitro characterization of viral fitness of therapy-resistant hepatitis B variants. Gastroenterology 2009;136(1): 168–76, e2.
149. Zoulim F. In vitro models for studying hepatitis B virus drug resistance. Semin Liver Dis 2006;26(2):171–80.
150. Yuen MF, Fung J, Wong DK, et al. Prevention and management of drug resistance for antihepatitis B treatment. Lancet Infect Dis 2009;9(4):256–64.
151. Fung SK, Chae HB, Fontana RJ, et al. Virologic response and resistance to adefovir in patients with chronic hepatitis B. J Hepatol 2006;44(2):283–90.
152. Lai CL, Dienstag J, Schiff E, et al. Prevalence and clinical correlates of YMDD variants during lamivudine therapy for patients with chronic hepatitis B. Clin Infect Dis 2003;36(6):687–96.
153. Benhamou Y, Bochet M, Thibault V, et al. Long-term incidence of hepatitis B virus resistance to lamivudine in human immunodeficiency virus-infected patients. Hepatology 1999;30(5):1302–6.
154. Litwin S, Toll E, Jilbert AR, et al. The competing roles of virus replication and hepatocyte death rates in the emergence of drug-resistant mutants: theoretical considerations. J Clin Virol 2005;34(Suppl 1):S96–107.
155. Chang ML, Chien RN, Yeh CT, et al. Virus and transaminase levels determine the emergence of drug resistance during long-term lamivudine therapy in chronic hepatitis B. J Hepatol 2005;43(1):72–7.
156. Zoulim F, Poynard T, Degos F, et al. A prospective study of the evolution of lamivudine resistance mutations in patients with chronic hepatitis B treated with lamivudine. J Viral Hepat 2006;13(4):278–88.

157. Locarnini S, Warner N. Major causes of antiviral drug resistance and implications for treatment of hepatitis B virus monoinfection and coinfection with HIV. Antivir Ther 2007;12(Suppl 3):H15–23.
158. Lok AS, Lai CL, Leung N, et al. Long-term safety of lamivudine treatment in patients with chronic hepatitis B. Gastroenterology 2003;125(6):1714–22.
159. Hadziyannis SJ, Tassopoulos NC, Heathcote EJ, et al. Long-term therapy with adefovir dipivoxil for HBeAg-negative chronic hepatitis B for up to 5 years. Gastroenterology 2006;131(6):1743–51.
160. Tenney DJ, Rose RE, Baldick CJ, et al. Long-term monitoring shows hepatitis B virus resistance to entecavir in nucleoside-naïve patients is rare through 5 years of therapy. Hepatology 2009;49(5):1503–14.
161. Nguyen MH, Keeffe EB. Chronic hepatitis B: early viral suppression and long-term outcomes of therapy with oral nucleos(t)ides. J Viral Hepat 2009;16(3):149–55.
162. Liaw YF, Gane E, Leung N, et al. 2-Year GLOBE trial results: telbivudine Is superior to lamivudine in patients with chronic hepatitis B. Gastroenterology 2009;136(2):486–95.
163. Lee YS, Suh DJ, Lim YS, et al. Increased risk of adefovir resistance in patients with lamivudine-resistant chronic hepatitis B after 48 weeks of adefovir dipivoxil monotherapy. Hepatology 2006;43(6):1385–91.
164. Das K, Xiong X, Yang H, et al. Molecular modeling and biochemical characterization reveal the mechanism of hepatitis B virus polymerase resistance to lamivudine (3TC) and emtricitabine (FTC). J Virol 2001;75(10):4771–9.
165. Sharon A, Chu CK. Understanding the molecular basis of HBV drug resistance by molecular modeling. Antiviral Res 2008;80(3):339–53.
166. Allen MI, Deslauriers M, Andrews CW, et al. Identification and characterization of mutations in hepatitis B virus resistant to lamivudine. Lamivudine Clinical Investigation Group. Hepatology 1998;27(6):1670–7.
167. Villet S, Pichoud C, Billioud G, et al. Impact of hepatitis B virus rtA181V/T mutants on hepatitis B treatment failure. J Hepatol 2008;48(5):747–55.
168. Delaney WE 4th, Yang H, Westland CE, et al. The hepatitis B virus polymerase mutation rtV173L is selected during lamivudine therapy and enhances viral replication in vitro. J Virol 2003;77(21):11833–41.
169. Yang H, Qi X, Sabogal A, et al. Cross-resistance testing of next-generation nucleoside and nucleotide analogues against lamivudine-resistant HBV. Antivir Ther 2005;10(5):625–33.
170. Angus P, Vaughan R, Xiong S, et al. Resistance to adefovir dipivoxil therapy associated with the selection of a novel mutation in the HBV polymerase. Gastroenterology 2003;125(2):292–7.
171. Fung SK, Andreone P, Han SH, et al. Adefovir-resistant hepatitis B can be associated with viral rebound and hepatic decompensation. J Hepatol 2005;43(6):937–43.
172. Yang H, Westland C, Xiong S, et al. In vitro antiviral susceptibility of full-length clinical hepatitis B virus isolates cloned with a novel expression vector. Antiviral Res 2004;61(1):27–36.
173. Kobashi H, Fujioka S, Kawaguchi M, et al. Two cases of development of entecavir resistance during entecavir treatment for nucleoside-naïve chronic hepatitis B. Hepatol Int 2009;3(2):403–10.
174. Tenney DJ, Levine SM, Rose RE, et al. Clinical emergence of entecavir-resistant hepatitis B virus requires additional substitutions in virus already resistant to Lamivudine. Antimicrob Agents Chemother 2004;48(9):3498–507.

175. Langley DR, Walsh AW, Baldick CJ, et al. Inhibition of hepatitis B virus polymerase by entecavir. J Virol 2007;81(8):3992–4001.
176. Tenney DJ, Rose RE, Baldick CJ, et al. Two-year assessment of entecavir resistance in Lamivudine-refractory hepatitis B virus patients reveals different clinical outcomes depending on the resistance substitutions present. Antimicrob Agents Chemother 2007;51(3):902–11.
177. Marcellin P, Heathcote EJ, Buti M, et al. Tenofovir disoproxil fumarate versus adefovir dipivoxil for chronic hepatitis B. N Engl J Med 2008;359(23):2442–55.
178. Sheldon J, Camino N, Rodes B, et al. Selection of hepatitis B virus polymerase mutations in HIV-coinfected patients treated with tenofovir. Antivir Ther 2005; 10(6):727–34.
179. Delaney WE, Ray AS, Yang H, et al. Intracellular metabolism and in vitro activity of tenofovir against hepatitis B virus. Antimicrob Agents Chemother 2006;50(7): 2471–7.
180. Fung S, Mazzulli T, Sherman M, et al. Presence of rtA194T at baseline does not reduce efficacy to tenofovir (TDF) in patients with lamivudine (LAM)-resistant chronic hepatitis B. In: Programs and abstracts of the 58th Annual Meeting of the American Association for the Study of Liver Disease (AASLD). San Francisco, October 31–November 4, 2008 [abstract: 880].
181. Markowitz JS, Martin P, Conrad AJ, et al. Prophylaxis against hepatitis B recurrence following liver transplantation using combination lamivudine and hepatitis B immune globulin. Hepatology 1998;28(2):585–9.
182. Gane EJ, Angus PW, Strasser S, et al. Lamivudine plus low-dose hepatitis B immunoglobulin to prevent recurrent hepatitis B following liver transplantation. Gastroenterology 2007;132(3):931–7.
183. Angus PW, Patterson SJ, Strasser SI, et al. A randomized study of adefovir dipivoxil in place of HBIG in combination with lamivudine as post-liver transplantation hepatitis B prophylaxis. Hepatology 2008;48(5):1460–6.
184. Bock CT, Tillmann HL, Torresi J, et al. Selection of hepatitis B virus polymerase mutants with enhanced replication by lamivudine treatment after liver transplantation. Gastroenterology 2002;122(2):264–73.
185. Fournier C, Zoulim F. Antiviral therapy of chronic hepatitis B: prevention of drug resistance. Clin Liver Dis 2007;11(4):869–92, ix.
186. Lampertico P, Vigano M, Manenti E, et al. Adefovir rapidly suppresses hepatitis B in HBeAg-negative patients developing genotypic resistance to lamivudine. Hepatology 2005;42(6):1414–9.
187. Fung J, Lai CL, Yuen JC, et al. Adefovir dipivoxil monotherapy and combination therapy with lamivudine for the treatment of chronic hepatitis B in an Asian population. Antivir Ther 2007;12(1):41–6.
188. van Bommel F, Wunsche T, Mauss S, et al. Comparison of adefovir and tenofovir in the treatment of lamivudine-resistant hepatitis B virus infection. Hepatology 2004;40(6):1421–5.
189. Sherman M, Yurdaydin C, Sollano J, et al. Entecavir for treatment of lamivudine-refractory, HBeAg-positive chronic hepatitis B. Gastroenterology 2006;130(7): 2039–49.
190. Seifer M, Patty A, Serra I, et al. Telbivudine, a nucleoside analog inhibitor of HBV polymerase, has a different in vitro cross-resistance profile than the nucleotide analog inhibitors adefovir and tenofovir. Antiviral Res 2009;81(2):147–55.
191. Villeneuve JP, Durantel D, Durantel S, et al. Selection of a hepatitis B virus strain resistant to adefovir in a liver transplantation patient. J Hepatol 2003;39(6): 1085–9.

192. Yim HJ, Hussain M, Liu Y, et al. Evolution of multi-drug resistant hepatitis B virus during sequential therapy. Hepatology 2006;44(3):703–12.
193. Brunelle MN, Jacquard AC, Pichoud C, et al. Susceptibility to antivirals of a human HBV strain with mutations conferring resistance to both lamivudine and adefovir. Hepatology 2005;41(6):1391–8.
194. Fung SK, Fontana RJ. Management of drug-resistant chronic hepatitis B. Clin Liver Dis 2006;10(2):275–302, viii.
195. Trojan J, Stuermer M, Teuber G, et al. Treatment of patients with lamivudine-resistant and adefovir dipivoxil-resistant chronic hepatitis B virus infection: is tenofovir the answer? Gut 2007;56(3):436–7 [author reply: 37].
196. Yatsuji H, Hiraga N, Mori N, et al. Successful treatment of an entecavir-resistant hepatitis B virus variant. J Med Virol 2007;79(12):1811–7.
197. Villet S, Ollivet A, Pichoud C, et al. Stepwise process for the development of entecavir resistance in a chronic hepatitis B virus infected patient. J Hepatol 2007; 46(3):531–8.
198. Gish RG, Trinh H, Leung N, et al. Safety and antiviral activity of emtricitabine (FTC) for the treatment of chronic hepatitis B infection: a two-year study. J Hepatol 2005;43(1):60–6.

Fungal Infections in Transplant and Oncology Patients

Anna K. Person, MD[a,*], Dimitrios P. Kontoyiannis, MD, ScD[b], Barbara D. Alexander, MD, MHS[c]

KEYWORDS

- Invasive fungal infection • Transplant • Solid-organ transplant
- Hematopoietic stem cell transplant • Oncology • Fungus

Invasive fungal infections (IFIs) in oncology and transplant populations have been associated with significant morbidity and mortality. Research in this area remains in flux; as epidemiologic patterns shift, more is being learned about optimal treatment and the unique risks that predispose these special populations to such potentially devastating infections. This article highlights recent advances and important factors to consider when treating transplant and oncology patients with IFIs.

EPIDEMIOLOGY OF IFIS

Despite high associated morbidity and mortality, the epidemiology of IFIs in high-risk populations has not previously been well defined. Incidence estimates have been primarily based on single-center, retrospective studies.[1–3] The Transplant Associated Infections Surveillance Program (TRANSNET), a network of 23 transplant centers in the United States, prospectively studied the epidemiology of IFIs among solid-organ and stem cell transplant populations over a 5-year period (March 2001 to March 2006) and provided the first true approximation of the burden of fungal disease among transplant populations in the United States. Based on TRANSNET data, the overall incidence of IFIs in the hematopoietic stem cell transplant (HSCT) population was 3.4%, somewhat lower than previous estimates (DP Kontoyiannis, unpublished data, July 2009). In addition, invasive aspergillosis (IA) surpassed invasive candidiasis (IC) as

This work was supported by Grant No. NIAID K24 AI072522 (BD Alexander) from the National Institutes of Health.

[a] Division of Infectious Diseases, Department of Medicine, Duke University Health System, Duke University School of Medicine, Box 102359, Durham, NC 27710, USA

[b] Department of Infectious Diseases, Infection Control and Employee Health, The University of Texas MD Anderson Cancer Center, 1515 Holcombe Boulevard, Houston, TX 77030, USA

[c] Division of Infectious Diseases, Department of Medicine, Duke University School of Medicine, PO Box 3035, Durham, NC 27710, USA

* Corresponding author.

E-mail address: perso006@mc.duke.edu

Infect Dis Clin N Am 24 (2010) 439–459
doi:10.1016/j.idc.2010.01.002

0891-5520/10/$ – see front matter © 2010 Elsevier Inc. All rights reserved.

the most common IFI encountered in the HSCT population: *Aspergillus* accounted for 43% of infections and *Candida* accounted for 28%, followed by other or unspecified molds including *Fusarium* and *Scedosporium* (16%), and zygomycetes (8%). Pneumocystosis, endemic fungal infections, and cryptococcosis were rarely encountered in the HSCT population. Consistent with previous reports,[4–7] mortality was high and 1-year survival was low for HSCT patients with IFI. Fusarium infections and IA were associated with the lowest 1-year survival (6% and 25%, respectively); however, survival among patients with zygomycosis (28%) and IC (34%) was not substantially better.

Among solid-organ transplant (SOT) recipients, *Candida* infections were significantly more common than *Aspergillus* infections. This distribution held true for all solid-organ groups except lung transplant recipients. In lung transplant recipients, *Aspergillus* was the most common fungal pathogen, and, when coupled with other molds, invasive mold infections were responsible for 70% of IFIs (PG Pappas, unpublished data, July 2009). This distribution has also been shown in other studies of SOT recipients.[8,9] Less common overall, but seen more frequently than in the HSCT population, were infections due to *Cryptococcus* and endemic fungi, causing 8% and 5% of IFIs, respectively. Zygomycetes were responsible for 2% of infections (PG Pappas, unpublished data, July 2009). The mortality associated with IFIs in the SOT population is high, but lower overall than in HSCT and oncology patients.

There are no recent, multicenter studies describing the incidence and clinical outcome of IFIs among the general oncology population, and it is difficult to obtain an accurate estimate of the frequency of fungal infections in this population from the published literature because most reports do not provide sufficient information regarding the patients' underlying disease. In general, compared with patients with solid tumors, patients with hematologic malignancies are at increased risk for fungal disease and response to IFI treatment is lower.[10] A 1992 international autopsy survey of patients with cancer identified fungal infections in 25% of patients with leukemia, 12% with lymphoma, and 5% with solid tumors. Overall, *Candida* was the most common fungal pathogen, responsible for 58% of fungal infections, whereas 30% of fungal infections were caused by *Aspergillus*.[11] A more recent single-center survey of autopsies performed on patients with hematologic malignancy confirmed the increased risk for IFI among patients with leukemia. Consistent with trends among transplant populations, the prevalence of IFI remained high and constant throughout the study period (1989–2003); although the rate of IC decreased, the prevalence of invasive mold infections increased.[12]

TYPES OF IFIS

Aspergillus

Aspergillus fumigatus is the most frequent species of *Aspergillus* causing clinical disease, perhaps due to specific virulence factors unique to the organism.[13] However, other species, most commonly *Aspergillus flavus*, *Aspergillus terreus*, and *Aspergillus niger*, are also implicated in invasive infections in humans. *A terreus* has been associated with amphotericin B resistance and a higher mortality[14] than other *Aspergillus* species, although the data to support this claim were primarily gleaned from patients treated with amphotericin B as initial therapy and before use of triazoles as first-line treatment of IA.[15]

In immunocompromised hosts, *Aspergillus* most commonly presents as invasive pulmonary aspergillosis, often with subsequent dissemination.[16–18] In lung transplant recipients, *Aspergillus* may also cause tracheobronchitis and bronchial anastomotic infection. However, pulmonary infections can present with fever, hemoptysis, cough, dyspnea, reduction in pulmonary function, pleuritic chest pain, respiratory failure, and altered mental status,[19] and the immunosuppressed patient may have few, or only subtle, clinical signs and symptoms present early in the course of infection. The distinction between colonization and infection with *Aspergillus* can be difficult. For example, *Aspergillus* can be recovered from the lower respiratory tract of many patients after lung transplant, but, based on a review of the literature, progression from colonization to infection in lung transplant recipients is rare.[20] In contrast, recovery of *Aspergillus* from lower respiratory tract specimens in patients with hematologic malignancy or undergoing HSCT has a high positive predictive value for invasive disease.[21]

Candida

The overall decrease in *Candida* infections and the shift from *Candida albicans* to non-*albicans* Candida as the most common infecting *Candida* species in the past 2 decades are notable. Data from Brazil collected between 1997 and 2003 document that 79% of episodes of candidemia in patients with hematological malignancies, and 52% in those with solid tumors, were caused by non-*albicans Candida* ($P = .034$).[22] Similarly, between 2001 and 2007 at MD Anderson Cancer Center, non-*albicans Candida* species were responsible for 75% of IC cases occurring in patients with hematologic malignancy or undergoing HSCT.[23] The routine use of azole prophylaxis in high-risk cancer populations has contributed to the decreased incidence of IC in these populations,[24,25] and likely accounts in part for the increasing frequency of infections caused by non-*albicans Candida*.[23,26,27] Although *C albicans* remains the most frequently isolated *Candida* species among SOT recipients, a shift toward more non-*albicans Candida* infections also seems to be occurring in this population.[28]

Infections due to *Candida* can manifest as candidemia, peritonitis, empyema, endopthalmitis, esophagitis, and urinary tract or anastomotic infections. In lung transplant recipients, *Candida* can also cause tracheobronchitis.[29] Presenting clinical signs may be fever, leukocytosis, and, less commonly, hypothermia.[30]

Hyaline Hyphomycetes

The other molds responsible for IFIs in immunosuppressed patients are a heterogeneous group of organisms. More than 30 non-*Aspergillus* hyalohyphomycetes have been implicated in human disease, including species of *Acremonium*, *Fusarium*, *Paecilomyces*, and *Scedosporium*.[31] These organisms are typically opportunistic, causing invasive disease following environmental exposures. Several of the non-*Aspergillus* hyalohyphomycetes are unique in their capability to sporulate in vivo, which permits recovery of the organisms from the bloodstream and dissemination to other organs, particularly skin.[32]

Recently, a shift toward more non-*Aspergillus* mold infections has been noticed in SOT recipients. In a prospective multicenter study, 53 invasive mold infections were reported from liver and heart transplant recipients. Pathogens included *Aspergillus* species in 70%, non-*Aspergillus* hyalohyphomycetes in 9%, phaeohyphomycetes in 9%, zygomycetes in 6%, and other or unidentified molds in 6% of patients. Dissemination was significantly more likely with infection due to a non-*Aspergillus* mold compared with *Aspergillus*.[17]

Zygomycetes

Zygomycetes cause devastating invasive disease in a variety of different hosts. In one review of 929 reported cases of zygomycosis, 36% were seen in patients with diabetes mellitus, 7% in SOT recipients, and 5% in bone marrow transplant recipients.

Among the bone marrow transplant group, slightly more than half (52%) had pulmonary zygomycosis, with 16% having infection in the sinuses. Outcome from zygomycosis varied based on the underlying condition, site of infection, and use of antifungal therapy. For patients with underlying malignancy, overall mortality was 66%.[33] Other studies cite mortalities up to 80% among those with hematologic malignancies.[34] The incidence of zygomycosis seems to be increasing in oncology centers and in HSCT populations specifically, possibly related to the use of voriconazole prophylaxis.[35–39]

Pneumocystis jiroveci

The risk of *Pneumocystis jiroveci* infection (previously *Pneumocystis carinii*) in HSCT and SOT recipients can be as high as 5% to 15% without prophylaxis.[40,41] In the era of routine *P jiroveci* prophylaxis, transplant recipients who develop infection typically do so after stopping their prophylactic regimen.[42] Similarly, patients with cancer who develop *Pneumocystis* infection typically do so in the absence of prophylaxis.[43] *Pneumocystis* has a worldwide distribution and the organism that infects humans has been recognized as unique and distinct from that infecting animals[44]; humans seem to acquire *Pneumocystis* only from other humans, but active pneumonia does not seem to be required for transmission to occur. Serologic data indicate that most humans are infected with *Pneumocystis* within the first 2 to 4 years of life.[45] Immunocompromised patients develop disease as a consequence of reinfection with a new strain, or possibly from reactivation of latent infection. However, it is believed that most cases of *P jiroveci* pneumonia develop following acquisition of a new strain shortly before clinical symptoms manifest.[46]

Particular attention was given to *P jiroveci* infection in SOT recipients in the 1980s given to high rates of infection in heart-lung transplant recipients.[47,48] However, in the era of routine prophylaxis for at least 6 months following the transplant procedure in all solid-organ groups,[41] *Pneumocystis* infections in the SOT population are rare. In one retrospective review of 32,757 kidney recipients transplanted between 2000 and 2004, the cumulative incidence was 0.4%. Patients receiving sirolimus as part of their immunosuppressive regimen had an increased risk of developing *P jiroveci* pneumonia that was associated with increased risk of graft loss and death.[49] The underlying mechanism by which sirolimus predisposes to *P jiroveci* infection is as yet undefined; however, it may ultimately be linked with the ability of sirolimus to cause interstitial pneumonia, a known side effect of the drug.

Cryptococcus

Cryptococcus neoformans and *Cryptococcus gatti*[50] represent the main pathogenic species in the genus *Cryptococcus*.[51] Although cryptococcosis has been most commonly encountered in the HIV-infected population,[52] a multicenter study reporting 306 cases of cryptococcosis in patients who are not infected with HIV found 0.7% of total cases occurred in HSCT recipients, 18% in SOT recipients, 9% in patients with hematologic malignancies, and 9% in patients with other malignancies.[53] Other studies in the United States have found similarly low rates of cryptococcal infection in the HSCT population,[1,5,54] most likely because of the use of routine fluconazole prophylaxis following HSCT. The overall mortality for cryptococcosis in the non-HIV population was 30%, attributable mortality 12%, and hematologic malignancy as an underlying diagnosis was associated with decreased survival.[53]

Cryptococcus infection most commonly involves the lungs and central nervous system, but cutaneous infection and disseminated disease also occur. In one study, heart transplant patients were more likely than other solid-organ groups to develop cryptococcosis, but kidney transplant recipients were most likely to have disseminated disease. This study also showed that serum cryptococcal antigen was not always helpful in identifying isolated pulmonary *Cryptococcus* infection; 82% of patients with cryptococcal pneumonia had a negative serum cryptococcal antigen.[55]

Endemic Fungi

Endemic fungi, including *Histoplasma capsulatum*, *Blastomyces dermatitidis*, and *Coccidioides immitus*, are present in the soil in certain geographic regions, and inhalation of conidia leads to systemic infection.[56] Disease may manifest after primary exposure or through reactivation of a latent focus when there is a decrease in cell-mediated immunity. Pulmonary involvement is common but clinical symptoms are nonspecific and may be subacute in onset.

Although endemic mycoses are rarely encountered in cancer and transplant populations, immunosuppression (defined as hematologic malignancy or treatment with immunosuppressive medications) has been identified as a risk for developing histoplasmosis. Among immunosuppressed patients with histoplasmosis, 74% had fatal or disseminated infections, compared with 7% of patients who were not immunosuppressed.[57] Histoplasmosis is the most frequent endemic mycosis reported in the SOT population[58,59] and it has been transmitted to SOT recipients via the transplanted allograft.[60] Information regarding *B dermatitidis* in transplant populations remains limited to individual case reports and small case series.[61] The largest series included 11 cases in SOT recipients; infection occurred a median of 26 months after SOT and rejection did not precede any case.[62] *B dermatitidis* pneumonia was frequently complicated by acute respiratory distress syndrome and accordingly high mortality (67%).[63] Even in endemic regions, *C immitus* infection is rarely encountered in the HSCT population,[64] and most descriptions are in SOT recipients.[65] As with the other endemic mycoses in the immunosuppressed population, dissemination is common, mortality is high (up to 72%), and infection can be transmitted via donated organs.[66]

TIMING OF IFIS

IFI Timeline: HSCT

Time to development of IFI after transplantation varies according to type of fungal infection, type of transplant, and the use/duration of antifungal prophylaxis. As shown in **Fig. 1**, the timeline for IFIs following HSCT is typically broken into 3 periods, early onset (≤40 days after HSCT), late onset (41–180 days after HSCT), and very late onset (>180 days after HSCT). In the TRANSNET cohort, 66% of *Candida* infections among autologous HSCT recipients occurred within the first 30 days (DP Kontoyiannis MD, unpublished data, July 2009). Similarly, in a single-center study of 655 allogeneic HSCT recipients transplanted between 1994 and 1997 and receiving routine fluconazole prophylaxis, the median time to development of candidemia was day 28 after transplant.[25] A recent multicenter report of IFIs occurring between 2004 and 2007 reported the median timing of IC after HSCT to be 77 days; IC tended to occur earlier after autologous HSCT (median 28 days) compared with allogeneic HSCT (median 108 days).[67] In general, early-onset IC following HSCT is influenced by the presence of neutropenia and mucosal injury (mucositis), whereas later onset is more often seen in allogeneic HSCT recipients owing to the development of graft-versus-host disease (GVHD) and the need for chronic central venous catheters.

Aspergillus and other mold infections tend to occur later after HSCT. In a single-center study of allogeneic HSCT recipients transplanted between 1993 and 1998, 30% of IA diagnoses (N = 187) were early, 53% late, and 17% very late onset following the procedure.[68] In the more recent TRANSNET cohort, 50% of IA cases among

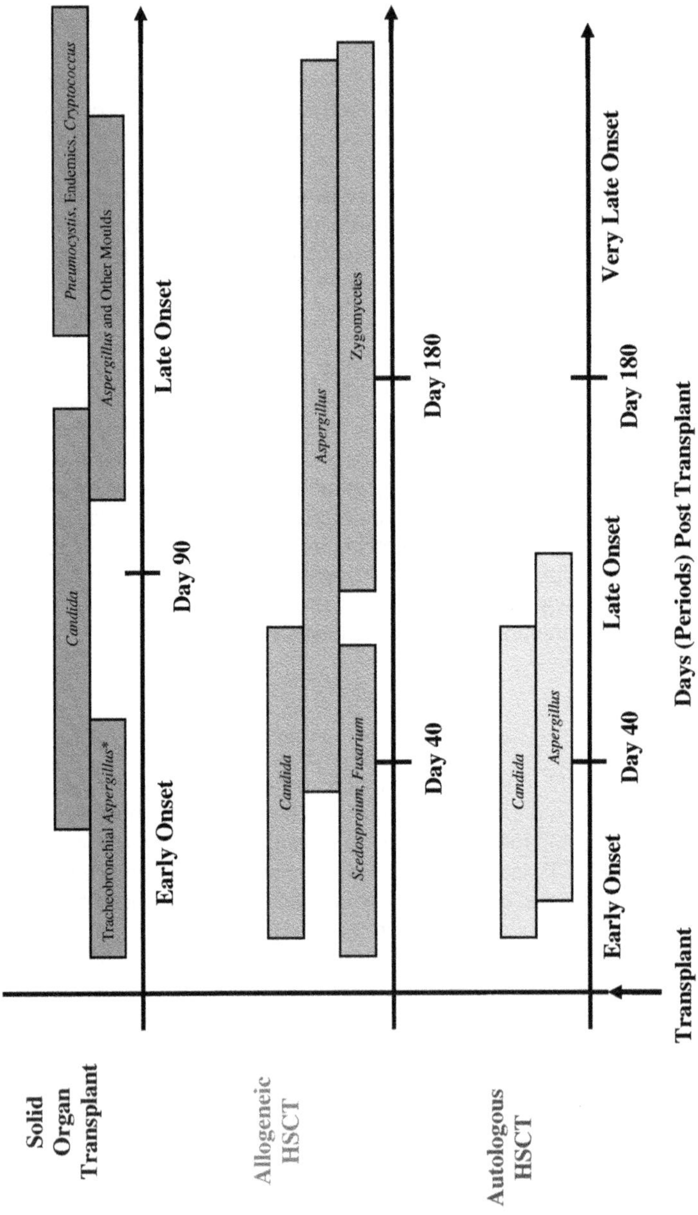

*Unique to lung transplant

Fig. 1. Timing of IFIs based on transplant type.

autologous HSCT recipients were early onset and 24% occurred more than 120 days after onset, whereas 22% of cases among allogeneic HSCT recipients were early onset and 47% occurred more than 120 days after transplant (DP Kontoyiannis, MD, unpublished data, July 2009). In general, IA occurs more frequently and is encountered later after allogeneic HSCT compared with autologous HSCT. Late IA has been associated with a higher mortality, possibly because of increased fungal burden accompanying a delay in diagnosis and the cumulative burden of immunosuppression in patients with chronic/refractory GVHD.[69]

The timing of non-*Aspergillus* mold infections such as zygomycetes, *Fusarium*, and *Scedosporium* seems to be organism specific. One large study of more than 5500 HSCT recipients showed that the majority (56%) of zygomycete infections occurred more than 90 days after transplant, and GVHD was associated with zygomycete infection. However, *Scedosporium* infections were more likely to occur within the first 30 days after transplant.[5] Similarly, nearly half (46%) of patients with fusariosis were neutropenic at the time of diagnosis, and the median time from transplant to diagnosis was 64 days.[6]

IFI Timeline: SOT

The timeline for infections following SOT has traditionally been divided into 3 phases: the first month, months 2 to 6, and more than 6 months after the transplant procedure.[70] Recent data regarding the epidemiology of IFIs following SOT suggest that the timing of fungal infections may no longer conform precisely with these risk windows.

Historically, infections due to *Candida* occurred early after SOT, typically during the transplant hospitalization.[9,71] However, TRANSNET data showed a somewhat later time to onset, with median time to diagnosis of IC of 103 days (PG Pappas MD, unpublished data, July 2009). In addition, a recent Australian study of candidemia in SOT recipients found that 54% of infections developed greater than 6 months after transplant, most of them in renal transplant recipients. Nearly all these patients were hospitalized at the time of diagnosis because of complications from various bacterial infections, and had been receiving broad-spectrum antibiotics.[72]

Most *Aspergillus* infections historically occurred within the first year following SOT.[20,73,74] Tracheobronchial or anastomotic *Aspergillus* infections typically occurred within the first 90 days after transplant, compared with invasive pulmonary aspergillosis that tended to occur later.[73,74] Most experts agree that the risk for IA is high enough immediately following lung transplant to warrant antifungal prophylaxis, and American Society of Transplantation guidelines recommend continuing prophylaxis following lung transplantation at least until bronchial anastomosis remodeling is complete.[75] A 2006 international survey of lung transplant centers revealed that 69% (30/43) used universal antifungal prophylaxis during the immediate posttransplant period as the anastomosis was healing, most commonly an aerosolized formulation of amphotericin B alone or in combination with itraconazole. The median durations of prophylaxis with aerosolized amphotericin B and itraconazole were 30 and 90 days, respectively.[76] In the current era of routine prophylaxis in high-risk organ transplant recipients, nearly one-half of *Aspergillus* infections in SOT recipients occur late (>90 days after SOT) and, as in the HSCT population, late-onset IA has been associated with a higher mortality compared with early-onset infection.[77]

Cryptococcus and the endemic mycoses tend to occur even later in the posttransplant period.[70] In one study of SOT recipients with cryptococcosis, the median time to diagnosis in lung, heart, and kidney transplant recipients was 210, 450, and 630 days, respectively.[55] In the TRANSNET cohort, median time to diagnosis of cryptococcosis was 575 days. Similarly, the median time to diagnosis of the endemic mycoses was 343 days (PG Pappas MD, unpublished data, July 2009), and *P jiroveci* infections are most often seen after routine prophylaxis is stopped, typically more than 180 days after transplant.[49,70,78]

RISK FACTORS DEVELOPING IFIS

Unique Risks for IFIs in HSCT Recipients

Many factors affect a patient's individual risk for fungal disease, including those associated with the host, the transplanted graft, and complications of the procedure. The influence of each factor fluctuates throughout the posttransplant course, creating a dynamic timeline. Host (eg, older age) and transplant variables (eg, human leukocyte antigen mismatch) tend to influence IFI risk early, whereas complications of the transplant procedure (eg, GVHD and cytomegalovirus [CMV] disease) tend to predominate later.[1,2,5,68] Certain biologic factors, such as malnutrition, iron overload, diabetes mellitus, and cytopenias, are influential throughout the posttransplant course.[79] Risk factors specific to early-onset IA have been identified as aplastic anemia, myelodysplastic syndrome, cord-blood transplantation, delayed neutrophil engraftment, and CMV disease. Risks for late-onset IA were multiple myeloma, neutropenia, GVHD, and CMV disease.[68] Iron overload has been shown to be a risk factor for severe bacterial infections in autologous HSCT recipients,[80] and also associated with IA and zygomycete infections.[81] Diabetes mellitus, voriconazole prophylaxis, and malnutrition have also been identified as risks for zygomycosis.[39]

Only a subset of patients who are at risk will actually develop IFI. This fact has led to a growing interest in host genetic differences that may contribute to the individual's risk of developing IFI. Recently, studies in HSCT populations have shown that polymorphisms in Toll-like receptor 4[82] and genetic variations within the plasminogen allele may influence susceptibility to IA after transplant.[83] More research is needed into host genetic influence on the risk of fungal disease following transplant.

Unique Risks for IFIs in Oncology Patients

In patients with acute leukemia, the risk for IC in published reports varies considerably. This is related to the status of leukemia (newly diagnosed, postremission, relapsed, or refractory to treatment), duration of neutropenia, and the types of antineoplastic agents used. Based on a study of patients from Brazil with cancer and with candidemia between 1997 and 2003, in comparison with patients with solid tumors, neutropenia and corticosteroid use were more frequent in the hematologic malignancy group. Only 22% of patients with solid tumors were neutropenic before candidemia. The presence of ileus and the use of anaerobicides were independent risk factors for candidemia in patients with solid cancers. Compared with candidemic patients without cancer, central venous catheters and gastrointestinal surgery were independently associated with candidemia in patients with solid tumor.[22]

Unique Risks for IFIs in SOT Recipients

Rejection and exogenous immunosuppressive agents, particularly high-dose steroids and antilymphocyte antibody treatment, lead to increased risk for IFIs in the SOT population.[84] However, within organ transplant groups, the risk for IFI is strongly influenced by medical and surgical factors including technical complexity. For example, prolonged operative time requiring multiple blood transfusions, reperfusion organ injury during transplantation, or multiple simultaneous organ transplants have all been associated with the development of fungal infections.[85] One study associated prolonged ischemia time with the development of IA in lung transplant recipients.[86] Liver transplant recipients have been shown to be at higher risk for IFIs if there is fulminant hepatic failure, a need to undergo retransplantation, or renal failure. Unique risks for renal transplant recipients include diabetes mellitus or need for prolonged hemodiaylsis before transplant.[87] Factors predisposing to IFI, primarily IC, in pancreas transplant recipients include older donor age, enteric (vs bladder) drainage, pancreas after kidney transplant (vs pancreas alone), the development of posttransplant pancreatitis, retransplantation, and preoperative peritoneal dialysis.[88]

Infection with certain viruses following SOT has also been associated with the development of IFIs. The most frequently implicated virus is CMV. In a prospective study of liver transplant recipients, 36% of patients with CMV disease developed IFIs within the first year after transplant, compared with 8% of those without CMV disease.[89] CMV prophylaxis seems to result in fewer IFIs, which further supports the association.

MANAGEMENT

Management of IFIs involves several components and is pathogen specific. Pharmacologic treatment requires consideration of first- and second-line therapies, potential drug interactions, and the value of combination therapies. The roles of immunomodulation, reversal of neutropenia, and surgery also need to be considered.

Aspergillus

Treatment of IA has evolved in the past decade, but few randomized controlled trials comparing various agents exist. The therapy of choice had historically been amphotericin B deoxycholate, its administration complicated by infusion reactions and renal dysfunction.[90] A randomized controlled trial documented superiority and decreased toxicity of voriconazole over amphotericin B deoxycholate. This landmark study also noted a 12-week survival advantage for patients treated with voriconazole.[91] As a result, voriconazole is now considered the drug of choice for IA.[92]

Complications of voriconazole therapy, as with other azoles, are mainly due to its drug interactions, which are particularly pertinent in transplant populations. Concomitant administration of cyclosporine, tacrolimus, or sirolimus with any azole requires preemptive dose adjustments of the immunosuppressants and subsequent close monitoring.[93] Voriconazole is metabolized through the cytochrome p450 system, and polymorphisms in the CYP2C19 gene can result in widely variable rates of drug metabolism.[94] In addition, response seems to be lower among patients with IA and low mean voriconazole plasma levels (<0.25 μg/mL). Because of these issues, voriconazole levels should be monitored during therapy.[95]

The appropriate choice for therapy in the setting of voriconazole intolerance or failure is a subject of debate. Current Infectious Diseases Society of America (IDSA) guidelines for treatment of IA include echinocandins (caspofungin and micafungin) as an option for salvage therapy, with lipid formulations of amphotericin B, itraconazole, and posaconazole.[92] Posaconazole, another triazole with activity against molds, is available in oral formulation only and shows moderate variability in absorption. In a salvage study for IA in patients previously treated with amphotericin products, favorable response was observed in 42%,[96] and among SOT recipients specifically, 58% had successful outcomes on treatment. As with voriconazole, drug interactions can frequently be seen with posaconazole, absorption is variable, and therapeutic drug level monitoring is encouraged. Treatment-related adverse events included nausea, vomiting, and increased liver function tests (the latter occurring in <3% of patients).[97]

Visual disturbances and certain rashes experienced with voriconazole are not seen with posaconazole treatment. Thus, in some patients intolerant to voriconazole, posaconazole is an acceptable alternative. However, whether failure to respond to voriconazole should prompt the switch to a different antifungal class is a different issue. Research has shown that mutations in the *Aspergillus cyp51A* gene produces clinically significant resistance to the triazoles and different mutations confer unique patterns of azole activity.[98] For example, some mutations lead to high minimal inhibitory concentrations (MICs) for itraconazole and posaconazole, but not voriconazole and ravuconazole, whereas others result in high MICs for all 4 drugs.[99] Thus, in cases of voriconazole failure, susceptibility testing is recommended before switching to another triazole.

Echinocandins, which act by inhibiting the synthesis of β-D-glucan in the cell wall, are generally well tolerated and offer an appealing option for treatment if intolerance to, or failure of, voriconazole develops. Caspofungin was studied alone or in combination in 90 patients with IA refractory to, or intolerant of, other licensed therapy. Favorable response was achieved in 45% and only 2 patients discontinued the drug because of adverse events.[100] Micafungin, in contrast with caspofungin, does not have a formal indication as salvage treatment of IA, but it has been studied for this use. In an open-label, multicenter study of micafungin in the treatment of IA, an overall favorable response rate of 36% was reported.[101] The main drawback to echinocandin therapy is the narrow spectrum of activity and lack of an oral preparation.

There is a need for better outcomes in IA. Although it seems that combination antifungal therapy as primary therapy for IA may confer some benefit, this has not yet been rigorously tested in a controlled trial, and the decision regarding what combination to use is based primarily on in vitro data, retrospective cohort outcomes, and animal data.[102] Only 1, small, prospective randomized trial of combination anti-*Aspergillus* therapy has been published to date. This study included only 30 patients with hematologic malignancy and IA. Patients were randomized to caspofungin plus liposomal amphotericin B (3 mg/kg/d) versus monotherapy with high-dose liposomal amphotericin B (10 mg/kg/d). The combination therapy group had a 66% (10/15) favorable response, which was statistically superior to the 27% (4/15) clinical response in the monotherapy group. However, 12-week survival was not statistically different and there was significantly more nephrotoxicity in patients treated with the high-dose monotherapy. Thus, it is unclear whether the superiority of combination therapy was caused by the lower dose of liposomal amphotericin B or the addition of caspofungin.[103] Another study compared 40 SOT recipients with IA who received caspofungin plus voriconazole as primary therapy with a historical cohort of 47 SOTs treated with a lipid formulation of amphotericin B. Survival at 90 days, the primary end point, was not significantly different between the 2 groups.[104]

A phase III prospective, randomized, double-blind trial comparing voriconazole monotherapy with combination voriconazole plus anidulafungin as primary therapy for IA is currently enrolling and should help definitively establish the efficacy of azole-echinocandin combination therapy for this disease. Until such data are available, combination therapy should be reserved for patients in whom voriconazole monotherapy has failed or is contraindicated, and for patients who are high risk with unusual or resistant isolates.

Candida

Several randomized control trials comparing various antifungals have been performed and are summarized in **Table 1**. In 2009, the IDSA revised its guidelines on the treatment of *Candida* infections, reflecting new data on the use of echinocandins and the

Table 1
Major prospective randomized controlled trials of IC

Author, Year	Comparators	Number Enrolled[a]	Proportion Candidemic (%)	*C albicans* Infections (%)	End of Therapy Success (%)	Significance (*P* Value)	Comments
Rex 1994[122]	Fluconazole	113	100	70	72	0.17	Non-neutropenic population
	Amphotericin B	111	100	63	80		Less toxicity with fluconazole
Rex 2003[123]	Fluconazole plus placebo	107	100	68	56	0.043	Higher APACHE II scores in fluconazole arm Mortality not improved with combination
	Fluconazole plus amphotericin B	112	100	68	69		Higher nephrotoxicity with combination
Kullberg 2005[124]	Voriconazole	248	100	43	70	0.42	Nonblinded, non-neutropenic population
	Amphotericin B followed by fluconazole	122	100	51	74		More renal toxicity and SAEs with AmB
Mora-Duarte 2002[125]	Caspofungin	109	83	36	73	0.09	No difference in mortality
	Amphotericin B	115	79	54	62		More drug-related adverse events with AmB
Kuse 2007[126]	Micafungin	264	83	39	74	NS	12% of study population neutropenic
	LAMB	267	84	43	70		
Reboli 2007[127]	Anidulafungin	127	91	64	76	NS	3% of study population neutropenic
	Fluconazole	118	87	59	60		Microbiologic response higher with anidulafungin
Pappas 2007[128]	Caspofungin	188	86	44	72	NS	9% of study population neutropenic
	Micafungin 100 mg	191	85	48	76		
	Micafungin 150 mg	199	84	51	71		

Abbrevations: AmB, amphotericin B; LAMB, liposomal amphotericin B; NS, not significant; SAEs, serious adverse events.
[a] Modified intent to treat population.

increasing prevalence of non-*albicans Candida* species. For non-neutropenic adults with candidemia, fluconazole, or an echinocandin is recommended as initial therapy. For candidemia in neutropenic patients, initial therapy with a lipid formulation of amphotericin B or an echinocandin is recommended, unless the patient has had limited prior azole exposure, in which case initial therapy with fluconazole is appropriate. Once the infecting pathogen has been identified, treatment can be further tailored. For *Candida glabrata*, treatment with an echinocandin is recommended unless the isolate has been confirmed as susceptible to fluconazole or voriconazole, in which case transition to either drug is appropriate. For *Candida krusei*, which is intrinsically resistant to fluconazole, therapy with a lipid formulation of amphotericin B, voriconazole, or an echinocandin is recommended.[105]

Zygomycetes

Treatment of invasive zygomycosis has evolved to some extent; perhaps most importantly, lipid formulations of amphotericin B have replaced amphotericin B deoxycholate as the cornerstone of primary therapy.[106] Prompt initiation of amphotericin B–based therapy (ie, initiating treatment within 6 days of diagnosis) has been shown to significantly improve outcome.[107] Although it cannot be recommended as primary therapy for zygomycosis on the basis of available data, posaconazole has been increasingly studied as a therapeutic alternative. In one retrospective review of patients who had intolerance to, or progression of, infection on an amphotericin B–based regimen, 66% had a complete or partial response to posaconazole.[108] The zygomycetes include many pathogenic molds, and the MIC of posaconazole varies considerably between these organisms.[109]

Most recently, echinocandins have been shown in vitro to exhibit immunomodulatory activity and synergistic activity in combination with amphotericin B against the zygomycetes.[110,111] Clinical data supporting the addition of an echinocandin to an amphotericin B–based regimen are limited to a retrospective review of 34 diabetic patients with rhino-orbital-cerebral zygomycosis.[112] Treatment was successful for all evaluable patients (n = 6) who received amphotericin B–caspofungin combination therapy, compared with 41% (14/34) in patients treated with amphotericin B monotherapy ($P = .19$). Whether the addition of an echinocandin offers a significant advantage to the patient awaits further clinical study.

Other Molds

Although correlation between in vitro antifungal susceptibility testing of molds and clinical outcomes is limited, information regarding intrinsic patterns of resistance for the various non-*Asperigllus* hyalohyphomycetes has emerged.[31] Many of these molds are intrinsically resistant to available antifungal agents. Susceptibility to amphotericin B and triazoles is variable for *Fusarium*, and the echinocandins offer no activity against this pathogen. Currently, most experts consider voriconazole as first-line therapy for *Fusarium*.[93] Species of *Scedosporium* are considered intrinsically resistant to polyene antifungals and as with *Fusarium*, third generation triazoles are considered first-line therapy for *Scedosporium apiospermum*,[113] however, *Scedosporium prolificans* is intrinsically resistant to all antifungal agents. Data to support the use of combination antifungal therapy for the management of the hyalohyphomycoses are currently limited to those obtained in vitro and case reports.

P jiroveci

Trimethoprim-sulfamethoxazole (TMP/SMX) remains the treatment of choice for *P jiroveci* pneumonia. Oral administration is appropriate for those able to take medication by mouth, given good bioavailability of the TMP/SMX. One of the most problematic side effects of TMP/SMX in the transplant population is cytopenia; all cell lines can be affected and patients must be monitored for this side effect. Duration of therapy for *P jiroveci* pneumonia is generally accepted to be 14 to 21 days. Although data have shown that adding prednisone to the treatment regimen accelerates clinical improvement and improves survival in patients infected with HIV with moderate or severe *P jiroveci* infection, no randomized data are available in cancer or transplant patients to support this practice. However, assuming the patient was not already on corticosteroids at the time symptomatic infection developed, most clinicians presume efficacy based on data from the HIV literature and would consider adding corticosteroids in transplant and other patients who do not have HIV with severe disease. If allergic to, or intolerant of, TMP/SMX, atovaquone, dapsone, or pentamidine have been used as alternative agents.[114]

Cryptococcosis

Treatment recommendations for cryptococcal disease in the transplant population are based largely on data extrapolated from clinical trials in other hosts and expert opinion. Current IDSA guidelines recommend amphotericin B plus flucytosine for 2 weeks, followed by fluconazole orally at 400 to 800 mg for up to 10 weeks, followed by a decreased dose of fluconazole (200 mg) for 6 to 12 months[115] for central nervous system or other severe disease. There are some data to suggest that, in SOT recipients with isolated pulmonary cryptococcosis, prolonged treatment with oral fluconazole is sufficient and induction therapy with amphotericin B may not be necessary.[116]

Several management issues unique to the transplant population need to be considered. Owing to concomitant use of calcineurin inhibitors, lipid formulations of amphotericin B are preferred. In addition, flucytosine levels need to be monitored closely to avoid toxicity and side effects.[117] A gradual decrease in corticosteroids is another common management strategy; however, development of immune reconstitution syndrome (IRIS) in this setting has been seen and may be difficult to distinguish from manifestations of the cryptococcal infection itself.

Other Management Strategies

Reducing immunosuppression requires a delicate balance between improving outcome from infection and inducing rejection of the graft or an accelerated inflammatory reaction. As noted, rapid reduction of immunosuppressive therapy in conjunction with initiation of antifungal therapy in SOT recipients may lead to the development of IRIS, the clinical manifestations of which mimic worsening disease.[118] Reversal of neutropenia is another strategy that is often used in managing IFIs. The updated 2008 IDSA guidelines for treatment of IA include considering the use of a granulocyte-macrophage colony stimulating factor in those with prolonged neutropenia.[92] Granulocyte infusions may also be used as a bridge to recovery from neutropenia, but data to support this practice are scant. In one study of neutropenic patients with hematologic malignancies and IFI refractory to treatment with amphotericin B, 15 patients received granulocyte transfusions from related donors and 8 of the 15 had favorable outcomes.[119]

Surgery

The role of surgery in the treatment of IFIs can be paramount, but its usefulness depends on the type of IFI present. The IDSA recommends that surgery be considered in patients with IA who have a solitary lung lesion before chemotherapy or HSCT, those with hemoptysis from a lung lesion, disease that invades the chest wall, or situations in which the infection involves the pericardium or great vessels.[92] For zygomycosis in particular, treatment often requires surgical intervention in addition to pharmacologic therapy.[120] In one review of 86 cases of pulmonary zygomycosis reported in the literature, mortality was higher (55%) in those not receiving adjuvant surgery compared with those who did (27%).[121] For infections with highly resistant fungi, particularly for localized infection, surgical debridement and debulking should be considered.

SUMMARY

Recent shifts in the epidemiology of IFIs among transplant and oncology populations have led to new recommendations on treatment; however, they have also brought new controversies. New pharmacologic therapies are being studied, alone and in combination, and guidelines for management of several IFIs have been changed accordingly. More information is being discovered about unique genetic factors that put some transplant recipients at greater risk than others for fungal infection. The role of immunomodulation continues to be investigated; as always, the delicate balance of maintaining some immune integrity while assuring protection of the graft remains critical. Despite advances in the field, further studies are needed. For transplant and oncology patients, the diagnosis and management of IFIs remain challenging, and improving outcomes depends on continued progress in all of these arenas.

REFERENCES

1. Martino R, Subira M, Rovira M, et al. Invasive fungal infections after allogeneic peripheral blood stem cell transplantation: incidence and risk factors in 395 patients. Br J Haematol 2002;116(2):475–82.
2. Fukuda T, Boeckh M, Carter RA, et al. Risks and outcomes of invasive fungal infections in recipients of allogeneic hematopoietic stem cell transplants after nonmyeloablative conditioning. Blood 2003;102(3):827–33.
3. Singh N. Antifungal prophylaxis for solid organ transplant recipients: seeking clarity amidst controversy. Clin Infect Dis 2000;31(2):545–53.
4. Gudlaugsson O, Gillespie S, Lee K, et al. Attributable mortality of nosocomial candidemia, revisited. Clin Infect Dis 2003;37(9):1172–7.
5. Marr KA, Carter RA, Crippa F, et al. Epidemiology and outcome of mould infections in hematopoietic stem cell transplant recipients. Clin Infect Dis 2002;34(7): 909–17.
6. Nucci M, Marr KA, Queiroz-Telles F, et al. Fusarium infection in hematopoietic stem cell transplant recipients. Clin Infect Dis 2004;38(9):1237–42.
7. Husain S, Munoz P, Forrest G, et al. Infections due to *Scedosporium apiospermum* and *Scedosporium prolificans* in transplant recipients: clinical characteristics and impact of antifungal agent therapy on outcome. Clin Infect Dis 2005; 40(1):89–99.
8. Pugliese F, Ruberto F, Cappannoli A, et al. Incidence of fungal infections in a solid organ recipients dedicated intensive care unit. Transplant Proc 2007; 39(6):2005–7.
9. Grossi P, Farina C, Fiocchi R, et al. Prevalence and outcome of invasive fungal infections in 1,963 thoracic organ transplant recipients: a multicenter retrospective study. Italian Study Group of Fungal Infections in Thoracic Organ Transplant Recipients. Transplantation 2000;70(1):112–6.
10. DiNubile MJ, Hille D, Sable CA, et al. Invasive candidiasis in cancer patients: observations from a randomized clinical trial. J Infect 2005;50(5):443–9.

11. Bodey G, Bueltmann B, Duguid W, et al. Fungal infections in cancer patients: an international autopsy survey. Eur J Clin Microbiol Infect Dis 1992;11(2):99–109.
12. Chamilos G, Luna M, Lewis RE, et al. Invasive fungal infections in patients with hematologic malignancies in a tertiary care cancer center: an autopsy study over a 15-year period (1989–2003). Haematologica 2006;91(7):986–9.
13. Latge JP. *Aspergillus fumigatus* and aspergillosis. Clin Microbiol Rev 1999; 12(2):323–6.
14. Lass-Florl C, Kofler G, Kropshofer G, et al. In vitro testing of susceptibility to amphotericin B is a reliable predictor of clinical outcome in invasive aspergillosis. J Antimicrob Chemother 1998;42:497–502.
15. Steinbach WJ, Perfect JR, Schell WA, et al. In vitro analyses, animal models, and 60 clinical cases of invasive *Aspergillus terreus* infection. Antimicrobial Agents Chemother 2004;48(9):3217–25.
16. Munoz P, Rodriguez C, Bouza E, et al. Risk factors of invasive aspergillosis after heart transplantation: protective role of oral itraconazole prophylaxis. Am J Transplant 2004;4(4):636–43.
17. Husain S, Alexander BD, Munoz P, et al. Opportunistic mycelial fungal infections in organ transplant recipients: emerging importance of non-*Aspergillus* mycelial fungi. Clin Infect Dis 2003;37(2):221–9.
18. Minari A, Husni R, Avery RK, et al. The incidence of invasive aspergillosis among solid organ transplant recipients and implications for prophylaxis in lung transplants. Transpl Infect Dis 2002;4(4):195–200.
19. Marr KA, Patterson T, Denning D. Aspergillosis. Pathogenesis, clinical manifestations, and therapy. Infect Dis Clin North Am 2002;16(4):878–83.
20. Mehrad B, Paciocco G, Martinez FJ, et al. Spectrum of *Aspergillus* infection in lung transplant recipients: case series and review of the literature. Chest 2001;119(1):169–75.
21. Perfect JR, Cox GM, Lee JY, et al. The impact of culture isolation of *Aspergillus* species: a hospital-based survey of aspergillosis. Clin Infect Dis 2001;33(11): 1824–33.
22. Pasqualotto AC, Rosa DD, Medeiros LR, et al. Candidaemia and cancer: patients are not all the same. BMC Infect Dis 2006;6:50.
23. Sipsas NV, Lewis RE, Tarrand J, et al. Candidemia in patients with hematologic malignancies in the era of new antifungal agents (2001–2007): stable incidence but changing epidemiology of a still frequently lethal infection. Cancer 2009.
24. Goodman JL, Winston DJ, Greenfield RA, et al. A controlled trial of fluconazole to prevent fungal infections in patients undergoing bone marrow transplantation. N Engl J Med 1992;326(13):845–51.
25. Marr KA, Seidel K, White TC, et al. Candidemia in allogeneic blood and marrow transplant recipients: evolution of risk factors after the adoption of prophylactic fluconazole. J Infect Dis 2000;181(1):309–16.
26. Van Burik JH, Leisenring W, Myerson D, et al. The effect of prophylactic fluconazole on the clinical spectrum of fungal diseases in bone marrow transplant recipients with special attention to hepatic candidiasis. An autopsy study of 355 patients. Medicine 1998;77:246–54.
27. Wingard JR. Importance of *Candida* species other than *C. albicans* as pathogens in oncology patients. Clin Infect Dis 1995;20(1):115–25.
28. Horn DL, Neofytos D, Anaissie EJ, et al. Epidemiology and outcomes of candidemia in 2019 patients: data from the prospective antifungal therapy alliance registry. Clin Infect Dis 2009;48(12):1695–703.

29. Palmer SM, Perfect JR, Howell DN, et al. Candidal anastomotic infection in lung transplant recipients: successful treatment with a combination of systemic and inhaled antifungal agents. J Heart Lung Transplant 1998;17(10):1029–33.
30. Fraser VJ, Jones M, Dunkel J, et al. Candidemia in a tertiary care hospital: epidemiology, risk factors, and predictors of mortality. Clin Infect Dis 1992; 15(3):414–21.
31. Alexander BD, Schell WA. Hyalohyphomycosis. In: Kauffman CA, Mandell GL, editors. Atlas of fungal infections. 2nd edition. Philadelphia: Current Medicine Group, Inc; 2006. p. 253–66.
32. Schell WA. New aspects of emerging fungal pathogens. A multifaceted challenge. Clin Lab Med 1995;15(2):365–87.
33. Roden MM, Zaoutis TE, Buchanan WL, et al. Epidemiology and outcome of zygomycosis: a review of 929 reported cases. Clin Infect Dis 2005;41(5):634–53.
34. Kontoyiannis DP, Wessel VC, Bodey GP, et al. Zygomycosis in the 1990s in a tertiary-care cancer center. Clin Infect Dis 2000;30(6):851–6.
35. Trifilio SM, Bennett CL, Yarnold PR, et al. Breakthrough zygomycosis after voriconazole administration among patients with hematologic malignancies who receive hematopoietic stem-cell transplants or intensive chemotherapy. Bone Marrow Transplant 2007;39(7):425–9.
36. Marty FM, Cosimi LA, Baden LR. Breakthrough zygomycosis after voriconazole treatment in recipients of hematopoietic stem-cell transplants. N Engl J Med 2004;350(9):950–2.
37. Siwek GT, Dodgson KJ, de Magalhaes-Silverman M, et al. Invasive zygomycosis in hematopoietic stem cell transplant recipients receiving voriconazole prophylaxis. Clin Infect Dis 2004;39(4):584–7.
38. Imhof A, Balajee SA, Fredricks DN, et al. Breakthrough fungal infections in stem cell transplant recipients receiving voriconazole. Clin Infect Dis 2004;39(5): 743–6.
39. Kontoyiannis DP, Lionakis MS, Lewis RE, et al. Zygomycosis in a tertiary-care cancer center in the era of *Aspergillus*-active antifungal therapy: a case-control observational study of 27 recent cases. J Infect Dis 2005;191(8): 1350–60.
40. Sepkowitz KA. Opportunistic infections in patients with and patients without Acquired Immunodeficiency Syndrome. Clin Infect Dis 2002;34(8):1098–107.
41. *Pneumocystis jiroveci* (formerly *Pneumocystis carinii*). Am J Transplant 2004; 4(Suppl 10):135–41.
42. De Castro N, Neuville S, Sarfati C, et al. Occurrence of *Pneumocystis jiroveci* pneumonia after allogeneic stem cell transplantation: a 6-year retrospective study. Bone Marrow Transplant 2005;36(10):879–83.
43. Torres HA, Chemaly RF, Storey R, et al. Influence of type of cancer and hematopoietic stem cell transplantation on clinical presentation of *Pneumocystis jiroveci* pneumonia in cancer patients. Eur J Clin Microbiol Infect Dis 2006;25(6): 382–8.
44. Kovacs JA, Halpern JL, Swan JC, et al. Identification of antigens and antibodies specific for *Pneumocystis carinii*. J Immunol 1988;140(6):2023–31.
45. Meuwissen JH, Tauber I, Leeuwenberg AD, et al. Parasitologic and serologic observations of infection with *Pneumocystis* in humans. J Infect Dis 1977; 136(1):43–9.
46. Stringer JR. *Pneumocystis*. Int J Med Microbiol 2002;292(5–6):391–404.
47. Dummer JS, Montero CG, Griffith BP, et al. Infections in heart-lung transplant recipients. Transplantation 1986;41(6):725–9.

48. Gryzan S, Paradis IL, Zeevi A, et al. Unexpectedly high incidence of *Pneumocystis carinii* infection after lung-heart transplantation. Implications for lung defense and allograft survival. Am Rev Respir Dis 1988;137(6):1268–74.
49. Neff RT, Jindal RM, Yoo DY, et al. Analysis of USRDS: incidence and risk factors for *Pneumocystis jiroveci* pneumonia. Transplantation 2009;88(1):135–41.
50. MacDougall L, Kidd SE, Galanis E, et al. Spread of *Cryptococcus gattii* in British Columbia, Canada, and detection in the Pacific Northwest, USA. Emerg Infect Dis 2007;13(1):42–50.
51. Chayakulkeeree M, Perfect JR. Cryptococcosis. Infect Dis Clin North Am 2006; 20(3):507–44, v-vi.
52. Mirza SA, Phelan M, Rimland D, et al. The changing epidemiology of cryptococcosis: an update from population-based active surveillance in 2 large metropolitan areas, 1992–2000. Clin Infect Dis 2003;36(6):789–94.
53. Pappas PG, Perfect JR, Cloud GA, et al. Cryptococcosis in human immunodeficiency virus-negative patients in the era of effective azole therapy. Clin Infect Dis 2001;33(5):690–9.
54. Baddley JW, Stroud TP, Salzman D, et al. Invasive mold infections in allogeneic bone marrow transplant recipients. Clin Infect Dis 2001;32(9):1319–24.
55. Vilchez R, Shapiro R, McCurry K, et al. Longitudinal study of cryptococcosis in adult solid-organ transplant recipients. Transpl Int 2003;16(5):336–40.
56. Kauffman CA. Endemic mycoses: blastomycosis, histoplasmosis, and sporotrichosis. Infect Dis Clin North Am 2006;20(3):645–62, vii.
57. Wheat LJ, Slama TG, Norton JA, et al. Risk factors for disseminated or fatal histoplasmosis. Analysis of a large urban outbreak. Ann Intern Med 1982; 96(2):159–63.
58. Peddi VR, Hariharan S, First MR. Disseminated histoplasmosis in renal allograft recipients. Clin Transplant 1996;10(2):160–5.
59. Freifeld AG, Iwen PC, Lesiak BL, et al. Histoplasmosis in solid organ transplant recipients at a large Midwestern university transplant center. Transpl Infect Dis 2005;7(3-4):109–15.
60. Limaye AP, Connolly PA, Sagar M, et al. Transmission of *Histoplasma capsulatum* by organ transplantation. N Engl J Med 2000;343(16):1163–6.
61. Serody JS, Mill MR, Detterbeck FC, et al. Blastomycosis in transplant recipients: report of a case and review. Clin Infect Dis 1993;16(1):54–8.
62. Bradsher RW, Chapman SW, Pappas PG. Blastomycosis. Infect Dis Clin North Am 2003;17(1):21–40, vii.
63. Gauthier GM, Safdar N, Klein BS, et al. Blastomycosis in solid organ transplant recipients. Transpl Infect Dis 2007;9(4):310–7.
64. Glenn TJ, Blair JE, Adams RH. Coccidioidomycosis in hematopoietic stem cell transplant recipients. Med Mycol 2005;43(8):705–10.
65. Blair JE, Logan JL. Coccidioidomycosis in solid organ transplantation. Clin Infect Dis 2001;33(9):1536–44.
66. Wright PW, Pappagianis D, Wilson M, et al. Donor-related coccidioidomycosis in organ transplant recipients. Clin Infect Dis 2003;37(9):1265–9.
67. Neofytos D, Horn D, Anaissie E, et al. Epidemiology and outcome of invasive fungal infection in adult hematopoietic stem cell transplant recipients: analysis of Multicenter Prospective Antifungal Therapy (PATH) Alliance registry. Clin Infect Dis 2009;48(3):265–73.
68. Marr KA, Carter RA, Boeckh M, et al. Invasive aspergillosis in allogeneic stem cell transplant recipients: changes in epidemiology and risk factors. Blood 2002;100(13):4358–66.

69. Upton A, Kirby KA, Carpenter P, et al. Invasive aspergillosis following hematopoietic cell transplantation: outcomes and prognostic factors associated with mortality. Clin Infect Dis 2007;44(4):531–40.
70. Fishman JA, Rubin RH. Infection in organ-transplant recipients. N Engl J Med 1998;338(24):1741–51.
71. Patel R. Infections in recipients of kidney transplants. Infect Dis Clin North Am 2001;15(3):901–52, xi.
72. van Hal SJ, Marriott DJ, Chen SC, et al. Candidemia following solid organ transplantation in the era of antifungal prophylaxis: the Australian experience. Transpl Infect Dis 2009;11(2):122–7.
73. Singh N, Husain S. *Aspergillus* infections after lung transplantation: clinical differences in type of transplant and implications for management. J Heart Lung Transplant 2003;22(3):258–66.
74. Sole A, Morant P, Salavert M, et al. *Aspergillus* infections in lung transplant recipients: risk factors and outcome. Clin Microbiol Infect 2005;11(5):359–65.
75. Fungal infections. Am J Transplant 2004;4(Suppl 10):110–34.
76. Husain S, Zaldonis D, Kusne S, et al. Variation in antifungal prophylaxis strategies in lung transplantation. Transpl Infect Dis 2006;8(4):213–8.
77. Singh N, Limaye AP, Forrest G, et al. Late-onset invasive aspergillosis in organ transplant recipients in the current era. Med Mycol 2006;44(5):445–9.
78. Zaas AK, Alexander BD. Prevention of fungal infections in lung transplant patients. Current Fungal Infection Reports 2008;2:103–11.
79. Garcia-Vidal C, Upton A, Kirby KA, et al. Epidemiology of invasive mold infections in allogeneic stem cell transplant recipients: biological risk factors for infection according to time after transplantation. Clin Infect Dis 2008;47(8): 1041–50.
80. Miceli MH, Dong L, Grazziutti ML, et al. Iron overload is a major risk factor for severe infection after autologous stem cell transplantation: a study of 367 myeloma patients. Bone Marrow Transplant 2006;37(9):857–64.
81. Maertens J, Demuynck H, Verbeken EK, et al. Mucormycosis in allogeneic bone marrow transplant recipients: report of five cases and review of the role of iron overload in the pathogenesis. Bone Marrow Transplant 1999;24(3):307–12.
82. Bochud PY, Chien JW, Marr KA, et al. Toll-like receptor 4 polymorphisms and aspergillosis in stem-cell transplantation. N Engl J Med 2008;359(17):1766–77.
83. Zaas AK. Plasminogen alleles influence susceptibility to invasive aspergillosis. PLoS Genet 2008;4(6):e1000101.
84. Issa NC, Fishman JA. Infectious complications of antilymphocyte therapies in solid organ transplantation. Clin Infect Dis 2009;48(6):772–86.
85. Gabardi S, Kubiak DW, Chandraker AK, et al. Invasive fungal infections and antifungal therapies in solid organ transplant recipients. Transpl Int 2007; 20(12):993–1015.
86. Iversen M, Burton CM, Vand S, et al. *Aspergillus* infection in lung transplant patients: incidence and prognosis. Eur J Clin Microbiol Infect Dis 2007;26(12): 879–86.
87. Singh N. Fungal infections in the recipients of solid organ transplantation. Infect Dis Clin North Am 2003;17(1):113–34, viii.
88. Benedetti E, Gruessner AC, Troppmann C, et al. Intra-abdominal fungal infections after pancreatic transplantation: incidence, treatment, and outcome. J Am Coll Surg 1996;183(4):307–16.
89. George MJ, Snydman DR, Werner BG, et al. The independent role of cytomegalovirus as a risk factor for invasive fungal disease in orthotopic liver transplant

recipients. Boston Center for Liver Transplantation CMVIG-Study Group. Cytogam, MedImmune, Inc. Gaithersburg, Maryland. Am J Med 1997;103(2):106–13.

90. Bowden R, Chandrasekar P, White MH, et al. A double-blind, randomized, controlled trial of amphotericin B colloidal dispersion versus amphotericin B for treatment of invasive aspergillosis in immunocompromised patients. Clin Infect Dis 2002;35(4):359–66.
91. Herbrecht R, Denning DW, Patterson TF, et al. Voriconazole versus amphotericin B for primary therapy of invasive aspergillosis. N Engl J Med 2002;347(6):408–15.
92. Walsh TJ, Anaissie EJ, Denning DW, et al. Treatment of aspergillosis: clinical practice guidelines of the Infectious Diseases Society of America. Clin Infect Dis 2008;46(3):327–60.
93. VFend. Package insert. New York: Pfizer Inc; 2008.
94. Weiss J, Ten Hoevel MM, Burhenne J, et al. CYP2C19 genotype is a major factor contributing to the highly variable pharmacokinetics of voriconazole. J Clin Pharmacol 2009;49(2):196–204.
95. Denning DW, Ribaud P, Milpied N, et al. Efficacy and safety of voriconazole in the treatment of acute invasive aspergillosis. Clin Infect Dis 2002;34(5):563–71.
96. Walsh TJ, Raad I, Patterson TF, et al. Treatment of invasive aspergillosis with posaconazole in patients who are refractory to or intolerant of conventional therapy: an externally controlled trial. Clin Infect Dis 2007;44(1):2–12.
97. Alexander BD, Perfect JR, Daly JS, et al. Posaconazole as salvage therapy in patients with invasive fungal infections after solid organ transplant. Transplantation 2008;86(6):791–6.
98. Pfaller MA, Messer SA, Boyken L, et al. In vitro survey of triazole cross-resistance among more than 700 clinical isolates of *Aspergillus* species. J Clin Microbiol 2008;46(8):2568–72.
99. Rodriguez-Tudela JL, Alcazar-Fuoli L, Mellado E, et al. Epidemiological cutoffs and cross-resistance to azole drugs in *Aspergillus fumigatus*. Antimicrobial Agents Chemother 2008;52(7):2468–72.
100. Maertens J, Glasmacher A, Herbrecht R, et al. Multicenter, noncomparative study of caspofungin in combination with other antifungals as salvage therapy in adults with invasive aspergillosis. Cancer 2006;107(12):2888–97.
101. Denning DW, Marr KA, Lau WM, et al. Micafungin (FK463), alone or in combination with other systemic antifungal agents, for the treatment of acute invasive aspergillosis. J Infect 2006;53(5):337–49.
102. Steinbach WJ, Stevens DA, Denning DW. Combination and sequential antifungal therapy for invasive aspergillosis: review of published in vitro and in vivo interactions and 6281 clinical cases from 1966 to 2001. Clin Infect Dis 2003;37(Suppl 3):S188–224.
103. Caillot D, Thiebaut A, Herbrecht R, et al. Liposomal amphotericin B in combination with caspofungin for invasive aspergillosis in patients with hematologic malignancies: a randomized pilot study (Combistrat trial). Cancer 2007;110(12):2740–6.
104. Singh N, Limaye AP, Forrest G, et al. Combination of voriconazole and caspofungin as primary therapy for invasive aspergillosis in solid organ transplant recipients: a prospective, multicenter, observational study. Transplantation 2006;81(3):320–6.
105. Pappas PG, Kauffman CA, Andes D, et al. Clinical practice guidelines for the management of candidiasis: 2009 update by the Infectious Diseases Society of America. Clin Infect Dis 2009;48(5):503–35.

106. Spellberg B, Walsh TJ, Kontoyiannis DP, et al. Recent advances in the management of mucormycosis: from bench to bedside. Clin Infect Dis 2009;48(12): 1743–51.
107. Chamilos G, Lewis RE, Kontoyiannis DP. Delaying amphotericin B-based frontline therapy significantly increases mortality among patients with hematologic malignancy who have zygomycosis. Clin Infect Dis 2008;47(4):503–9.
108. van Burik JA, Hare RS, Solomon HF, et al. Posaconazole is effective as salvage therapy in zygomycosis: a retrospective summary of 91 cases. Clin Infect Dis 2006;42(7):e61–5.
109. Almyroudis NG, Sutton DA, Fothergill AW, et al. In vitro susceptibilities of 217 clinical isolates of zygomycetes to conventional and new antifungal agents. Antimicrobial Agents Chemother 2007;51(7):2587–90.
110. Lamaris GA, Lewis RE, Chamilos G, et al. Caspofungin-mediated beta-glucan unmasking and enhancement of human polymorphonuclear neutrophil activity against *Aspergillus* and non-*Aspergillus* hyphae. J Infect Dis 2008;198(2): 186–92.
111. Perkhofer S, Locher M, Cuenca-Estrella M, et al. Posaconazole enhances the activity of amphotericin B against hyphae of zygomycetes in vitro. Antimicrobial Agents Chemother 2008;52(7):2636–8.
112. Reed C, Bryant R, Ibrahim AS, et al. Combination polyene-caspofungin treatment of rhino-orbital-cerebral mucormycosis. Clin Infect Dis 2008;47(3):364–71.
113. Perfect JR, Marr KA, Walsh TJ, et al. Voriconazole treatment for less-common, emerging, or refractory fungal infections. Clin Infect Dis 2003; 36(9):1122–31.
114. Kovacs JA, Masur H. Evolving health effects of Pneumocystis: one hundred years of progress in diagnosis and treatment. JAMA 2009;301(24):2578–85.
115. Saag MS, Graybill RJ, Larsen RA, et al. Practice guidelines for the management of cryptococcal disease. Infectious Diseases Society of America. Clin Infect Dis 2000;30(4):710–8.
116. Singh N, Alexander BD, Lortholary O, et al. *Cryptococcus neoformans* in organ transplant recipients: impact of calcineurin-inhibitor agents on mortality. J Infect Dis 2007;195(5):756–64.
117. Dromer F, Mathoulin-Pelissier S, Launay O, et al. Determinants of disease presentation and outcome during cryptococcosis: the CryptoA/D study. PLoS Med 2007;4(2):e21.
118. Singh N, Lortholary O, Alexander BD, et al. An immune reconstitution syndrome-like illness associated with *Cryptococcus neoformans* infection in organ transplant recipients. Clin Infect Dis 2005;40(12):1756–61.
119. Dignani MC, Anaissie EJ, Hester JP, et al. Treatment of neutropenia-related fungal infections with granulocyte colony-stimulating factor-elicited white blood cell transfusions: a pilot study. Leukemia 1997;11(10):1621–30.
120. Ribes JA, Vanover-Sams CL, Baker DJ. Zygomycetes in human disease. Clin Microbiol Rev 2000;13(2):236–301.
121. Lee FY, Mossad SB, Adal KA. Pulmonary mucormycosis: the last 30 years. Arch Intern Med 1999;159(12):1301–9.
122. Rex JH, Bennett JE, Sugar AM, et al. A randomized trial comparing fluconazole with amphotericin B for the treatment of candidemia in patients without neutropenia. Candidemia Study Group and the National Institute. N Engl J Med 1994; 331(20):1325–30.
123. Rex JH, Pappas PG, Karchmer AW, et al. A randomized and blinded multicenter trial of high-dose fluconazole plus placebo versus fluconazole plus

amphotericin B as therapy for candidemia and its consequences in nonneutropenic subjects. Clin Infect Dis 2003;36(10):1221–8.
124. Kullberg BJ, Sobel JD, Ruhnke M, et al. Voriconazole versus a regimen of amphotericin B followed by fluconazole for candidaemia in non-neutropenic patients: a randomised non-inferiority trial. Lancet 2005;366(9495):1435–42.
125. Mora-Duarte J, Betts R, Rotstein C, et al. Comparison of caspofungin and amphotericin B for invasive candidiasis. N Engl J Med 2002;347(25):2020–9.
126. Kuse ER, Chetchotisakd P, da Cunha CA, et al. Micafungin versus liposomal amphotericin B for candidaemia and invasive candidosis: a phase III randomised double-blind trial. Lancet 2007;369(9572):1519–27.
127. Reboli AC, Rotstein C, Pappas PG, et al. Anidulafungin versus fluconazole for invasive candidiasis. N Engl J Med 2007;356(24):2472–82.
128. Pappas PG, Rotstein CM, Betts RF, et al. Micafungin versus caspofungin for treatment of candidemia and other forms of invasive candidiasis. Clin Infect Dis 2007;45(7):883–93.

Parasitic Infections in Solid Organ Transplant Recipients

Patricia Muñoz, MD, PhD[a,b,*], Maricela Valerio, MD[a], Daniel Puga, MD[a], Emilio Bouza, MD, PhD[a,b]

KEYWORDS

- Solid organ transplant • Parasitic infections • Malaria
- Leishmaniasis • Babesiosis • Chagas disease
- Toxoplasmosis • Microsporidiosis

Parasitic infections in solid organ transplant (SOT) are increasingly reported.[1] More organ donors harboring tissue parasites, expanding transplant programs in developing nations, and greater numbers of SOT recipients traveling to endemic areas explain this increase.

Current challenges include delayed diagnosis due to low clinical suspicion and atypical presentations, suboptimal implementation of prophylactic measures, and complicated management because of drug toxicity and interactions.[1]

This article brings parasitic infections into the spotlight and focuses on reviewing current experience in the prevention, presentation, diagnosis, and management of parasitic infection in SOT recipients. For practical purposes, parasites are classified into 3 groups: nonintestinal protozoa, intestinal protozoa, and helminthes.

NONINTESTINAL PROTOZOA

Toxoplasmosis

Microorganism and pathogenesis

Toxoplasma gondii is a ubiquitous, obligate intracellular protozoan that infects humans after ingesting oocysts from soil contaminated with feline excrements or undercooked meat, through vertical transmission or blood transfusion.[2] These parasites cannot complete their reproductive cycle without felines; therefore, cats represent the main

This work was partially supported by Fundación para la Investigación Biomédica del Hospital Gregorio Marañón.

[a] Department of Clinical Microbiology and Infectious Diseases, Hospital General Universitario Gregorio Marañón Doctor Esquerdo 46, Madrid 28007, Spain

[b] Facultad de Medicina, Universidad Complutense de Madrid, Avenue Complutense s/n, Ciudad Universitaria, Madrid 28040, Spain

* Corresponding author. Department of Clinical Microbiology and Infectious Diseases, Hospital General Universitario Gregorio Marañón Doctor Esquerdo 46, Madrid 28007, Spain.

E-mail address: pmunoz@micro.hggm.es

Infect Dis Clin N Am 24 (2010) 461–495
doi:10.1016/j.idc.2010.01.009
0891-5520/10/$ – see front matter © 2010 Elsevier Inc. All rights reserved.

reservoir of infection. *T gondii* persists in human tissues causing latent infection that is asymptomatic in 80% to 90% of cases in normal population.[3] Prevalence in different countries and continents is variable, ranging from 3% to 50%, and related to hygiene and diet.[4]

Transplant recipients may also acquire infection through an infected allograft, mainly when a transplanted organ is the heart and when donor-recipient mismatch (donor seropositive/receptor seronegative [D+/R−]) exists.[5] In this situation, the risk of transmission is greater than 50% in heart transplant (HT) recipients, less than 20% in liver transplant (LT) recipients, and less than 1% in kidney transplant (KT), intestinal transplant, and renal/pancreas transplant recipients.[6] Reactivation of latent infection has also been described in seropositive recipients.[7–12] Nowadays toxoplasmosis in SOT is decreasing due to the widespread use of trimethoprim-sulfamethoxazole (TMP-SMX) prophylaxis.[13]

Clinical picture

Unlike the general population, most SOT recipients with acute toxoplasmosis are symptomatic, developing fever (80%), myocarditis, encephalitis, or choroiditis.[14] Other possible manifestations include skin rash, pneumonitis, generalized lymphadenopathy, testicular masses, or disseminated infection involving brain, heart, lungs, eyes, liver, pancreas, adrenal glands, or kidneys.

T gondii is responsible for 4% to 29% of central nervous system (CNS) lesions in transplant recipients.[15] Symptoms include headache, impaired consciousness, and coma. MRI may reveal periventricular calcifications, affecting primarily the cerebral cortex and basal ganglia and, more rarely, deep-seated ring-enhanced lesions.[2,12]

Retinochoroiditis is usually described 3 to 6 months after transplantation and can lead to extensive macular scarring.[11,16] Yellow and white retinal patches can be seen on fundoscopy.[2] Pulmonary involvement is characterized by bilateral interstitial pneumonia, hypoxemia, and lactic dehydrogenase elevation.[9,17] Chest radiograph findings may mimic *Pneumocystis jiroveci* (bilateral interstitial lung infiltration) or appear as bilateral nodular infiltrates or simply pleural effusion.[17]

Hematologic manifestations of toxoplasmosis include anemia, thrombocytopenia, leukopenia and, in some cases, hemophagocytic syndrome.[18–22] Occasionally the infection is devastating with multiorganic failure and disseminated infection at autopsy.[7,23] In HT recipients, signs and symptoms may simulate organ rejection and in this case visualizing tachyzoites on endomyocardial biopsy is essential for correct diagnosis.

Diagnosis

Three pillars of diagnosis are serology, direct visualization of the microorganism, and polymerase chain reaction (PCR). Seroconversion (from negative to positive) or a 4-fold increase in IgG levels is indicative of active toxoplasmosis. Seroconversion may occur up to 6 weeks after infection in SOT recipients, so clinical suspicion should remain high in mismatched recipients. Asymptomatic seroconversion in a previously seronegative recipient should always prompt treatment in a transplant recipient.[24]

Early diagnosis of disseminated toxoplasmosis can be achieved by identifying tachyzoites with Giemsa or Wright stains in bronchoalveolar lavage (BAL) or bone marrow aspirates. PCR assays can be performed in blood, BAL fluid, or other samples.[25–27] Quantitative real-time PCR on plasma is a highly sensitive and rapid method that may lead to early initiation of specific therapy and increased survival.[7,28] Some investigators also recommend using plasma PCR as a guide to decide when to interrupt anti-*Toxoplasma* prophylaxis.[29]

Treatment

The preferred regime is pyrimethamine (25 to 50 mg/d) in association with folinic acid (5 to 10 mg/d) plus sulfadiazine (1.0 to 1.5 g 4 times a day) for 4 to 6 weeks after resolution of all signs and symptoms.[11,30] Adverse events are common and include bone marrow suppression (due to pyrimethamine), nausea, rash, psychiatric alterations, and nephrotoxicity due to crystalluria (caused by sulfadiazine). Patients with sulfadiazine intolerance can be treated with pyrimethamine (25 to 50 mg/d) and clindamycin (600 mg 4 times a day).[9]

Alternative therapies include TMP-SMX (10 mg/kg/d of the TMP component divided in 2 doses), pyrimethamine (25 to 50 mg/d) plus atovaquone (1500 mg every 12 h), pyrimethamine (25 to 50 mg/d) plus clarithromycin (500 mg every 12 h), pyrimethamine (25 to 50 mg/d) plus azithromycin (900 mg–1200 mg every day) or pyrimethamine (25 to 50 mg/d) plus dapsone (100 mg/d).[31]

Prognosis and prophylaxis

Mortality of disseminated toxoplasmosis in immunocompromised hosts approaches 100% if left untreated.[4,8] Mortality is associated to low clinical suspicion and delayed diagnosis.[12]

Prophylaxis is required for D+/R− HT recipients and the preferred regimen is a double-strength tablet of TMP-SMX 3 times a week during 6 months after transplantation.[32] This regime has the same efficacy as the classic scheme with pyrimethamine and sulfadiazine.[33] Patients with TMP-SMX intolerance may be treated with dapsone (50 mg/d) plus pentamidine (50 mg/wk).[34,35] Despite a lower incidence of toxoplasmosis, in KT and LT recipients mismatched patients should also receive prophylaxis.[22]

Seroconversion during TMP-SMX prophylaxis is a rare event. Seronegative patients who have completed prophylaxis may seroconvert and develop fatal disseminated toxoplasmosis after stopping prophylaxis; therefore, postprophylaxis serologic follow-up is recommended.[4] During the first 6 months after transplantation, SOT-seronegative recipients should undertake precautions avoiding raw meat consumption and exposure to cats.[36]

Leishmaniasis

Microorganism and pathogenesis

Leishmaniasis is caused by a protozoa of the *Leishmania* genus, which is transmitted from wild or domestic animal reservoirs (usually canine) to humans by the bite of a female *Phlebotomus* sand fly.[1,37] The sand flies inject promastigotes into the bloodstream which are carried by circulating macrophages where they transform into amastigotes that multiply in the cell. The infected macrophage eventually ruptures, releasing the amastigotes, which infect other mononuclear phagocytic cells. Infected circulating monocytes are sucked by the vector, where they reproduce as promastigotes, thereby completing the life cycle.[1]

Different species of *Leishmania* are prevalent in different areas of the world. For example, *L donovani* complex (*L donovani*, *L infantum*, and *L chagasi*) is endemic in Mediterranean areas, Middle East and India, Pakistan, China, sub-Saharan Africa, and Latin America whereas *L mexicana* is endemic in Latin America and Texas. There are 3 main forms of leishmaniasis: visceral, mucocutaneous, and cutaneous. Clinical expression depends on the infecting *Leishmania* species and on the host's immune response.[37] Visceral forms, known as kala-azar (black fever in Hindi) are produced by *L donovani* complex, whereas cutaneous forms are produced by *L tropica*, *L mexicana*, or *L major*, among others.[38] Mucocutaneous forms are associated to *L braziliensis* complex.

The overall prevalence of leishmaniasis is estimated to be 12 million cases worldwide[39] but only 62 cases of leishmaniasis have been published in SOT recipients: 49 (79%) in KT, 6 (9.6%) in LT, 3 (4.8%) in HT, 2 (3.2%) in lung transplant, and 1 each (1.6%) in a bone marrow and KT plus pancreas transplant recipient.[40] Active leishmaniasis arises in SOT recipients mainly through reactivation of a prior latent infection associated to postransplant immunosuppression,[1] although transfusion or allograft-related leishmaniasis have also been reported.[41,42]

Clinical picture

Visceral (kala-azar) leishmaniasis and cutaneous leishmaniasis have been reported in transplant recipients. Visceral leishmaniasis in SOT recipients is usually a late disease (median of 32 months after transplantation)[37] and is characterized by fever (84%), splenomegaly (58%), hepatomegaly (27%), weight loss (21%), leukopenia (88%), anemia (77%), thrombocytopenia (68%), pancytopenia (57%), and hypogammaglobulinemia.[40,43] Interstitial pneumonitis,[44] diarrhea, ascites, acute renal failure, high erythrocyte sedimentation rate, and γ-globulin levels have also been reported.[37] Superinfections by bacteria, mycobacteria, viruses, or fungi are common in SOT recipients with visceral leishmaniasis and are sometimes the direct cause of death.[4,45]

Cutaneous leishmaniasis is characterized by the presence of a sore at the bite site, which heals within several months, leaving a scar. *L braziliensis* has been reported to cause simultaneous cutaneous, visceral, and ocular leishmaniasis in KT recipients, which constitutes an exception to the classical species determined pattern of infection.[38,42,46,47]

Diagnosis

Diagnosis usually relies on the visualization of amastigotes in bone marrow smears, generally with Wright-Giemsa stain. The microorganism can also be detected in and cultured from peripheral blood, bone marrow aspirates, spleen, liver, lymph nodes, and skin lesions.[44] BAL provides the diagnosis in 85% of patients with lung involvement.[44] Serology is positive in 75% to 90% of the SOT recipients with leishmaniasis.[40,43] Quantitative PCR in bone marrow or blood specimens is a sensitive diagnostic tool and may be useful in the follow-up to monitor treatment response.

Treatment

Pentavalent antimonials used to be the standard treatment for visceral leishmaniasis, but have now been displaced by liposomal amphotericin B (4 mg/kg/d on days 1 to 5, 10, 17, 24, 31, and 38).[48] Although cure rates are similar with the 2 drugs,[40] side effects, such as pancreatitis and interaction with cyclosporine metabolites associated with antimonials, have pushed them to second-line treatment.[37,49] Some investigators prefer a sequential combination of liposomal amphotericin B and oral miltefosine (2.5 mg/kg by mouth daily for 28 days).[50]

Ketoconazole plus allopurinol during 21 days and itraconazole are other alternatives in cutaneous leishmaniasis but are not frequently used due to moderate efficacy. When using azoles, interaction with cyclosporine and tacrolimus should be kept in mind.[47,51]

Prognosis and prophylaxis

Early diagnosis is a key prognostic factor in SOT patients and mortality is higher when treatment is delayed, reaching 27.7% in some series.[43,52] Close follow-up is essential because relapse is common (30%) 2 months to 1 year after completing antileishmanial treatment.[43,51] The need for secondary prophylaxis is not well established in SOT patients, but some investigators have administered fluconazole, antimonials, or liposomal amphotericin B.[41,53]

SOT recipients should avoid exposure and caring directly for domestic animals, at least early after transplantation.[52] A clinical history to assess travel to endemic areas should always be performed and in endemic countries *Leishmania* serologic pretransplantation donor and recipient screening is advisable.

Malaria

Microorganism and pathogenesis

Malaria is a vector-borne disease caused by *Plasmodium*, which is a prevalent protozoon in tropical and subtropical regions. Transmission occurs primarily through the bite of an infective female *Anopheles* mosquito. Vertical transmission, blood and platelet transfusions and bone marrow and organ transplantation are also possible sources of infection. *P falciparum, P ovale, P vivax, P malariae*, and, recently, *P knowlesi*, have been recognized to cause malaria in humans.[54]

Overall, malaria is present in 109 countries (http://www.who.int), mainly in Southeast Asia, Latin America, and sub-Saharan Africa. The World Health Organization (WHO) reported 247 million cases of malaria in 2006, causing nearly 1 million deaths, mostly among African children. To the best of the authors' knowledge, 40 cases of malaria in SOT recipients have been reported to date. Malaria is more common in KT recipients (27 cases, 67.5%),[6,55–69] followed by LT (9 cases, 22.5%)[67,69–76] and HT patients (4 cases, 10%).[67,69,77] In some endemic countries, such as the Philippines, the frequency of malaria in renal transplant has been estimated to be 1.2%.[78]

One study showed that malaria in transplant patients is mainly transmitted via the allograft (77.5%) followed by blood transfusion (7.5%) and mosquito bites (2.5%). In the remaining 12.5% the source of infection was unclear. The most common species causing malaria in SOT is *P falciparum* (48.5%), followed by *P vivax* (30.3%).

Clinical picture

Clinical manifestations of malaria in SOT recipients are often nonspecific and include fever, chills, myalgia, headache, cough, nausea, vomiting, and diarrhea.[79] Many non-immunocompromised patients and SOT recipients do not necessarily express the classically described malaria fever patterns (every 48 hours in *P vivax* and *P ovale* infections and every 72 hours in *P malariae* infection). Different studies showed a mean interval between transplant and onset of symptoms of 10 to 21 days.[55,68]

Malaria due to *P falciparum* causes most lethal infections and may course with severe hemolytic anemia, hyperthermia, and seizures that may occur several days after the onset of symptoms. Hypoglycemia is common and can lead to coma. Other complications include acute abdominal pain, renal insufficiency, rapidly fatal noncardiogenic pulmonary edema, and acute respiratory distress syndrome, appearing generally in later stages of the disease.[80] Radiologic signs of lung or cerebral malaria are generally nonspecific. Chest radiograph may reveal lobar consolidation, diffuse interstitial edema, and pleural effusion.[80] Cranial CT usually shows cerebral edema, and on MRI diffuse edema and multifocal cortical or subcortical lesions that enhance with gadolinium can be seen. In fatal cases of cerebral malaria transtentorial herniation can be detected on CT or MRI.[81,82]

In KT recipients, reported complications include acute renal failure, nephrotic syndrome, and intravascular coagulation.[55,66] LT recipients may present elevated aminotransferases and cholestasis.[70,83] There are few cases of malaria in HT recipients, but cases of severe disease with fatal outcome despite treatment have been reported.[77]

Diagnosis

Diagnosis is made by microscopic examination of Giemsa-stained thick or thin blood smears. Microscopy allows quantification of parasitemia, which is related to the prognosis and is useful for monitoring response to treatment. In expert hands, sensitivity is excellent, allowing the detection of densities as low as 5 to 10 parasites/μL.[84] Hyperparasitemia is defined by the WHO as a parasite density greater than or equal to 500,000/mm^3 (10% parasitemia) and is associated with severe anemia, hypoglycemia, cerebral malaria, and renal failure.[31] Diagnostic errors occur more commonly in patients with low-density parasitemia (10 to 100 parasites/μL).[85] Given the cyclic nature of parasitemia, smears should be evaluated every 6 to 12 hours before malaria is ruled out. The first smear is positive in 95% of the cases.[86]

Rapid diagnostic tests are useful because they do not require expertise in microscopic examination. Different types of dipstick tests are commercially available; sensitivity ranges from 77% to 100% and specificity from 83% to 100%.[31] These tests provide species identification as well. A nested, multiplex real-time PCR can detect parasites down to a level of 1 to 5 parasites/μL of blood. PCR can also detect mixed-species infections.[87,88]

Detection of malaria antibodies is of no value for diagnosing acute disease and is used for epidemiologic studies.

Treatment

Choice of treatment in SOT follows the same rules as in the general population and depends on the infecting *Plasmodium* species and the geographic location. *P falciparum* is responsible for the most complicated and lethal form of malaria and is frequently resistant to chloroquine. The WHO now recommends artemisinin-based combination therapy (ACTs) for treating uncomplicated malaria. The ACTs combine an artemisinin-derivative with another longer-lasting drug reducing the risk of developing resistance.[89] Updated guidelines for the treatment of malaria can be consulted at http://apps.who.int/malaria/treatmentguidelines.html. A main issue regarding malaria treatment in SOT recipients is drug interaction, because chloroquine may increase cyclosporine levels and doxycycline and mefloquine may increase cyclosporine and tacrolimus levels. Serum levels of immunosuppressant medications should be carefully monitored before initiating and after stopping malaria prophylaxis and treatment.[68,90]

Another concern in LT recipients is the hepatotoxic effects of some antimalarial drugs (quinine, mefloquine, artemisin, artesunate, artemotil, atovaquone, and tetracycline) that can even be fatal in LT recipients.[67] Quinine must always be adjusted to hepatic dysfunction.

Prognosis and prophylaxis

The authors' review of the literature shows that overall malaria mortality in SOT recipients was 10%, although it reached 40% in some series.[78] Prognosis is influenced by the type of transplantation (worse for LT and HT recipients), the infecting *Plasmodium* species, the immunosuppressive therapy, and delayed treatment.[55,69]

SOT recipients traveling from malaria-free areas to disease hot spots are especially vulnerable to infection and chemoprophylaxis is strongly recommended.[60,91] The prophylactic regimen chosen must take into account the geographic region that will be visited, past medical history of the patient, and possible interactions with immunosuppressive therapy. Travelers to chloroquine-resistant malarial endemic regions need prophylaxis with atovaquone-proguanil, mefloquine, or doxycycline.[92] Patients living in endemic areas may benefit from a short-term prophylaxis course (proguanil hydrochloride [200 mg/daily]) for 4 weeks after transplantation.[60] The use of long-lasting insecticides and bed nets to avoid mosquito bites is also advisable. Only 25% of all the SOT recipients that traveled to malaria-endemic areas adhered to mosquito prevention measures.[91]

As migration of populations around the world increases, individuals infected with malaria are more likely to be encountered as potential organ and blood donors. To rule out malaria in donors recently traveling to or emigrating from endemic areas, a meticulous history, thick blood films, and PCR (to exclude cases with low parasitemia) should be obtained.[13]

Babesiosis

Epidemiology/life cycle/microbiologic facts

Babesiosis is caused by a protozoon of the genus, *Babesia*. Although more than 100 species have been reported, only a few have been identified as causing human infections. The 2 main species responsible of human infection are *B microti* and *B divergens*. *B microti* is endemic mainly in the northeast coastal region of United States, and cases of babesiosis caused by *B divergens* have been reported mostly in Europe.[93] *Babesia* infects erythrocytes of wild and domestic animals and is transmitted to humans by a deer tick (*Ixodes scapularis*), which is considered the definitive host. This tick is also the vector of Lyme disease and ehrlichiosis. Once inoculated in the human, *Babesia* sporozoites infect red blood cells and undergo asexual replication (budding) causing erythrocyte lysis. Multiplication of the blood stage parasites is responsible for the clinical manifestations of the disease. Humans are, for all practical purposes, dead-end hosts and there is probably little, if any, subsequent transmission that occurs from ticks feeding on infected persons. Babesiosis may also be acquired by blood and pooled platelet transfusions.[94,95] Human babesiosis is a rare condition and, to the best of the authors' knowledge, only 6 cases have been described in SOT (4 in KT, 1 in LT, and 1 in HT) recipients who acquired the diseases by blood transfusion, tick bite, or unknown mechanisms.[96–100]

Clinical picture

Incubation period is shorter in transfusion acquired infections (1–9 weeks) than in those acquired by tick bites (1–12 weeks).[101,102]

Clinical manifestations mimic those of malaria with malaise, fever, myalgias, arthralgias, and dark urine. Mild splenomegaly and hepatomegaly are also common.[103,104] Laboratory markers include hemolytic anemia, leukocytosis, thrombocytopenia, hemoglobinuria, and elevated liver enzymes.

In normal hosts, infection is usually self-limited, but splenectomy and other types of immunosuppression facilitate the possibility of severe disease.[98,105] SOT patients, in particular those with concomitant asplenia, constitute a group at risk for severe evolution. They may present with disseminated intravascular coagulation, congestive heart failure, acute respiratory distress syndrome, splenic infarcts or rupture, and renal failure.[106–108] Hemophagocytic syndrome has been described in asplenic KT recipients[97,99] and fatal cases of babesiosis with jaundice, intravascular hemolysis, and liver enzymes elevation in asplenic LT recipients.[109]

Diagnosis

Babesiosis must be ruled out in all transplant recipients with a malaria-like syndrome. A history of no travel to endemic areas should not exclude this potential diagnosis. The main diagnostic method is microscopic examination of thin blood smears (Wright or

Giemsa stains) but it requires expertise. Thick blood smears are not recommended, because babesial parasites may be too small to be visualized. Identification of the parasite may require multiple blood smears over several days if low numbers of red blood cells are parasitized (particularly at the onset of symptoms).[102] *B microti* appears as an oval ring and may be mistaken for *P falciparum* trophozoites, although the former does not produce hemozooin.

Serologic indirect immunofluorescence tests may detect IgM or IgG antibodies and prove useful for screening in blood donors and asymptomatic individuals, but unfortunately they are not universally available.[102] Titers greater than or equal to 1:64 are considered positive by most laboratories. IgM titers greater than or equal to 1:64 suggest acute infection whereas IgG titers greater than or equal to 1:1024 reflect active or recent infection. Other diagnostic methods include PCR-based amplification of the babesial 18S ribosomal RNA gene and could be especially useful in cases with low parasitemia.

Treatment

Treatment depends on the clinical severity and the involved species. In *B microti* mild forms, the preferred regimen is a well-tolerated combination of atovaquone (750 mg orally twice a day) plus azithromycin (500–1000 mg orally on day 1 and thereafter 250 mg/d) for a total of 7 to 10 days. In severe forms, clindamycin (300–600 mg intravenously 4 times a day or 600 mg orally 3 times a day) plus quinine (650 mg orally 3 or 4 times a day) for a total of 7 to 10 days is the treatment of choice.[110] In nonresolving cases, repeating a course of 1 of the regimens for 7 to 10 days could be effective.[111] In cases of *B divergens* infection, intravenous clindamycin (600 mg 3 or 4 times a day) plus oral quinine (650 mg 3 times a day) for a total of 7 to 10 days is the preferred treatment.[111,112] Persistent and relapsing babesiosis, occurring in immunosuppressed patients, may require prolonged treatment ($\geq$6 weeks).[113] Partial or complete red cell exchange transfusion may be required as salvage therapy of severe babesiosis with renal, hepatic, pulmonary involvement, anemia (hemoglobin $\leq$10 g/dL), and more than 10% of parasitemia.[114]

Prognosis and prophylaxis

SOT recipients traveling to endemic regions must adhere to standard recommendations to avoid tick bites. In the United States, saving the tick and submitting it to a laboratory allows for PCR identification of *Borrellia*, *Babesia*, *Ehrlichia*, *Bartonella*, and *Rickettsia*. There is no role for antimicrobial prophylaxis in SOT recipients. There is not a screening recommendation of blood donations to exclude babesiosis in most areas of the world.

American Trypanosomiasis

Epidemiology/life cycle/microbiologic facts

Chagas disease (also known as American trypanosomiasis) is produced by the hemoflagellate protozoan, *Trypanosoma cruzi*, and is transmitted by the triatominae insect, or kissing bug. In Latin America, the estimated prevalence is 13 to 18 million people are infected with the disease.[115] Chagas disease also occurs in nonendemic areas where it may be acquired through congenital transmission, blood or platelet transfusion, and organ transplantation.[115,116] In nonendemic countries, with a high percentage of immigrants from endemic regions, the risk of transmission through blood transfusion is present. This was demonstrated by 2 studies in southern California where a 0.1% of blood donors and 0.25% of solid organ donors presented anti–*T cruzi* antibodies.[117,118]

Acute Chagas disease in SOT recipients may result from blood transfusions or allograft transmission or as a reactivation of a chronic infection in the context of immunosuppression. Transmission of *T cruzi* by KT, HT, and LT from donors infected with the parasite has been reported.[119–122] Newly acquired *T cruzi* infection is of special concern in SOT recipients because of their limited immunologic ability to respond.[123]

Heart failure due to chronic Chagas disease is an important cause of HT in Latin America, representing approximately 22% of all the HTs in countries, such as Brazil.[124] Reactivation of Chagas disease is possible in these patients, especially after rejection or severe immunosuppression.[123]

Clinical picture

The majority of infected persons are asymptomatic and remain undiagnosed.[125] The heart, gastrointestinal tract, and CNS are the main target organs in *T cruzi* infection, but the parasite can be found in other organs and tissues,[126,127] including bone,[128] cartilage, and cornea.[129]

Acute and chronic Chagas disease present 2 distinct clinical syndromes. In the acute phase patients may have fever, malaise, lymph node swelling, and hepatosplenomegaly. Life-threatening myocarditis or meningoencephalitis can also occur. In the chronic phase, 60% to 70% of infected individuals remain asymptomatic, but the rest may progress to megaesophagus, megacolon, or cardiomegaly within 10 to 30 years.[17]

Clinical symptoms of Chagas disease in HT recipients with allograft-acquired infection include myocarditis, diarrhea, abdominal rash, and fever. In some cases, acute Chagas can be confused with organ rejection.[125] Endomyocardial biopsy may reveal amastigotes, and trypomastigotes may be found in a thin blood smear.[125]

Reactivation of Chagas disease in HT recipients occurs early after transplant. Clinical manifestations are myocarditis, fever, and rash and outcome is usually poor. This could be due to accelerated amastigotes reproduction leading to increased parasitemia and tissue invasion.[130]

Chagas disease in KT and LT recipients is mainly related to allograft transmission, appearing generally during the first year after transplantation. Clinical manifestations include myocarditis, panniculitis and encephalitis. Asymptomatic parasitemia is the most frequent event, however.

Diagnosis

Early diagnosis and timely treatment of Chagas disease in immunosuppressed patients is essential for a favorable prognosis.[130] The main diagnostic test for acute infection is detection of trypanosomes by microscopic examination. Circulating parasites are motile and can be seen in wet preparations of blood or buffy coat viewed under a cover slip or in microhematocrit tubes. Giemsa-stain smears are also useful. The parasite can be visualized in samples of endomyocardial biopsy, lymph nodes, pericardial fluid, cerebrospinal fluid, and, rarely, bone marrow aspirates.[31] Xenodiagnosis and culture are not practical and are now rarely used.

In the immunocompetent host, serologic tests are useful in diagnosing chronic phases[13]; this does not always apply to the immunocompromised host because seroconversion does not always occur.[119] Moreover, serology has high number of false-negative results (41%). PCR may substantially improve diagnosis in this scenario. Unfortunately PCR is not universally available.[131]

Treatment

Benznidazole or nifurtimox are used in the acute phase of Chagas disease and in cases of reactivation. Benznidazole (5 to 7 mg/kg per day for 60 days) is the drug of choice. Alternative treatment is nifurtimox (8 to 10 mg/kg per day for 90 to 120 days). Both drugs should be administered in divided doses at 8- to 12-hour intervals.[31] Adverse effects of benznidazole are rash, polineurophathy, myelotoxicity, and hepatotoxicity.

The role of antiparasitic therapy in the chronic phase of Chagas heart disease is uncertain.[31] A potential benefit of treating chronic disease is parasitemia suppression, which might improve prognosis and delay ventricular failure and is, therefore, advisable for certain patients.[132] When treating chronic disease, benznidazole (5 mg/kg per day for 30 days) is used.[133]

Prognosis and prophylaxis

Fatality rate in immunocompetent patients is about 5% in the acute phase and unknown in chronic disease because it is difficult to assess.[134]

Chemoprophylaxis is indicated for patients with chagasic cardiomyopathy who undergo cardiac transplantation to prevent disease reactivation. These patients should be carefully followed-up (with serology and parasitemia) to detect a posttransplant reactivation.

Routine serologic testing of organ and blood donors should be performed in all endemic areas of Chagas disease. Latin American immigrants that became blood donors or organ donors/recipients should also be screened. Any organ or tissue from a seropositive donor must be regarded as potentially infectious. The risk may depend on factors, such as donor parasite load and the specific organ or tissue involved. *T cruzi*–positive donor organs may be transplanted into –negative recipients when no alternative exists, especially in circumstances of organ scarcity and a high prevalence of positive Chagas serology in the general population.[130] The use of a heart from a patient with chronic infection is an absolute contraindication given the risk of development of chagasic myocarditis due to the immunosuppression. There is no consensus about renal, pulmonary, and hepatic grafts of seropositive donors but in some countries of Latin America they are used for transplant. Close follow-up with serologic and parasitologic methods starting in the first week posttransplant is recommended. Immediate treatment with benznidazole for 30 to 60 days or nifurtimox for 90 to 120 days should be started upon finding evidence of infection.

SOT recipients traveling to Latin America and those who are permanent residents of endemic areas should be advised to avoid rural areas where the triatomine insect dwells. Slaughterhouse workers, landscapers, hunters, and forestry workers are all at increased risk for Chagas disease. SOT recipients must avoid all these occupational activities during the first 6 months after transplantation.[36]

Free-Living Amebas

There are several species of free-living amebas with a wide distribution in the environment. Infection is rare but severe diseases in humans are mainly caused by *Acanthamoeba castellani*, *Naegleria fowleri*, and *Balamuthia mandrillaris*. When swimming in freshwater (rivers, lakes, and swimming pools), amebas can access the olfactory or corneal epithelium and reach the CNS triggering infection. In most cases, infection is acquired through use of contaminated contact lens cleaning solutions.

Acanthamebiasis typically complicates corneal transplant, leading to keratitis, corneal opacities, and perforation. In other cases, it produces granulomatous amebic encephalitis. Disseminated acanthamebiasis is a rare disease that occurs predominantly in patients with HIV infection. Few cases have been reported in transplant patients: 1 bone marrow, 1 peripheral stem cell, and 1 KT recipient.[1] The KT recipient developed an unusual presentation with osteomyelitis and widespread cutaneous lesions. A fatal outcome was inevitable and autopsy provided the diagnosis.[135]

Naegleria fowleri is a rare but rapidly lethal cause of meningoencephalitis. In SOT recipients no cases of this infection have been described. One case of amebic meningoencephalitis diagnosed post mortem, however, was reported in a liver and kidney donor; fortunately, none of the recipients developed the disease.[136]

INTESTINAL PROTOZOOS

Microsporidiosis

Epidemiology/life cycle/microbiologic facts

Microsporidia are unicellular, spore forming, and obligate intracellular parasites. *Microsporidia* phylum includes 1200 species but only 14 of them infect human beings. The most prevalent species are *Enterocytozoon bieneusi* and *Encephalitozoon* spp.[137] Zoonotic transmission can result from contact with domestic, farm, and wild animals.[138] Contaminated irrigation waters are responsible for food and water transmission.[139] Cases of sexual transmission of *Encephalitozoon* species may also occur.[140] After ingestion, the organism replicates in the small intestine villus epithelium, reducing villus height and surface area, generating malabsorption and diarrhea.[141]

Microsporidiosis has a worldwide distribution but it is an uncommon disease in immunocompetent hosts, with most cases described in HIV patients.[142] To the best of the authors' knowledge, in transplant recipients a total of 18 cases have been reported, 3 in BMT recipients and 15 in SOT. The majority of them were produced by *E bieneusi*.[143–158] More than half of the cases are reported in KT recipients (8); the others were liver (4) and heart, heart/lung, and pancreas/kidney (1 each).[143–155,158] It is unknown if the infection is donor related or acquired by the host in the posttransplant period.[1] *Microsporidia* infection emerges a median of 16 months after transplant and it has been associated with aggressive immunosuppression in the setting of allograft rejection.[150]

Clinical picture

Immunocompetent individuals are usually asymptomatic, although children or travelers who are immunologically naive to *Microsporidia* may develop self-limited diarrhea.[159,160] Clinical presentation in SOT recipients resembles microsporidiosis in the HIV population, consisting of chronic diarrhea with massive weight loss and sometimes fever.[147] In some cases it also produces a focal infection of the biliary tract leading to cholangitis or cholecystitis.[161] Disseminated microsporidiosis affecting ileum, colon, liver, CNS, upper and lower respiratory tracts, and the grafted kidney has been described.[143,144,146] Dissemination may occur after infection of the peritoneal cavity, as described in a pancreas/kidney recipient with duodenal-vesicular anastomoses leakeage.[145] *Encephalitozoon* species and *E cuniculi* are the more common microorganisms related to invasive disease.[145] Mortality of disseminated microsporidiosis in transplant recipients is high (33%).

Fluctuating serum levels of tacrolimus due to intestinal malabsorption may complicate the management of these patients.[151] Some transplant recipients may only respond when immunosuppression is reduced. In 2 renal transplant recipients, symptoms disappeared and stool analysis became negative only after mycophenolate mofetil was replaced by azathioprine.[147]

Diagnosis

Microsporidia spores can be detected in stool or tissue specimens. Transmission electron microscopy (TEM) is the diagnostic gold standard and also allows species identification.[162] Because TEM is time consuming, however, light microscopy with a modified trichrome stain is more commonly used. With this method, microsporidia spores appear pink against a blue-green background. Fluorescent brighteners (Calcofluor White, Uvitex 2B, and Fungi-Fluor) that target the chitinous spore wall are also available but are not useful for species identification. These stains can be used in stool samples, intestinal fluid, and paraffin biopsy sections. Because the kidney is a common site of disseminated infection in KT recipients, examination of urine samples is likely to improve detection of systemic infections.[142] Immunofluorescent antibody staining may be used for species-specific identification (sensitivity 83%, specificity 96%).[163–165]

Serologic assays have been developed and used for epidemiologic studies but are not useful in immunosuppressed patients because of high number of false-negative results.[166]

PCR-based methods amplifying microsporidial ribosomal DNA genes may also improve sensitivity and specificity, but this technique is limited to research laboratories.[142,167]

Treatment

E intestinalis infections usually respond to albendazole treatment (400 mg 2 times per day for 2–4 weeks). *E bieneusi* response to albendazole is variable, however.[168] Recently, some investigators reported that a 7-day course of fumagillin was successful in renal and LT recipients. The mechanisms by which fumagillin inhibits microsporidial replication are poorly understood but it has proved effective in the treatment of *E bieneusi* infection.[169,170] Thrombocytopenia and neutropenia are well-known side-effects that fortunately resolve after drug withdrawal.[149]

Alternative drugs are metronidazole and nitazoxanide. In some cases metronidazole provides transient clinical improvement but fails to achieve clearance of the organism or permanent symptomatic relief.[171]

Prognosis and prophylaxis

Chlorine and ozone successfully disinfect *E intestinalis*–contaminated water.[142] General hygienic measures, such as washing vegetables with chlorine before consuming and drinking bottled water, could prevent microsporidiosis in SOT recipients.

Cryptosporidiosis

Epidemiology/life cycle/microbiologic facts

Cryptosporidiosis is caused by intracellular protozoa belonging to the phylum Apicomplexa. The most prevalent species producing gastrointestinal infection in humans are *C parvum* followed by *C hominis* and *C meleagridis*.[172,173]

Infection is acquired through person-to-person contact, contact with animals, or ingesting contaminated water or food. Oocyst ingestion is followed by excystation and release of sporozoites on contact with bile salts. Sporozoites enter the brush border surface of intestinal epithelium and develop into merozoites capable of replicating asexually or sexually. Oocysts result from sexual reproduction, some sporulate and persist, whereas others are excreted in stools. Systemic dissemination essentially does not occur but occasional biliary tract or respiratory tract infections in immunocompromised patients may result from migration through the intestinal luminal surface.[174]

Prevalence ranges from 1% to 3% in industrialized countries and approximately 10% in developing countries.[175] *Cryptosporidium* is considered a pathogen of significant public health importance due to its low infective dose and its resistance to chlorination.[176] Large outbreaks have been reported in United States (430,000 people with diarrhea) due to contamination of municipal water supply.[177]

Cryptosporidiosis cases have been reported in 25 KT, 7 LT, and 7 intestinal and 1 kidney plus pancreas transplant recipients and 7 nonspecified SOTs.

Clinical picture

Clinical manifestations begin after an incubation period of 7 to 10 days. Immunocompetent hosts develop self-limited diarrhea, but in immunocompromised hosts infection can be severe leading to life-threatening diarrhea with severe malabsorption and body weight loss.[178] Other symptoms include nausea, vomiting, crampy abdominal pain (50%), and fever (36%).[179] Some LT recipients developed sclerosing cholangitis, a rare but dangerous extraintestinal complication that may require bile duct anastomoses, and, in the worst cases, retransplantation due to biliary cirrhosis.[180,181]

Tacrolimus levels should be monitored, because diarrhea affects its absorption. The concomitant use of mycophenolate mofetil may exacerbate diarrhea.

Diagnosis

Diagnosis is made by microscopic examination of the stools. Multiple samples should be examined because oocyst shedding may occur intermittently.[175] Modified Ziehl-Neelsen stain reveals 4- to 6-μ red oocysts. Direct imunofluorescence using monoclonal antibodies is considered the gold standard. Several enzyme-linked immunosorbent assay (ELISA) methods are available for detection of fecal cryptosporidial antigen with sensitivity in diarrheal specimens ranging from 83% to 95%. PCR testing for *Cryptosporidium* is useful for detecting the pathogen in water supplies and asymptomatic carriers.[174]

Treatment

There is limited experience in treating this infection in SOT. Although newer drugs active against *Cryptosporidium* exist, they are only authorized in the United States for treatment of immunocompetent hosts. Currently, the use of fluid and electrolyte replacement and of antimotility agents is the cornerstone of treatment in immunocompromised host.[176]

Cryptosporidium can be treated with nitazoxanide, paramomycin, or azithromycin. Clinical response is variable, however, and intestinal protozoa can be difficult to eradicate. A systematic review and meta-analysis evaluated the efficacy of treatment in HIV patients. Nitaxozanide reduced parasite load, duration, and frequency of diarrhea. The review concluded, however, that no drug effectively eradicated *Cryptosporidiosis* in these patients.[176] Hong and colleagues[182] reported a case of severe *cryptosporidiosis* in a KT recipient successfully managed with combined therapy (nitazoxanide, paramomycin, and azithromycin) plus immunosuppressor dose reduction. In transplant patients, antimicrobial therapy with concurrent reduction in immunosuppression may optimize immunologic status and potentially lead to infection resolution.[183]

Prognosis and prophylaxis

The absence of effective therapy highlights the importance of preventive interventions in this group of patients. Veterinary personnel, animal handlers, dog owners, and individuals who practice oral-anal sex or anal-genital sex are at particularly high risk of developing cryptosporidiosis.[175] SOT recipients should be aware of these potentials risks.

In the United Kingdom and United States, authorities recommend that immunocompromised people boil their drinking water. This seems suitable for HIV patients, children with severe combined immunodeficiency syndrome, and people with CD40 ligand deficiency. Some investigators consider that the recommendation for SOT recipients lacks supporting evidence. When traveling to endemic countries, SOT recipients should be advised to drink bottled water.[184]

Cyclosporiasis

Epidemiology/life cycle/microbiologic facts

Cyclospora cayetanensis is a coccidian protozoan, considered an emergent cause of gastroenteric disease. Humans are the only known hosts of *C cayetanensis*. No zoonotic reservoirs have been identified. Life cycle begins with ingestion of a sporulated oocyst in contaminated water or food. *Cyclospora* oocysts release sporozoites in the gut that invade the epithelial cells of the jejunum surviving as obligate intracellular parasites. Sporozoites undergo asexual reproduction in the cell, producing merozoites. The merozoites penetrate new cells to form gametes and after sexual reproduction develop zygotes. These zygotes fabricate a resilient wall and become unsporulated oocysts. Oocysts mature within the small intestine and when excreted require 2 to 3 days of maturation outside the host to become infectious, making direct person-to-person spread of infection impossible.[168]

Cyclosporiasis is endemic in developing countries, such as Egypt, Guatemala, Nepal, Nigeria, Peru, Turkey, and Venezuela, constituting a public health issue related to water and sanitation. In these countries, cyclosporiasis produces a self-limited diarrhea in immunocompetent individuals.[185–190] Several outbreaks in the United States, Canada, and Europe have been reported mainly related to food imported from endemic countries (fruits and vegetables).[191–194] Travelers returning from Haiti, Guatemala, Mexico, Morocco, Pakistan, and Puerto Rico have also developed cyclosporiasis.[190]

Prevalence varies depending on the population studied; in China, the infection rate in immunocompetent hosts is 0.25% but reaches 9.3% in immunocompromised patients.[195] Prevalence in the general population in United States and Europe is less than 1% and in the United Kingdom 0.1%.[196,197] No cases of cyclosporiasis have been reported in SOT recipients, which suggests that cyclosporiasis may be underdiagnosed.

Clinical picture

Cyclosporiasis incubation period is 1 week and, if untreated, lasts for a few days to a month.[190] Clinical manifestations of cyclosporiasis range from asymptomatic infection to watery diarrhea, fatigue, abdominal pain, weight loss, anorexia, and, in some cases, flu-like symptoms. *Cyclosporiasis* can mimic celiac disease and irritable bowel syndrome.[198] *C cayetanensis* has been associated with various complications, including biliary disease, cholecystitis, Guillian-Barré syndrome, and reactive arthritis after prolonged infection.[199–202]

In HIV patients and SOT recipients, cyclosporiasis may be more severe and chronic, and, in some cases, life-threatening.[203,204]

Diagnosis

Cyclospora oocysts can be secreted intermittently and shed in low numbers, so at least 3 stool samples should be tested to rule it out. *Cyclospora* oocysts have an 8- to 10-μm diameter and may be detected with a modified Ziehl Neelsen or safranin methylene blue stain.[205] Some investigators report that acid-fast stool examination with light microscopy has 50% sensitivity and 100% specificity when compared with PCR.[206] Fluorescence microscopy is another highly sensitive method used to detect autofluorescent oocysts.[207] Electron microscopy is also useful identifying *C cayetanensis* in gastrointestinal biopsies of HIV and transplant patients.[208]

Highly sensitive PCR methods have been designed mainly for the food industry but have no role in routine diagnosis of human infections for the time being.[206,209]

Treatment

Infection usually responds to a 7-day course of TMP-SMX with a standard dose of 160/800 mg of oral TMP-SMX taken twice a day. Higher doses are used in immunocompromised patients (160/800 mg of oral TMP-SMX 4 times a day for 10 days). Symptoms usually resolve within 24 to 48 hours. In immunosuppressed patients the recurrence rate is higher but it may be prevented by using secondary TMP-SMX prophylaxis.[210,211]

Nitazoxanide (500 mg twice daily for 3 days) is considered an effective alternative but more clinical evidence is needed[212]

Prognosis and prophylaxis

Recommendations for SOT recipients are to avoid untreated drinking water and swimming in rivers or springs, when traveling to endemic countries. SOT recipients should be advised that eating raw or uncooked bivalves, which are filter feeders that concentrate pathogens from waters can lead to infection.[213] SOT recipients should avoid direct contact with soil and ownership of dogs, chicken or other fowls, guinea pigs, and rabbits.[186] No specific prophylaxis has been studied or recommended.

Amebiasis

Amebiasis is a protozooal infection caused by *Entamoeba histolytica* that causes gastrointestinal infection and hepatic abscess. Amebiasis is acquired by ingestion of water or food contaminated with *E histolytica* cysts. It is highly endemic in Africa, Asia, and Latin America.

Only 1 case of severe *E histolytica* enterocolitis in an LT recipient has been published.[214] The patient had been drinking unboiled water from a well during a 6-month period. Diagnosis of intestinal amebiasis is done by microscopic examination of feces where cysts or trophozoites can be observed. Other diagnostic methods include detection of fecal *E histolytica* antigen, PCR in feces, and serologic tests. All of them are more sensitive than microscopic examination methods. Metronidazole is the drug of choice and eliminates infection in up to 90% of patients in 10 days.[215] In the sole SOT recipient with reported amebiasis the infection was eradicated after 6 weeks of metronidazole.[214] Screening of donors in endemic countries is not systematic, due to the high prevalence of the disease. When traveling to endemic regions, SOT recipients should be encouraged to drink only bottled water.

HELMINTHS

Strongyloidiasis

Epidemiology/life cycle/microbiologic facts

Strongyloidiasis is caused by a nematode called *Strongyloides stercoralis*. Free-living filariform larvae in soil penetrate the skin. The filariform larvae migrate hematogenously to the lungs, enter the alveolar sacs, and ascend the tracheobronchial tree, where they are swallowed. The larvae finish the maturation process in the intestinal mucosa of the duodenum and jejunum, where they produce eggs that develop into rhabditiform larvae. The rhabditiform larvae migrate back into the intestinal lumen and are excreted into stool or become autoinfective, penetrating the colonic mucosa or perianal skin.[31] That is, *S stercoralis* can complete its life cycle entirely within the human host and this autoinfective cycle allows the nematode to perpetuate itself in the host indefinitely.[216]

Strongyloidiasis is endemic in tropical and subtropical regions and emergent in United States, Asia, Africa, Latin America, and some regions of Europe. Infections in

SOT recipients may occur in patients from endemic regions and in patients traveling to endemic areas. To the best of the authors' knowledge, 54 cases of strongyloidiasis have been reported in SOT (46 KTs, 2 HTs, 2 LTs, and 1 lung, 1 heart plus kidney, 1 pancreas, and 1 intestinal transplant).[217–231,45,232–254]

Clinical picture

Clinical manifestations range from asymptomatic eosinophilia to mild gastrointestinal, pulmonary, or cutaneous symptoms to full-blown systemic infections (hyperinfection syndrome and disseminated strongyloidiasis).[223] Severe systemic involvement is usually associated with suppression of the host's immune response and, in the case of solid organ recipients, symptoms usually develop in the first 6 months posttransplant.

Eosinophilia is present in 50% to 80% of the cases and may be a key clue in paucisymptomatic patients. It may be absent, however, in immunosuppressed patients.[255,256]

In patients with chronic strongyloidiasis, larvae migration may cause serpiginous and erythematous tracks developing usually on buttocks. These manifestations are known as larva currens and occur in association with autoinfection. Gastrointestinal chronic infection may lead to upper abdominal pain, anorexia, nausea and vomiting, or enterocolitis and malabsorption. Löffler-like syndrome rarely emerges when the larva migrates through the lungs and infiltrates pulmonary vasculature; classical symptoms are cough, throat irritation, wheezing, dyspnoea, and hemoptysis. In chronically infected individuals, pulmonary manifestations mimicking recurrent bacterial pneumonia or asthma occur. Pulmonary edema, hemorrhage, and secondary bacterial pneumonia have also been reported.[257]

The likelihood of developing the hyperinfection syndrome is increased in immunosuppressed patients with depressed cell-mediated immunity, underlying malignancy (leukemia and lymphoma), HIV infection, malnutrition and hemopoietic stem cell transplant, or SOT.[216,222,258–260] In hyperinfection syndrome, overwhelming parasite load occurs with massive dissemination of larvae to internal organs from the gastrointestinal tract. Manifestations include severe gastrointestinal symptoms (nausea, vomiting, diarrhea, abdominal pain, and paralytic ileus), pulmonary symptoms (dyspnea, hemoptysis, cough, and wheezing), and fever. Gastrointestinal complications of hyperinfection syndrome are colonic ulceration, peritonitis, and intestinal obstruction.[222] Hyperinfection syndrome has been described in renal, heart, and pancreas transplant recipients.[219,223,224] Corticosteroid therapy is a common denominator of hyperinfection syndrome.[257] Disseminated strongyloidiasis organs, such as lungs, liver, heart, CNS, and endocrine glands, may be affected with massive tissue invasion, inducing inflammation that may result in symptomatic dysfunction. Sepsis, meningitis, or encephalitis caused by enteric bacteria originating from the gastrointestinal tract may occur and septic shock is a common cause of death.[224]

Nucci and colleagues[261] reviewed 343 patients with hematologic malignancies showing that the use of corticosteroids was one of the predictive factors for disseminated strongyloidiasis (odds ratio 2.29). Most investigators hypothesize that corticosteroids may precipitate dissemination of *S stercoralis* accelerating the life cycle of the nematode.[262,263]

Strongyloidiasis has not been described in SOT recipients receiving cyclosporine A (CyA). Some investigators have attributed this observation to the potential antiparasitic activity of CyA.[221,225] Tacrolimus, however, does not have antihelminthic activity.[264]

Diagnosis

Diagnosis of uncomplicated strongyloidiasis is usually made by detecting rhabditiform larvae in concentrated stool (on the third to fourth week after initial infection).[265] More specific techniques, such as Baerman or the Harada-Mori concentration techniques, are recommended when the clinical suspicion is high.[266,267] The agar plate culture method is one of the best techniques for the detection of *S stercoralis* infection. The parasite can also be isolated in duodenojejunal fluid after endoscopy or string test.[268] Endoscopic changes include thickened folds and mucosal erosions on the stomach, edema, erythematous spots, and subepithelial hemorrhages in the duodenum and even megaduodenum.[269] Colonic findings include edema, aphthous, or serpiginous ulcers and erosions. A biopsy can reveal larvae affecting the mucosa.[270]

In disseminated infections, other specimens, such as sputum, BAL fluid, pleural fluid, peritoneal fluid, and surgical drainage fluid, must also be analyzed in search for filariform larvae.[271–273]

Serologic tests, such as ELISA, have been evaluated in immunocompetent patients with sensitivity and specificity ranging from 70% to 90% and 85% to 95%, respectively.[224] ELISA, however, can be falsely negative in immunocompromised hosts, and the anti-*Strongyloides* antibody can persist for years after treatment.[271] False-positive results are explained by cross-reaction with filariae and other nematodes.

Outcome and treatment

Prognosis of uncomplicated strongyloidiasis is favorable although relapse is common in the era of thiabendazol (30%).[274] Disseminated syndromes have an overall mortality of 50% to 75%.[234] Mortality is increased with concomitant immunosuppression, bacteremia, and delayed diagnosis.[263]

Uncomplicated infections are treated with ivermectin (200 μg/kg) in a single dose[275] or with a second dose 2 weeks apart,[276] to prevent relapse. Alternative drugs include albendazole (400 mg by mouth twice daily for 3 days) or thiabendazole (25 mg/kg 2 times a day for 2 days) but have lower efficacy than ivermectin.[257] Disseminated syndromes require prolonged treatment (5–7 days of ivermectin or a combination of ivermectin and albendazole). Serologic studies and serial determinations of eosinophilia may be used to monitor response. Some investigators recommend monthly 5-day treatment courses for at least 6 months before treatment is definitely discontinued.[219]

Prophylaxis

Chronic carriage is common among environmentally exposed individuals and has been found to persist for up to 30 years. Accordingly, patients awaiting transplantation with risk of prior exposure should undergo screening before transplantation.[224] In endemic areas, cadaveric donor screening for *Strongyloides* is mandatory.[225] If positive, they should be treated before transplant and closely followed-up to exclude reactivations. Regarding specific prophylaxis for *S stercoralis* in SOT recipients, some investigators recommend administration of preemptive therapy to all transplant candidates who have traveled to or resided in an area of endemic infection.[219]

Schistosomiasis

Epidemiology/life cycle

Schistosomiasis is due to infection by trematode blood flukes of the genus *Schistosoma*. Species responsible for human infection are: *S haematobium*, *S mansoni*, *S japonicum*, *S mekongi*, and *S intercalatum*. Infection results from contact with

Schistosoma cercariae contaminated water or through blood transfusion or organ transplantation.[1,277]

S haematobium lives in the venous plexus of urinary tract, whereas the adult worms of *S mansoni*, *S japonicum*, *S mekongi*, and *S intercalatum* reside in intestinal veins, laying hundreds of ova per day that drain to the liver via the portal circulation. Ova trapped in the microcirculation induce inflammation, granuloma formation, and fibrosis.

Schistosomiasis is endemic in Southeast Asia, South America, Africa, and the Middle East, affecting 200 to 250 million people worldwide.[278] Schistosomiasis after SOT may be due to allograft transmission, reactivation of latent disease, or reinfection. Renal or hepatic failure due to schistosomiasis may be an indication for transplantation, and reactivation may arise under immunosuppression.[279] In highly endemic countries, such as Egypt, posttransplant reinfection affects 23% of the KT recipients.[280] Few cases of schistosomiasis in LT recipients have been reported.[279,281]

Clinical picture

The clinical profile of schistosomiasis in SOT is not significantly different from natural infection in immunocompetent individuals.[1] Acute phase is usually asymptomatic and is more frequent in nonimmune individuals. Acute infection presents as swimmer's itch or Katayama fever. Chronic complications require intense exposure and are common in patients from endemic regions. The major manifestations vary according to the infecting species and anatomic location.

S mansoni, *S japonicum*, *S intercalatum*, *S mekongi*, and rarely *S haematobium* cause intestinal infections. Most common symptoms include nausea, vomiting, abdominal pain, diarrhea, hepatomegaly, splenomegaly, and eosinophilia.[282] Colitis due to *S mansoni* has been reported in a Sudanese KT recipient 6 years after transplantation.[283] Liver schistosomiasis occurs with *S mansoni*, *S japonicum*, and *S mekongi*. Infection can lead to acute inflammatory hepatic reaction and in later stages portal hypertension and its complications. Two patients born in endemic areas suffered reactivation of a latent infection (early gastric ulcer and liver involvement 15 months after transplantation).[279]

S haematobium causes urinary schistosomiasis, which may present with hematuria, dysuria, increased urinary frequency, and anemia. In later stages, fibrosis and calcification of the bladder and ureters can occur, resulting in hydroureter and hydronephrosis. Anatomic obstruction can lead to chronic renal failure and increased risk of squamous cell carcinoma of the bladder. Kidney injury may also result from deposition of circulating complexes with any *Schistosoma* species. Recrudescence of *S mansoni* glomerulopathy is common after KT.[284,285] In schistosomiasis, other organs can be affected when eggs embolize, causing neurologic complications (spinal cord, cerebral, or cerebellar) and pulmonary manifestations, such as pulmonary hypertension.

Diagnosis

Diagnosis is made by demonstration of parasite eggs in urine or stool specimens in a microscopic examination. *S haematobium* eggs are usually found in urine but may also be present in feces. Eggs of *S mansoni*, *S japonicum*, *S haematobium*, and *S mekongi* are found in stool specimens. Determination of the intensity of infection is performed by quantitative sampling of defined amounts of stool (Kato-Katz technique) or urine (syringe filtration). Schistosomiasis may also be diagnosed by finding eggs in rectal, intestinal, liver, or bladder biopsies.[31] Serology has a sensitivity of 85% and is a more specific diagnostic tool in patients who reside in schistosome-free countries and travel to endemic areas. These patients often have light egg excretion because the burden of infection is low. Seroconversion is generally 4 to 8 weeks after infection and occurs before eggs become detectable in the stool or urine. Circulating antibody titers can remain high for long periods, even after successful treatment, making differentiation between reactivation or reinfection difficult.[279]

In liver schistosomiasis, periportal fibrosis around portal vein tributaries and splenomegaly may be seen on ultrasound. In urinary tract involvement, an ultrasound may reveal structural bladder defects (polyps or tumors) and hydronephrosis. Ureter strictures may also be detected by intravenous pyelogram.[31]

Treatment

Praziquantel (40 mg/kg in 1 or 2 doses) is the standard treatment, but infections due to *S japonicum* and *S mekongi* require 60 mg/kg in 2 or 3 doses. Praziquantel increases cell membrane permeability to calcium ions, resulting in parasite paralysis and consequent dislodgment from their site of action. It also interferes with ovipositioning.

In endemic countries, such as Egypt, potential donors or recipients who had active schistosomal infection are treated with praziquantel (60 mg/kg given in 2 divided doses on the same day). After 1 month, microscopic examination and serologic tests are repeated and, if positive, another course of praziquantel is given.[278] Cyclosporine may decrease the metabolism of praziquantel, resulting in potential nephrotoxicity, so CyA level monitoring is required.[286] Some reports suggest that CyA has antischistosomal properties (especially against *S mansoni*) with a 45% reduction in worm burden.[287]

Prognosis and prophylaxis

In endemic countries, patients infected with schistosomiasis can be considered suitable donors and recipients.[286] This was demonstrated by a large 10-year follow-up study in KT recipients in Egypt that compared 136 *Schistosoma*-infected cases with 107 controls. Schistosomiasis had no significant impact on patient or graft outcomes or in the rate of acute or chronic rejection.[286] Based on case reports, transplanting a liver from a donor with a history of well-treated schistosomiasis is not contraindicated.[277] Pungpapong and colleagues[288] reported 3 LT cases in which allograft schistosomiasis was diagnosed in the posttransplant biopsy, all of them were treated successfully with praziquantel and remained asymptomatic after 35 weeks of follow-up.

All recipients from high-risk areas should undergo pretransplant stool and serology screening. Patients who have a positive result must receive preoperative praziquantel. Recipients of donors with schistosomiasis need to be treated with praziquantel also.[278] Primary infections should be prevented in SOT recipients traveling to endemic areas and immigrants returning to their origin countries because of risk of reinfection.

Echinococcosis

Epidemiology/life cycle/clinical presentation

Echinococcal disease is a zoonosis caused by infection with the metacestode stage of the tapeworm *Echinococcus*, which belongs to the family Taeniidae. Echinococcosis is more predominant in rural areas where canines may ingest contaminated offal from livestock. Domestic dogs and other canines are definite hosts; humans are intermediate hosts. Humans become infected by ingesting eggs, with resulting release of oncospheres in the intestine and the development of cysts in various organs. Four species of *Echinococcus* produce infection in humans; *E granulosus* and *E multilocularis* are the most common, causing cystic echinococcosis and alveolar echinococcosis (AE), respectively. The 2 other species, *E vogeli* and *E oligarthrus*, cause polycystic echinococcosis but are rarely associated with human infection.

E granulosus has a worldwide distribution (Mediterranean, South America, Russia, China, Australia, and Africa) and produces cystic echinococcosis, which is mostly asymptomatic. In symptomatic cases, clinical presentation depends on anatomic site, size, and number of the hydatid cysts. These cysts may create a mass effect obstructing blood or lymphatic flow. Rupture of the cyst and secondary bacterial infection is also possible. Most affected organs are liver and lungs; other localizations include kidney, muscle, bone, brain, heart, and pancreas.

E multilocularis infection produces AE. Its life cycle is similar to that of *E granulosus* but it has a more aggressive clinical presentation marked by invasion and greater destruction due to its perpetual proliferative phase. AE is prevalent in North America (Alaska and Northern Canada), Central Europe (Germany, Swiss, Austria, and France), Turkey, Russia, China, and Japan.[289] *E multilocularis* infections are less likely to be asymptomatic, although the clinical manifestations are frequently nonspecific. Common clinical manifestations include malaise, weight loss, and right upper quadrant discomfort due to hepatomegaly. If left untreated, more than 90% of patients die within 10 years of the onset of clinical symptoms.

Diagnosis

Diagnosis of cystic echinococcosis and AE is made by a combination of imaging and serology (ELISA). In *E granulosus* infection, diagnosis is suspected when incidentally finding a cystic lesion in a chest radiograph, ultrasonography, CT scan, or MRI. In cystic echinococcosis, hepatic ultrasound reveals infoldings of the inner cyst wall, separation of the hydatid membrane from the cyst wall, or hydatid sand. In AE, ultrasound may reveal lesions with an irregular contour that may be confused with neoplasic disease.

Serologic assays are more sensitive and specific for *E multilocularis* compared with *E granulosus* but may be negative in cases where the cyst remains unruptured.

Percutaneous aspiration, fine needle or biopsy guided by ultrasound or CT, may be the last option when other diagnostic methods are inconclusive. They should not be performed routinely due to risk of anaphylaxis and secondary spread of the infection.

E granulosus and SOT

In some cases, a liver cyst enlarges leading to terminal liver failure and LT. Moreno-González and colleagues[290,291] reported their experience with 6 patients with liver infestation by *E granulosus* that required LT. Four patients survived transplantation and 2 died from associated complications. No recurrences of hydatid cysts after LT were seen. A case of a patient with liver hydatidosis who underwent an HT has been reported in which immunosuppression had no effect on the size of the cyst.[292]

In endemic countries, cases of liver grafts with hydatid cysts have been reported. If the cyst is solitary, calcified, and does not fistulate to the biliary tree, it may be resected, and the liver can be used for transplantation.[293]

E multilocularis and SOT

No cases of allograft transmission of *E multilocularis* have been reported. Patients with incurable AE can benefit from an LT. Bresson-Hadni and colleagues[289] performed a long-term evaluation in 15 patients with AE who received LT and reported these outcomes: 4 recurrences and 2 deaths due to dissemination of residual foci to the lungs and brain.

Treatment with albendazole (15 mg/kg per day in 2 divided doses) is recommended for a minimum of 2 years after transplantation even in cases of apparent curative surgery.[294]

In AE, the affected organ cannot be used for transplantation, and disease at other sites, mainly lungs and CNS, should be ruled out.

Filariasis

Filariae are a group of nematodes capable of affecting subcutaneous tissue or lymphatic vessels. Most important species related to human infection are *Wuchereria bancrofti*, *Brugia malayi*, *Onchocerca volvolus*, and *Loa loa*. Filariasis is an arthropod-borne infection endemic in some areas of the tropics. To the best of the authors' knowledge only 1 case of possible transmission of *W bancrofti* via a living-donor renal transplant from India has been reported.[295] The KT recipient was asymptomatic and diagnosis was made incidentally on perioperative biopsy. Due to the lack of data regarding SOT recipients no recommendations can be given except avoiding insect bites when traveling to endemic areas.

SUMMARY

Parasitic infections are rare but potentially life threatening in SOT recipients. Parasitic infection in the SOT recipient rises in parallel to increased travel and chances of receiving blood or organs from infected donors. Clinicians attending SOT recipients should be familiar with the potential pathogens, their geographic distribution, and pathogenesis to identify the patients at risk of developing a parasitic infection. Rapid diagnosis and treatment is of paramount importance to achieve a successful outcome. Management of parasitic infections is usually the same as in the immunocompetent host, but clinicians must pay special attention to drug interactions because many antiparasitics may affect the metabolism of immunosuppressors. Each transplant center needs to develop a policy, taking into account local epidemiology, establishing criteria for suitable donors and requiring donor/receptor pretransplant screening and recipient postoperative prophylaxis. SOT recipients should be encouraged to adhere to universal recommendations to minimize exposition to endemic parasitosis. The most effective approach to reducing SOT recipient parasite infection may be maximizing disease eradication in endemic areas. Targeting these areas will bring substantial relief to affected peoples who, it must be remembered, bear the brunt of these diseases.

ACKNOWLEDGMENTS

We thank Dr Pablo Martín-Rabadán for reviewing the manuscript.

REFERENCES

1. Barsoum RS. Parasitic infections in organ transplantation. Exp Clin Transplant 2004;2(2):258–67.
2. Nasser QJ, Power RE, Eng MP, et al. Toxoplasmosis after a simultaneous pancreas and kidney transplantation. Transplant Proc 2004;36(9):2843–4.
3. Remington JS. Toxoplasmosis in the adult. Bull N Y Acad Med 1974;50(2):211–27.
4. Gourishankar S, Doucette K, Fenton J, et al. The use of donor and recipient screening for toxoplasma in the era of universal trimethoprim sulfamethoxazole prophylaxis. Transplantation 2008;85(7):980–5.
5. Derouin F, Pelloux H. Prevention of toxoplasmosis in transplant patients. Clin Microbiol Infect 2008;14(12):1089–101.

6. Alkhunaizi AM, Al-Tawfiq JA, Al-Shawaf MH. Transfusion-transmitted malaria in a kidney transplant recipient. How safe is our blood transfusion? Saudi Med J 2008;29(2):293–5.
7. Campbell AL, Goldberg CL, Magid MS, et al. First case of toxoplasmosis following small bowel transplantation and systematic review of tissue-invasive toxoplasmosis following noncardiac solid organ transplantation. Transplantation 2006;81(3):408–17.
8. Renoult E, Georges E, Biava MF, et al. Toxoplasmosis in kidney transplant recipients: report of six cases and review. Clin Infect Dis 1997;24(4):625–34.
9. Giordano LF, Lasmar EP, Tavora ER, et al. Toxoplasmosis transmitted via kidney allograft: case report and review. Transplant Proc 2002;34(2):498–9.
10. Rogers NM, Peh CA, Faull R, et al. Transmission of toxoplasmosis in two renal allograft recipients receiving an organ from the same donor. Transpl Infect Dis 2008;10(1):71–4.
11. Gallino A, Maggiorini M, Kiowski W, et al. Toxoplasmosis in heart transplant recipients. Eur J Clin Microbiol Infect Dis 1996;15(5):389–93.
12. Wulf MW, van Crevel R, Portier R, et al. Toxoplasmosis after renal transplantation: implications of a missed diagnosis. J Clin Microbiol 2005;43(7):3544–7.
13. Angelis M, Cooper JT, Freeman RB. Impact of donor infections on outcome of orthotopic liver transplantation. Liver Transpl 2003;9(5):451–62.
14. Derouin F, Debure A, Godeaut E, et al. *Toxoplasma* antibody titers in renal transplant recipients. Pretransplant evaluation and posttransplant follow-up of 73 patients. Transplantation 1987;44(4):515–8.
15. Singh N, Husain S. Infections of the central nervous system in transplant recipients. Transpl Infect Dis 2000;2(3):101–11.
16. Conrath J, Mouly-Bandini A, Collart F, et al. *Toxoplasma gondii* retinochoroiditis after cardiac transplantation. Graefes Arch Clin Exp Ophthalmol 2003;241(4):334–8.
17. Martinez-Giron R, Esteban JG, Ribas A, et al. Protozoa in respiratory pathology: a review. Eur Respir J 2008;32(5):1354–70.
18. Bergin M, Menser MA, Procopis PG, et al. Central nervous system toxoplasmosis and hemolytic-uremic syndrome. N Engl J Med 1987;317(24):1540–1.
19. Michelson AD, Lammi AT. Haemolytic anaemia associated with acquired toxoplasmosis. Aust Paediatr J 1984;20(4):333–5.
20. Blatrix C, Baufine-Ducrocq H, Couzineau P, et al. [Toxoplasmosis causing immunologic hemolytic anemia]. Presse Med 1967;75(7):333–6 [in French].
21. Segall L, Moal MC, Doucet L, et al. Toxoplasmosis-associated hemophagocytic syndrome in renal transplantation. Transpl Int 2006;19(1):78–80.
22. Hebraud B, Kamar N, Borde JS, et al. Unusual presentation of primary toxoplasmosis infection in a kidney-transplant patient complicated by an acute left-ventricular failure. NDT Plus 2008;1(6):429–32.
23. Mayes JT, O'Connor BJ, Avery R, et al. Transmission of *Toxoplasma gondii* infection by liver transplantation. Clin Infect Dis 1995;21(3):511–5.
24. Sluiters JF, Balk AH, Essed CE, et al. Indirect enzyme-linked immunosorbent assay for immunoglobulin G and four immunoassays for immunoglobulin M to *Toxoplasma gondii* in a series of heart transplant recipients. J Clin Microbiol 1989;27(3):529–35.
25. Jacobs F, Depierreux M, Goldman M, et al. Role of bronchoalveolar lavage in diagnosis of disseminated toxoplasmosis. Rev Infect Dis 1991;13(4):637–41.
26. Feron D, Goldman M, Jacobs F, et al. Bone marrow aspiration as a diagnostic tool for acute toxoplasmosis in a kidney transplant recipient. Transplantation 1990;50(6):1054–5.

27. Rostaing L, Baron E, Fillola O, et al. Toxoplasmosis in two renal transplant recipients: diagnosis by bone marrow aspiration. Transplant Proc 1995;27(2):1733–4.
28. Vaessen N, Verweij JJ, Spijkerman IJ, et al. Fatal disseminated toxoplasmosis after liver transplantation: improved and early diagnosis by PCR. Neth J Med 2007;65(6):222–3.
29. Caner A, Doskaya M, Karasu Z, et al. Incidence and diagnosis of active toxoplasma infection among liver transplant recipients in Western Turkey. Liver Transpl 2008;14(10):1526–32.
30. Montoya JG, Liesenfeld O. Toxoplasmosis. Lancet 2004;363(9425):1965–76.
31. Mandell GL, Bennett JE, Dolin R. Sixth editionIn: Douglas, and Bennett's principles and practice of infectious diseases, vol. 2. Philadelphia (PA): Elsevier Churchill Livingston; 2005.
32. Munoz P, Arencibia J, Rodriguez C, et al. Trimethoprim-sulfamethoxazole as toxoplasmosis prophylaxis for heart transplant recipients. Clin Infect Dis 2003; 36(7):932–3 [author reply 933].
33. Baran DA, Alwarshetty MM, Alvi S, et al. Is toxoplasmosis prophylaxis necessary in cardiac transplantation? Long-term follow-up at two transplant centers. J Heart Lung Transplant 2006;25(11):1380–2.
34. Murri R, Ammassari A, Pezzotti P, et al. Incidence and determinants of bacterial infections in HIV-positive patients receiving anti- *Pneumocystis carinii/ Toxoplasma gondii* primary prophylaxis within a randomized clinical trial. J Acquir Immune Defic Syndr 2001;27(1):49–55.
35. Girard PM, Landman R, Gaudebout C, et al. Dapsone-pyrimethamine compared with aerosolized pentamidine as primary prophylaxis against Pneumocystis carinii pneumonia and toxoplasmosis in HIV infection. The PRIO Study Group. N Engl J Med 1993;328(21):1514–20.
36. Kotton CN. Zoonoses in solid-organ and hematopoietic stem cell transplant recipients. Clin Infect Dis 2007;44(6):857–66.
37. Frapier JM, Abraham B, Dereure J, et al. Fatal visceral leishmaniasis in a heart transplant recipient. J Heart Lung Transplant 2001;20(8):912–3.
38. Tavora ER, Lasmar EP, Orefice J, et al. Unusual manifestations of leishmaniasis in renal transplant. Transplant Proc 2002;34(2):502–3.
39. Choi CM, Lerner EA. Leishmaniasis as an emerging infection. J Investig Dermatol Symp Proc 2001;6(3):175–82.
40. Basset D, Faraut F, Marty P, et al. Visceral leishmaniasis in organ transplant recipients: 11 new cases and a review of the literature. Microbes Infect 2005; 7(13):1370–5.
41. Horber FF, Lerut JP, Reichen J, et al. Visceral leishmaniasis after orthotopic liver transplantation: impact of persistent splenomegaly. Transpl Int 1993;6(1):55–7.
42. Golino A, Duncan JM, Zeluff B, et al. Leishmaniasis in a heart transplant patient. J Heart Lung Transplant 1992;11(4 Pt 1):820–3.
43. Berenguer J, Gómez-Campderá F, Padilla B, et al. Visceral leishmaniasis (Kala-Azar) in transplant recipients: case report and review. Transplantation 1998; 65(10):1401–4.
44. Jokipii L, Salmela K, Saha H, et al. Leishmaniasis diagnosed from bronchoalveolar lavage. Scand J Infect Dis 1992;24(5):677–81.
45. Venizelos PC, Lopata M, Bardawil WA, et al. Respiratory failure due to *Strongyloides stercoralis* in a patient with a renal transplant. Chest 1980;78(1):104–6.
46. Gontijo CM, Pacheco RS, Orefice F, et al. Concurrent cutaneous, visceral and ocular leishmaniasis caused by *Leishmania (Viannia) braziliensis* in a kidney transplant patient. Mem Inst Oswaldo Cruz 2002;97(5):751–3.

47. Fernandes IM, Baptista MA, Barbon TR, et al. Cutaneous leishmaniasis in kidney transplant recipient. Transplant Proc 2002;34(2):504–5.
48. Drugs for parasitic infections. Med Lett Drugs Ther 1998;40(1021):28.
49. Moulin B, Ollier J, Bouchouareb D, et al. Leishmaniasis: a rare cause of unexplained fever in a renal graft recipient. Nephron 1992;60(3):360–2.
50. Sundar S, Rai M, Chakravarty J, et al. New treatment approach in Indian visceral leishmaniasis: single-dose liposomal amphotericin B followed by short-course oral miltefosine. Clin Infect Dis 2008;47(8):1000–6.
51. Llorente S, Gimeno L, Navarro MJ, et al. Therapy of visceral leishmaniasis in renal transplant recipients intolerant to pentavalent antimonials. Transplantation 2000;70(5):800–1.
52. Morales P, Torres JJ, Salavert M, et al. Visceral leishmaniasis in lung transplantation. Transplant Proc 2003;35(5):2001–3.
53. Hernandez-Perez J, Yebra-Bango M, Jimenez-Martinez E, et al. Visceral leishmaniasis (kala-azar) in solid organ transplantation: report of five cases and review. Clin Infect Dis 1999;29(4):918–21.
54. Daneshvar C, Davis TM, Cox-Singh J, et al. Clinical and laboratory features of human *Plasmodium knowlesi* infection. Clin Infect Dis 2009;49(6):852–60.
55. Turkmen A, Sever MS, Ecder T, et al. Posttransplant malaria. Transplantation 1996;62(10):1521–3.
56. Hung CC, Chang SC, Chen YC, et al. *Plasmodium vivax* infection in a renal transplant recipient: report of a case. J Formos Med Assoc 1994;93(10):888–9.
57. Tan HW, Ch'ng SL. Drug interaction between cyclosporine A and quinine in a renal transplant patient with malaria. Singapore Med J 1991;32(3):189–90.
58. Holzer BR, Gluck Z, Zambelli D, et al. Transmission of malaria by renal transplantation. Transplantation 1985;39(3):315–6.
59. Lefavour GS, Pierce JC, Frame JD. Renal transplant-associated malaria. JAMA 1980;244(16):1820–1.
60. Anteyi EA, Liman HM, Gbaji A. Malaria prophylaxis in post renal transplant recipients in the tropics: is it necessary? Cent Afr J Med 2003;49(5–6):63–6.
61. Johnston ID. Possible transmission of malaria by renal transplantation. Br Med J (Clin Res Ed) 1981;282(6266):780.
62. Bemelman F, De Blok K, De Vries P, et al. *Falciparum* malaria transmitted by a thick blood smear negative kidney donor. Scand J Infect Dis 2004;36(10):769–71.
63. Nuesch R, Cynke E, Jost MC, et al. Thrombocytopenia after kidney transplantation. Am J Kidney Dis 2000;35(3):537–8.
64. Geddes CC, Henderson A, Mackenzie P, et al. Outcome of patients from the west of Scotland traveling to Pakistan for living donor kidney transplants. Transplantation 2008;86(8):1143–5.
65. Yenen OS, Keskin K, Cavuslu S, et al. A case of *Plasmodium vivax* infection transmitted by renal allograft. Nephrol Dial Transplant 1994;9(12):1805–6.
66. Cruz I, Mody V, Callender C, et al. Malaria infection in transplant recipient. J Natl Med Assoc 1978;70(2):105–7.
67. Fischer L, Sterneck M, Claus M, et al. Transmission of malaria tertiana by multi-organ donation. Clin Transplant 1999;13(6):491–5.
68. Einollahi B. *Plasmodium falciparum* infection transmitted by living kidney donation: a case report from Iran. Ann Transplant 2008;13(4):75–8.
69. Chiche L, Lesage A, Duhamel C, et al. Posttransplant malaria: first case of transmission of *Plasmodium falciparum* from a white multiorgan donor to four recipients. Transplantation 2003;75(1):166–8.

70. Seth AK, Puri P, Chandra A, et al. Mixed Plasmodium falciparum and *Plasmodium vivax* malaria in orthotopic liver transplant recipient. Transplantation 2009;88(2):288.
71. Menichetti F, Bindi ML, Tascini C, et al. Fever, mental impairment, acute anemia, and renal failure in patient undergoing orthotopic liver transplantation: post-transplantation malaria. Liver Transpl 2006;12(4):674–6.
72. Mejia GA, Alvarez CA, Pulido HH, et al. Malaria in a liver transplant recipient: a case report. Transplant Proc 2006;38(9):3132–4.
73. Talabiska DG, Komar MJ, Wytock DH, et al. Post-transfusion acquired malaria complicating orthotopic liver transplantation. Am J Gastroenterol 1996;91(2): 376–9.
74. Crafa F, Gugenheim J, Fabiani P, et al. Possible transmission of malaria by liver transplantation. Transplant Proc 1991;23(5):2664.
75. Pandey D, Lee KH, Wong SY, et al. Malaria after living donor liver transplantation: report of two cases. Hepatobiliary Pancreat Dis Int 2008;7(2):210–3.
76. Wiwanitkit V. Malaria due to liver transplantation: summary of reports. Rev Esp Enferm Dig 2009;101(4):302.
77. Babinet J, Gay F, Bustos D, et al. Transmission of *Plasmodium falciparum* by heart transplant. BMJ 1991;303(6816):1515–6.
78. Gueco I, Saniel M, Mendoza M, et al. Tropical infections after renal transplantation. Transplant Proc 1989;21(1 Pt 2):2105–7.
79. Shah S, Filler S, Causer LM, et al. Malaria surveillance–United States, 2002. MMWR Surveill Summ 2004;53(1):21–34.
80. Vijayan VK. Parasitic lung infections. Curr Opin Pulm Med 2009;15(3):274–82.
81. Patankar TF, Karnad DR, Shetty PG, et al. Adult cerebral malaria: prognostic importance of imaging findings and correlation with postmortem findings. Radiology 2002;224(3):811–6.
82. Looareesuwan S, Wilairatana P, Krishna S, et al. Magnetic resonance imaging of the brain in patients with cerebral malaria. Clin Infect Dis 1995; 21(2):300–9.
83. Barsoum RS. Malarial acute renal failure. J Am Soc Nephrol 2000;11(11): 2147–54.
84. Moody A. Rapid diagnostic tests for malaria parasites. Clin Microbiol Rev 2002; 15(1):66–78.
85. Kilian AH, Metzger WG, Mutschelknauss EJ, et al. Reliability of malaria microscopy in epidemiological studies: results of quality control. Trop Med Int Health 2000;5(1):3–8.
86. White NJ. The treatment of malaria. N Engl J Med 1996;335(11):800–6.
87. Boonma P, Christensen PR, Suwanarusk R, et al. Comparison of three molecular methods for the detection and speciation of *Plasmodium vivax* and *Plasmodium falciparum.* Malar J 2007;6:124.
88. Shokoples SE, Ndao M, Kowalewska-Grochowska K, et al. Multiplexed real-time PCR assay for discrimination of *Plasmodium* species with improved sensitivity for mixed infections. J Clin Microbiol 2009;47(4):975–80.
89. Sinclair D, Zani B, Donegan S, et al. Artemisinin-based combination therapy for treating uncomplicated malaria. Cochrane Database Syst Rev 2009;(3): CD007483.
90. Kotton CN, Ryan ET, Fishman JA. Prevention of infection in adult travelers after solid organ transplantation. Am J Transplant 2005;5(1):8–14.
91. Boggild AK, Sano M, Humar A, et al. Travel patterns and risk behavior in solid organ transplant recipients. J Travel Med 2004;11(1):37–43.

92. Freedman DO. Clinical practice. Malaria prevention in short-term travelers. N Engl J Med 2008;359(6):603–12.
93. Villar BF, White DJ, Benach JL. Human babesiosis. Prog Clin Parasitol 1991;2: 129–43.
94. Dodd RY. Transmission of parasites by blood transfusion. Vox Sang 1998; 74(Suppl 2):161–3.
95. Grabowski EF, Giardina PJ, Goldberg D, et al. Babesiosis transmitted by a transfusion of frozen-thawed blood. Ann Intern Med 1982;96(4):466–7.
96. Lux JZ, Weiss D, Linden JV, et al. Transfusion-associated babesiosis after heart transplant. Emerg Infect Dis 2003;9(1):116–9.
97. Gupta P, Hurley RW, Helseth PH, et al. Pancytopenia due to hemophagocytic syndrome as the presenting manifestation of babesiosis. Am J Hematol 1995; 50(1):60–2.
98. Perdrizet GA, Olson NH, Krause PJ, et al. Babesiosis in a renal transplant recipient acquired through blood transfusion. Transplantation 2000;70(1):205–8.
99. Slovut DP, Benedetti E, Matas AJ. Babesiosis and hemophagocytic syndrome in an asplenic renal transplant recipient. Transplantation 1996;62(4):537–9.
100. Evenson DA, Perry E, Kloster B, et al. Therapeutic apheresis for babesiosis. J Clin Apheresis 1998;13(1):32–6.
101. Leiby DA. Babesiosis and blood transfusion: flying under the radar. Vox Sang 2006;90(3):157–65.
102. Vannier E, Gewurz BE, Krause PJ. Human babesiosis. Infect Dis Clin North Am 2008;22(3):469–88, viii-ix.
103. Hatcher JC, Greenberg PD, Antique J, et al. Severe babesiosis in Long Island: review of 34 cases and their complications. Clin Infect Dis. 2001;32(8):1117–25.
104. White DJ, Talarico J, Chang HG, et al. Human babesiosis in New York State: Review of 139 hospitalized cases and analysis of prognostic factors. Arch Intern Med 1998;158(19):2149–54.
105. Krause PJ, Spielman A, Telford SR 3rd, et al. Persistent parasitemia after acute babesiosis. N Engl J Med 1998;339(3):160–5.
106. Florescu D, Sordillo PP, Glyptis A, et al. Splenic infarction in human babesiosis: two cases and discussion. Clin Infect Dis 2008;46(1):e8–11.
107. Froberg MK, Dannen D, Bernier N, et al. Case report: spontaneous splenic rupture during acute parasitemia of *Babesia microti*. Ann Clin Lab Sci 2008; 38(4):390–2.
108. Kuwayama DP, Briones RJ. Spontaneous splenic rupture caused by *Babesia microti* infection. Clin Infect Dis 2008;46(9):e92–5.
109. Berman KH, Blue DE, Smith DS, et al. Fatal case of babesiosis in postliver transplant patient. Transplantation 2009;87(3):452–3.
110. Wittner M, Rowin KS, Tanowitz HB, et al. Successful chemotherapy of transfusion babesiosis. Ann Intern Med 1982;96(5):601–4.
111. Wormser GP, Dattwyler RJ, Shapiro ED, et al. The clinical assessment, treatment, and prevention of lyme disease, human granulocytic anaplasmosis, and babesiosis: clinical practice guidelines by the Infectious Diseases Society of America. Clin Infect Dis 2006;43(9):1089–134.
112. Raoult D, Soulayrol L, Toga B, et al. Babesiosis, pentamidine, and cotrimoxazole. Ann Intern Med 1987;107(6):944.
113. Krause PJ, Gewurz BE, Hill D, et al. Persistent and relapsing babesiosis in immunocompromised patients. Clin Infect Dis 2008;46(3):370–6.
114. Powell VI, Grima K. Exchange transfusion for malaria and *Babesia* infection. Transfus Med Rev 2002;16(3):239–50.

115. Control of Chagas disease. Report of a WHO Expert Committee. World Health Organ Tech Rep Ser 1991;811:1–95.
116. Schmunis GA. *Trypanosoma cruzi*, the etiologic agent of Chagas' disease: status in the blood supply in endemic and nonendemic countries. Transfusion 1991;31(6):547–57.
117. Kerndt PR, Waskin HA, Kirchhoff LV, et al. Prevalence of antibody to *Trypanosoma cruzi* among blood donors in Los Angeles, California. Transfusion 1991; 31(9):814–8.
118. Nowicki MJ, Chinchilla C, Corado L, et al. Prevalence of antibodies to *Trypanosoma cruzi* among solid organ donors in Southern California: a population at risk. Transplantation 2006;81(3):477–9.
119. Ferraz AS, Figueiredo JF. Transmission of Chagas' disease through transplanted kidney: occurrence of the acute form of the disease in two recipients from the same donor. Rev Inst Med Trop Sao Paulo 1993;35(5):461–3.
120. Riarte A, Luna C, Sabatiello R, et al. Chagas' disease in patients with kidney transplants: 7 years of experience 1989–1996. Clin Infect Dis 1999;29(3):561–7.
121. de Faria JB, Alves G. Transmission of Chagas' disease through cadaveric renal transplantation. Transplantation 1993;56(6):1583–4.
122. Vazquez MC, Sabbatiello R, Schiavelli R, et al. Chagas disease and transplantation. Transplant Proc 1996;28(6):3301–3.
123. Kun H, Moore A, Mascola L, et al. Transmission of *Trypanosoma cruzi* by heart transplantation. Clin Infect Dis 2009;48(11):1534–40.
124. Campos SV, Strabelli TM, Amato Neto V, et al. Risk factors for Chagas' disease reactivation after heart transplantation. J Heart Lung Transplant 2008;27(6):597–602.
125. Centers for Disease Control and Prevention (CDC). Chagas disease after organ transplantation—Los Angeles, California, 2006. MMWR Morb Mortal Wkly Rep 2006;55(29):798–800.
126. Carvalho MF, de Franco MF, Soares VA. Amastigotes forms of *Trypanosoma cruzi* detected in a renal allograft. Rev Inst Med Trop Sao Paulo 1997;39(4):223–6.
127. Arias LF, Duque E, Ocampo C, et al. Detection of amastigotes of *Trypanosoma cruzi* in a kidney graft with acute dysfunction. Transplant Proc 2006;38(3):885–7.
128. Morocoima A, Rodriguez M, Herrera L, et al. *Trypanosoma cruzi*: experimental parasitism of bone and cartilage. Parasitol Res 2006;99(6):663–8.
129. Herrera L, Martinez C, Carrasco H, et al. Cornea as a tissue reservoir of *Trypanosoma cruzi*. Parasitol Res 2007;100(6):1395–9.
130. Souza FF, Castro ESO, Marin Neto JA, et al. Acute chagasic myocardiopathy after orthotopic liver transplantation with donor and recipient serologically negative for *Trypanosoma cruzi*: a case report. Transplant Proc 2008;40(3):875–8.
131. Salomone OA, Basquiera AL, Sembaj A, et al. *Trypanosoma cruzi* in persons without serologic evidence of disease, Argentina. Emerg Infect Dis 2003; 9(12):1558–62.
132. Bern C, Montgomery SP, Herwaldt BL, et al. Evaluation and treatment of chagas disease in the United States: a systematic review. JAMA 2007;298(18):2171–81.
133. Viotti R, Vigliano C, Lococo B, et al. Long-term cardiac outcomes of treating chronic Chagas disease with benznidazole versus no treatment: a nonrandomized trial. Ann Intern Med 2006;144(10):724–34.
134. Kirchhoff LV, Gam AA, Gilliam FC. American trypanosomiasis (Chagas' disease) in Central American immigrants. Am J Med 1987;82(5):915–20.
135. Steinberg JP, Galindo RL, Kraus ES, et al. Disseminated acanthamebiasis in a renal transplant recipient with osteomyelitis and cutaneous lesions: case report and literature review. Clin Infect Dis 2002;35(5):e43–9.

136. Kramer MH, Lerner CJ, Visvesvara GS. Kidney and liver transplants from a donor infected with *Naegleria fowleri*. J Clin Microbiol 1997;35(4):1032–3.
137. Didier ES. Microsporidiosis: an emerging and opportunistic infection in humans and animals. Acta Trop 2005;94(1):61–76.
138. Mathis A, Weber R, Deplazes P. Zoonotic potential of the microsporidia. Clin Microbiol Rev 2005;18(3):423–45.
139. Calvo M, Carazo M, Arias ML, et al. [Prevalence of Cyclospora sp., Cryptosporidium sp, microsporidia and fecal coliform determination in fresh fruit and vegetables consumed in Costa Rica]. Arch Latinoam Nutr 2004;54(4):428–32 [in Spanish].
140. Schwartz DA, Visvesvara G, Weber R, et al. Male genital tract microsporidiosis and AIDS: prostatic abscess due to Encephalitozoon hellem. J Eukaryot Microbiol 1994;41(5):61S.
141. Weber R, Deplazes P, Schwartz D. Diagnosis and clinical aspects of human microsporidiosis. Contrib Microbiol 2000;6:166–92.
142. Didier ES, Weiss LM. Microsporidiosis: current status. Curr Opin Infect Dis 2006; 19(5):485–92.
143. Latib MA, Pascoe MD, Duffield MS, et al. Microsporidiosis in the graft of a renal transplant recipient. Transpl Int 2001;14(4):274–7.
144. Gamboa-Dominguez A, De Anda J, Donis J, et al. Disseminated *Encephalitozoon cuniculi* infection in a Mexican kidney transplant recipient. Transplantation 2003;75(11):1898–900.
145. Carlson JR, Li L, Helton CL, et al. Disseminated microsporidiosis in a pancreas/kidney transplant recipient. Arch Pathol Lab Med 2004;128(3):e41–3.
146. Mohindra AR, Lee MW, Visvesvara G, et al. Disseminated microsporidiosis in a renal transplant recipient. Transpl Infect Dis 2002;4(2):102–7.
147. Guerard A, Rabodonirina M, Cotte L, et al. Intestinal microsporidiosis occurring in two renal transplant recipients treated with mycophenolate mofetil. Transplantation 1999;68(5):699–707.
148. Kelkar R, Sastry PS, Kulkarni SS, et al. Pulmonary microsporidial infection in a patient with CML undergoing allogeneic marrow transplant. Bone Marrow Transplant 1997;19(2):179–82.
149. Lanternier F, Boutboul D, Menotti J, et al. Microsporidiosis in solid organ transplant recipients: two *Enterocytozoon bieneusi* cases and review. Transpl Infect Dis 2009;11(1):83–8.
150. Gumbo T, Hobbs RE, Carlyn C, et al. Microsporidia infection in transplant patients. Transplantation 1999;67(3):482–4.
151. Goetz M, Eichenlaub S, Pape GR, et al. Chronic diarrhea as a result of intestinal microsposidiosis in a liver transplant recipient. Transplantation 2001;71(2): 334–7.
152. Sax PE, Rich JD, Pieciak WS, et al. Intestinal microsporidiosis occurring in a liver transplant recipient. Transplantation 1995;60(6):617–8.
153. Rabodonirina M, Bertocchi M, Desportes-Livage I, et al. *Enterocytozoon bieneusi* as a cause of chronic diarrhea in a heart-lung transplant recipient who was seronegative for human immunodeficiency virus. Clin Infect Dis 1996;23(1):114–7.
154. Sing A, Tybus K, Heesemann J, et al. Molecular diagnosis of an *Enterocytozoon bieneusi* human genotype C infection in a moderately immunosuppressed human immunodeficiency virus seronegative liver-transplant recipient with severe chronic diarrhea. J Clin Microbiol 2001;39(6):2371–2.
155. Metge S, Van Nhieu JT, Dahmane D, et al. A case of *Enterocytozoon bieneusi* infection in an HIV-negative renal transplant recipient. Eur J Clin Microbiol Infect Dis 2000;19(3):221–3.

156. Orenstein JM, Russo P, Didier ES, et al. Fatal pulmonary microsporidiosis due to *Encephalitozoon cuniculi* following allogeneic bone marrow transplantation for acute myelogenous leukemia. Ultrastruct Pathol 2005;29(3–4):269–76.
157. Teachey DT, Russo P, Orenstein JM, et al. Pulmonary infection with microsporidia after allogeneic bone marrow transplantation. Bone Marrow Transplant 2004; 33(3):299–302.
158. Mahmood MN, Keohane ME, Burd EM. Pathologic quiz case: a 45-year-old renal transplant recipient with persistent fever. Arch Pathol Lab Med 2003;127(4):e224–6.
159. Tumwine JK, Kekitiinwa A, Bakeera-Kitaka S, et al. Cryptosporidiosis and microsporidiosis in ugandan children with persistent diarrhea with and without concurrent infection with the human immunodeficiency virus. Am J Trop Med Hyg 2005;73(5):921–5.
160. Wichro E, Hoelzl D, Krause R, et al. Microsporidiosis in travel-associated chronic diarrhea in immune-competent patients. Am J Trop Med Hyg 2005; 73(2):285–7.
161. Didier ES. Microsporidiosis. Clin Infect Dis 1998;27(1):1–7 quiz 8.
162. Walker M, Kublin JG, Zunt JR. Parasitic central nervous system infections in immunocompromised hosts: malaria, microsporidiosis, leishmaniasis, and African trypanosomiasis. Clin Infect Dis 2006;42(1):115–25.
163. Conteas CN, Sowerby T, Berlin GW, et al. Fluorescence techniques for diagnosing intestinal microsporidiosis in stool, enteric fluid, and biopsy specimens from acquired immunodeficiency syndrome patients with chronic diarrhea. Arch Pathol Lab Med 1996;120(9):847–53.
164. Fedorko DP, Hijazi YM. Application of molecular techniques to the diagnosis of microsporidial infection. Emerg Infect Dis 1996;2(3):183–91.
165. van Gool T, Snijders F, Reiss P, et al. Diagnosis of intestinal and disseminated microsporidial infections in patients with HIV by a new rapid fluorescence technique. J Clin Pathol 1993;46(8):694–9.
166. Didier ES. Immunology of microsporidiosis. Contrib Microbiol 2000;6:193–208.
167. Fedorko DP, Nelson NA, Didier ES, et al. Speciation of human microsporidia by polymerase chain reaction single-strand conformation polymorphism. Am J Trop Med Hyg 2001;65(4):397–401.
168. Huston CD, Petri Jr. WA. Emerging and reemerging intestinal protozoa. Curr Opin Gastroenterol 2001;17(1):17–23.
169. Molina JM, Tourneur M, Sarfati C, et al. Fumagillin treatment of intestinal microsporidiosis. N Engl J Med 2002;346(25):1963–9.
170. Didier ES. Effects of albendazole, fumagillin, and TNP-470 on microsporidial replication in vitro. Antimicrobial Agents Chemother 1997;41(7):1541–6.
171. Sun T, Kaplan MH, Teichberg S, et al. Intestinal microsporidiosis. Report of five cases. Ann Clin Lab Sci 1994;24(6):521–32.
172. Cama VA, Bern C, Sulaiman IM, et al. *Cryptosporidium* species and genotypes in HIV-positive patients in Lima, Peru. J Eukaryot Microbiol 2003;50(Suppl):531–3.
173. Tzipori S, Widmer G. A hundred-year retrospective on cryptosporidiosis. Trends Parasitol 2008;24(4):184–9.
174. Guerrant RL. Cryptosporidiosis: an emerging, highly infectious threat. Emerg Infect Dis 1997;3(1):51–7.
175. Hoepelman AI. Current therapeutic approaches to cryptosporidiosis in immunocompromised patients. J Antimicrob Chemother 1996;37(5):871–80.
176. Abubakar I, Aliyu SH, Arumugam C, et al. Treatment of cryptosporidiosis in immunocompromised individuals: systematic review and meta-analysis. Br J Clin Pharmacol 2007;63(4):387–93.

177. MacKenzie WR, Schell WL, Blair KA, et al. Massive outbreak of waterborne *Cryptosporidium* infection in Milwaukee, Wisconsin: recurrence of illness and risk of secondary transmission. Clin Infect Dis 1995;21(1):57–62.
178. Hunter PR, Nichols G. Epidemiology and clinical features of *Cryptosporidium* infection in immunocompromised patients. Clin Microbiol Rev 2002;15(1):145–54.
179. Fayer R, Ungar BL. *Cryptosporidium* spp. and cryptosporidiosis. Microbiol Rev 1986;50(4):458–83.
180. Campos M, Jouzdani E, Sempoux C, et al. Sclerosing cholangitis associated to cryptosporidiosis in liver-transplanted children. Eur J Pediatr 2000;159(1-2): 113–5.
181. Denkinger CM, Harigopal P, Ruiz P, et al. *Cryptosporidium parvum*-associated sclerosing cholangitis in a liver transplant patient. Transpl Infect Dis 2008; 10(2):133–6.
182. Hong DK, Wong CJ, Gutierrez K. Severe cryptosporidiosis in a seven-year-old renal transplant recipient: case report and review of the literature. Pediatr Transplant 2007;11(1):94–100.
183. Tran MQ, Gohh RY, Morrissey PE, et al. *Cryptosporidium* infection in renal transplant patients. Clin Nephrol 2005;63(4):305–9.
184. Jelinek T, Lotze M, Eichenlaub S, et al. Prevalence of infection with *Cryptosporidium parvum* and *Cyclospora cayetanensis* among international travellers. Gut 1997;41(6):801–4.
185. Alakpa GE, Clarke SC, Fagbenro-Beyioku AF. C *yclospora cayetanensis* infection: vegetables and water as possible vehicles for its transmission in Lagos, Nigeria. Br J Biomed Sci 2003;60(2):113–4.
186. Bern C, Hernandez B, Lopez MB, et al. Epidemiologic studies of C *yclospora cayetanensis* in Guatemala. Emerg Infect Dis 1999;5(6):766–74.
187. el-Karamany EM, Zaher TI, el-Bahnasawy MM. Role of water in the transmission of cyclosporiarsis in Sharkia Governorate, Egypt. J Egypt Soc Parasitol 2005; 35(3):953–62.
188. Madico G, McDonald J, Gilman RH, et al. Epidemiology and treatment of *Cyclospora cayetanensis* infection in Peruvian children. Clin Infect Dis 1997;24(5): 977–81.
189. Chacin-Bonilla L, Barrios F, Sanchez Y. Epidemiology of *Cyclospora cayetanensis* infection in San Carlos Island, Venezuela: strong association between socio-economic status and infection. Trans R Soc Trop Med Hyg 2007;101(10): 1018–24.
190. Sancak B, Akyon Y. [Microsporidia: general characteristics, infections and laboratory diagnosis]. Mikrobiyol Bul 2005;39(4):513–22 [in Turkish].
191. Curry A, Smith HV. Emerging pathogens: *Isospora, Cyclospora* and microsporidia. Parasitology 1998;117(Suppl):S143–59.
192. Drenaggi D, Cirioni O, Giacometti A, et al. Cyclosporiasis in a traveler returning from South America. J Travel Med 1998;5(3):153–5.
193. Herwaldt BL. *Cyclospora cayetanensis*: a review, focusing on the outbreaks of cyclosporiasis in the 1990s. Clin Infect Dis 2000;31(4):1040–57.
194. Ho AY, Lopez AS, Eberhart MG, et al. Outbreak of cyclosporiasis associated with imported raspberries, Philadelphia, Pennsylvania, 2000. Emerg Infect Dis 2002;8(8):783–8.
195. Wang KX, Li CP, Wang J, et al. Cyclospore cayetanensis in Anhui, China. World J Gastroenterol Dec 2002;8(6):1144–8.
196. Wurtz R. *Cyclospora*: a newly identified intestinal pathogen of humans. Clin Infect Dis 1994;18(4):620–3.

197. Soave R. Cyclospora: an overview. Clin Infect Dis 1996;23(3):429–35 [quiz: 436–27].
198. Pinge-Suttor V, Douglas C, Wettstein A. *Cyclospora* infection masquerading as coeliac disease. Med J Aust 2004;180(6):295–6.
199. Connor BA, Johnson EJ, Soave R. Reiter syndrome following protracted symptoms of *Cyclospora* infection. Emerg Infect Dis 2001;7(3):453–4.
200. Zar FA, El-Bayoumi E, Yungbluth MM. Histologic proof of acalculous cholecystitis due to *Cyclospora cayetanensis*. Clin Infect Dis. 2001;33(12):E140–1.
201. Richardson RF Jr, Remler BF, Katirji B, et al. Guillain-Barre syndrome after *Cyclospora* infection. Muscle Nerve 1998;21(5):669–71.
202. Sifuentes-Osornio J, Porras-Cortes G, Bendall RP, et al. *Cyclospora cayetanensis* infection in patients with and without AIDS: biliary disease as another clinical manifestation. Clin Infect Dis 1995;21(5):1092–7.
203. Ferreira MS. Infections by protozoa in immunocompromised hosts. Mem Inst Oswaldo Cruz 2000;95(Suppl 1):159–62.
204. Aksoy U, Tuncay S. [Short communication: investigation of intestinal coccidia in patients with diarrhea]. Mikrobiyol Bul 2007;41(1):127–31 [in Turkish].
205. Abou EL, Naga IF. Studies on a newly emerging protozoal pathogen: Cyclospora cayetanensis. J Egypt Soc Parasitol 1999;29(2):575–86.
206. Helmy MM, Rashed LA, Abdel-Fattah HS. Co-infection with *Cryptosporidium parvum* and *Cyclospora cayetanensis* in immunocompromised patients. J Egypt Soc Parasitol 2006;36(2):613–27.
207. Varea M, Clavel A, Doiz O, et al. Fuchsin fluorescence and autofluorescence in *Cryptosporidium, Isospora* and *Cyclospora* oocysts. Int J Parasitol 1998;28(12): 1881–3.
208. Field AS. Light microscopic and electron microscopic diagnosis of gastrointestinal opportunistic infections in HIV-positive patients. Pathology 2002;34(1):21–35.
209. Lewthwaite P, Gill GV, Hart CA, et al. Gastrointestinal parasites in the immunocompromised. Curr Opin Infect Dis 2005;18(5):427–35.
210. Yazar S, Yalcln S, Sahin I. Human cyclosporiosis in Turkey. World J Gastroenterol 2004;10(12):1844–7.
211. Pape JW, Verdier RI, Boncy M, et al. *Cyclospora* infection in adults infected with HIV. Clinical manifestations, treatment, and prophylaxis. Ann Intern Med 1994; 121(9):654–7.
212. Fox LM, Saravolatz LD. Nitazoxanide: a new thiazolide antiparasitic agent. Clin Infect Dis. 2005;40(8):1173–80.
213. Negm AY. Human pathogenic protozoa in bivalves collected from local markets in Alexandria. J Egypt Soc Parasitol 2003;33(3):991–8.
214. Palau LA, Kemmerly SA. First report of invasive amebiasis in an organ transplant recipient. Transplantation 1997;64(6):936–7.
215. Aucott JN, Ravdin JI. Amebiasis and “nonpathogenic” intestinal protozoa. Infect Dis Clin North Am 1993;7(3):467–85.
216. Keiser PB, Nutman TB. *Strongyloides stercoralis* in the Immunocompromised Population. Clin Microbiol Rev 2004;17(1):208–17.
217. Lichtenberger P, Rosa-Cunha I, Morris M, et al. Hyperinfection strongyloidiasis in a liver transplant recipient treated with parenteral ivermectin. Transpl Infect Dis 2009;11(2):137–42.
218. Stone WJ, Schaffner W. *Strongyloides* infections in transplant recipients. Semin Respir Infect 1990;5(1):58–64.
219. DeVault GA Jr, King JW, Rohr MS, et al. Opportunistic infections with S *trongyloides stercoralis* in renal transplantation. Rev Infect Dis 1990;12(4):653–71.

220. Patel G, Arvelakis A, Sauter BV, et al. *Strongyloides* hyperinfection syndrome after intestinal transplantation. Transpl Infect Dis 2008;10(2):137–41.
221. Palau LA, Pankey GA. *Strongyloides* hyperinfection in a renal transplant recipient receiving cyclosporine: possible Strongyloides stercoralis transmission by kidney transplant. Am J Trop Med Hyg 1997;57(4):413–5.
222. Schaeffer MW, Buell JF, Gupta M, et al. *Strongyloides* hyperinfection syndrome after heart transplantation: case report and review of the literature. J Heart Lung Transplant 2004;23(7):905–11.
223. Ben-Youssef R, Baron P, Edson F, et al. *Stronglyoides stercoralis* infection from pancreas allograft: case report. Transplantation 2005;80(7):997–8.
224. El Masry HZ, O'Donnell J. Fatal *Strongyloides* hyperinfection in heart transplantation. J Heart Lung Transplant 2005;24(11):1980–3.
225. Said T, Nampoory MR, Nair MP, et al. Hyperinfection strongyloidiasis: an anticipated outbreak in kidney transplant recipients in Kuwait. Transplant Proc 2007;39(4):1014–5.
226. Mokaddas EM, Shati S, Abdulla A, et al. Fatal strongyloidiasis in three kidney recipients in Kuwait. Med Princ Pract 2009;18(5):414–7.
227. Balagopal A, Mills L, Shah A, et al. Detection and treatment of *Strongyloides* hyperinfection syndrome following lung transplantation. Transpl Infect Dis 2009;11(2):149–54.
228. Vilela EG, Clemente WT, Mira RR, et al. *Strongyloides stercoralis* hyperinfection syndrome after liver transplantation: case report and literature review. Transpl Infect Dis 2009;11(2):132–6.
229. Mizuno S, Iida T, Zendejas I, et al. *Strongyloides* hyperinfection syndrome following simultaneous heart and kidney transplantation. Transpl Int 2009;22(2):251–3.
230. Morrell MR, Dallas J, Kollef MH. A 50-year-old woman with abdominal pain and respiratory failure 3 months after kidney transplantation. Chest 2008;134(2):442–6.
231. Soman R, Vaideeswar P, Shah H, et al. A 34-year-old renal transplant recipient with high-grade fever and progressive shortness of breath. J Postgrad Med 2002;48(3):191–6.
232. Skandrani K, Richardet JP, Duvoux C, et al. [Hepatic transplantation for severe ductopenia related to ingestion of thiabendazole]. Gastroenterol Clin Biol 1997;21(8-9):623–5 [in French].
233. German JC, Flores JH, Chiesura G, et al. [Fatal strongyloidiasis in an immunodepressed patient following renal transplantation]. Rev Hosp Clin Fac Med Sao Paulo 1992;47(1):31–3 [in Spanish].
234. Morgan JS, Schaffner W, Stone WJ. Opportunistic strongyloidiasis in renal transplant recipients. Transplantation 1986;42(5):518–24.
235. van der Woude FJ, Kager PA, Weits J, et al. *Strongyloides stercoralis* hyperinfection as a consequence of immunosuppressive treatment. Neth J Med 1985;28(8):315–7.
236. Zuidema PJ. [Hyperinfection with Strongyloides stercoralis following kidney transplantation]. Ned Tijdschr Geneeskd 1984;128(6):261–3 [in Dutch].
237. Narasimhan N, Piering WF, Kauffman HM, et al. Kidney transplant recipient with disseminated *Strongyloides*. Transplantation 1983;36(4):472–3.
238. Fowler CG, Lindsay I, Levin J, et al. Recurrent hyperinfestation with Strongyloides stercoralis in a renal allograft recipient. Br Med J (Clin Res Ed) 1982;285(6352):1394.
239. Vishwanath S, Baker RA, Mansheim BJ. *Strongyloides* infection and meningitis in an immunocompromised host. Am J Trop Med Hyg 1982;31(4):857–8.

240. White JV, Garvey G, Hardy MA. Fatal strongyloidiasis after renal transplantation: a complication of immunosuppression. Am Surg 1982;48(1):39–41.
241. Hoy WE, Roberts NJ Jr, Bryson MF, et al. Transmission of strongyloidiasis by kidney transplant? Disseminated strongyloidiasis in both recipients of kidney allografts from a single cadaver donor. JAMA 1981;246(17):1937–9.
242. Muller J, Konigshausen T, Sandmann W, et al. [Fatal infection due to Strongyloides stercoralis after kidney transplantation]. Med Welt 1981;32(32–33): 1210–1 [in German].
243. Weller IV, Copland P, Gabriel R. *Strongyloides stercoralis* infection in renal transplant recipients. Br Med J (Clin Res Ed) 1981;282(6263):524.
244. Leapman SB, Rosenberg JB, Filo RS, et al. *Strongyloides stercoralis* in chronic renal failure: safe therapy with thiabendazole. Southampt Med J 1980;73(10):1400–2.
245. Briner J, Eckert J, Frei D, et al. [Strongyloidiasis following kidney transplantation]. Schweiz Med Wochenschr 1978;108(42):1632–7 [in German].
246. Meyers AM, Shapiro DJ, Milne FJ, et al. *Strongyloides stercoralis* hyperinfection in a renal allograft recipient. S Afr Med J 1976;50(33):1301–2.
247. Tarr PE, Miele PS, Peregoy KS, et al. Case report: rectal adminstration of ivermectin to a patient with *Strongyloides* hyperinfection syndrome. Am J Trop Med Hyg 2003;68(4):453–5.
248. Fisher D, McCarry F, Currie B. Strongyloidiasis in the Northern Territory. Under-recognised and under-treated? Med J Aust 1993;159(2):88–90.
249. Cook GA, Rodriguez H, Silva H, et al. Adult respiratory distress secondary to strongyloidiasis. Chest Dec 1987;92(6):1115–6.
250. Boram LH, Keller KF, Justus DE, et al. Strongyloidiasis in immunosuppressed patients. Am J Clin Pathol Dec 1981;76(6):778–81.
251. Huston JM, Eachempati SR, Rodney JR, et al. Treatment of *Strongyloides stercoralis* hyperinfection-associated septic shock and acute respiratory distress syndrome with drotrecogin alfa (activated) in a renal transplant recipient. Transpl Infect Dis 2009;11(3):277–80.
252. Avagnina MA, Elsner B, Iotti RM, et al. *Strongyloides stercoralis* in Papanicolaou-stained smears of ascitic fluid. Acta Cytol 1980;24(1):36–9.
253. Valar C, Keitel E, Dal Pra RL, et al. Parasitic infection in renal transplant recipients. Transplant Proc 2007;39(2):460–2.
254. Prasad N, Ram R, Satti Reddy V, et al. Non-fatal gastric mucormycosis in a renal transplant patient and review of the literature. Transpl Infect Dis 2006;8(4): 237–41.
255. Genta RM. Global prevalence of strongyloidiasis: critical review with epidemiologic insights into the prevention of disseminated disease. Rev Infect Dis 1989; 11(5):755–67.
256. Nutman TB, Ottesen EA, Ieng S, et al. Eosinophilia in Southeast Asian refugees: evaluation at a referral center. J Infect Dis 1987;155(2):309–13.
257. Fardet L, Genereau T, Cabane J, et al. Severe strongyloidiasis in corticosteroid-treated patients. Clin Microbiol Infect 2006;12(10):945–7.
258. Chu E, Whitlock WL, Dietrich RA. Pulmonary hyperinfection syndrome with *Strongyloides stercoralis*. Chest 1990;97(6):1475–7.
259. Safdar A, Malathum K, Rodriguez SJ, et al. Strongyloidiasis in patients at a comprehensive cancer center in the United States. Cancer 2004;100(7): 1531–6.
260. Orlent H, Crawley C, Cwynarski K, et al. Strongyloidiasis pre and post autologous peripheral blood stem cell transplantation. Bone Marrow Transplant 2003;32(1):115–7.

261. Nucci M, Portugal R, Pulcheri W, et al. Strongyloidiasis in patients with hematologic malignancies. Clin Infect Dis 1995;21(3):675–7.
262. Genta RM. Dysregulation of strongyloidiasis: a new hypothesis. Clin Microbiol Rev 1992;5(4):345–55.
263. Siddiqui AA, Berk SL. Diagnosis of *Strongyloides stercoralis* infection. Clin Infect Dis 2001;33(7):1040–7.
264. Nolan TJ, Schad GA. Tacrolimus allows autoinfective development of the parasitic nematode *Strongyloides stercoralis*. Transplantation 1996;62(7):1038.
265. Beal CB, Viens P, Grant RG, et al. A new technique for sampling duodenal contents: demonstration of upper small-bowel pathogens. Am J Trop Med Hyg 1970;19(2):349–52.
266. Rosenblatt JE. Clinical importance of adequately performed stool ova and parasite examinations. Clin Infect Dis 2006;42(7):979–80.
267. Martin-Rabadan P, Munoz P, Palomo J, et al. Strongyloidiasis: the Harada-Mori test revisited. Clin Microbiol Infect 1999;5(6):374–6.
268. Sreenivas DV, Kumar A, Kumar YR, et al. Intestinal strongyloidiasis—a rare opportunistic infection. Indian J Gastroenterol 1997;16(3):105–6.
269. Thompson BF, Fry LC, Wells CD, et al. The spectrum of GI strongyloidiasis: an endoscopic-pathologic study. Gastrointest Endosc 2004;59(7):906–10.
270. Overstreet K, Chen J, Rodriguez JW, et al. Endoscopic and histopathologic findings of *Strongyloides stercoralis* infection in a patient with AIDS. Gastrointest Endosc 2003;58(6):928–31.
271. Abdalla J, Saad M, Myers JW, et al. An elderly man with immunosuppression, shortness of breath, and eosinophilia. Clin Infect Dis. 2005;40(10):1464 1535–1466.
272. Smith B, Verghese A, Guiterrez C, et al. Pulmonary strongyloidiasis. Diagnosis by sputum gram stain. Am J Med 1985;79(5):663–6.
273. Harris RA Jr, Musher DM, Fainstein V, et al. Disseminated strongyloidiasis. Diagnosis made by sputum examination. JAMA 1980;244(1):65–6.
274. Liu LX, Weller PF. Strongyloidiasis and other intestinal nematode infections. Infect Dis Clin North Am 1993;7(3):655–82.
275. Igual-Adell R, Oltra-Alcaraz C, Soler-Company E, et al. Efficacy and safety of ivermectin and thiabendazole in the treatment of strongyloidiasis. Expert Opin Pharmacother 2004;5(12):2615–9.
276. Zaha O, Hirata T, Kinjo F, et al. Efficacy of ivermectin for chronic strongyloidiasis: two single doses given 2 weeks apart. J Infect Chemother 2002;8(1):94–8.
277. Kayler LK, Rudich SM, Merion RM. Orthotopic liver transplantation from a donor with a history of schistosomiasis. Transplant Proc 2003;35(8):2974–6.
278. Shokeir AA. Renal transplantation: the impact of schistosomiasis. BJU Int 2001;88(9):915–20.
279. Hoare M, Gelson WT, Davies SE, et al. Hepatic and intestinal schistosomiasis after orthotopic liver transplant. Liver Transpl 2005;11(12):1603–7.
280. Sobh MA, el-Agroudy AE, Moustafa FE, et al. Impact of schistosomiasis on patient and graft outcome after kidney transplantation. Nephrol Dial Transplant 1992;7(8):858–64.
281. Ahmed K, Safdar K, Kemmer N, et al. Intestinal schistosomiasis following orthotopic liver transplantation: a case report. Transplant Proc 2007;39(10):3502–4.
282. Bica I, Hamer DH, Stadecker MJ. Hepatic schistosomiasis. Infect Dis Clin North Am 2000;14(3):583–604, viii.

283. Mudawi HM, Elhassan EA, Baraka OZ, et al. Schistosomal colitis without granuloma formation in a kidney transplant recipient. Nat Clin Pract Gastroenterol Hepatol 2006;3(12):700–4.
284. Azevedo LS, de Paula FJ, Ianhez LE, et al. Renal transplantation and schistosomiasis *mansoni*. Transplantation 1987;44(6):795–8.
285. Falcao HA, Gould DB. Immune complex nephropathy i schistosomiasis. Ann Intern Med 1975;83(2):148–54.
286. Mahmoud KM, Sobh MA, El-Agroudy AE, et al. Impact of schistosomiasis on patient and graft outcome after renal transplantation: 10 years' follow-up. Nephrol Dial Transplant 2001;16(11):2214–21.
287. Caffrey CR, Gsell C, Ruppel A. *Schistosoma japonicum* is less sensitive to cyclosporin A in vivo than Schistosoma mansoni. J Parasitol 1999;85(4):736–9.
288. Pungpapong S, Krishna M, Abraham SC, et al. Clinicopathologic findings and outcomes of liver transplantation using grafts from donors with unrecognized and unusual diseases. Liver Transpl 2006;12(2):310–5.
289. Bresson-Hadni S, Koch S, Beurton I, et al. Primary disease recurrence after liver transplantation for alveolar echinococcosis: long-term evaluation in 15 patients. Hepatology 1999;30(4):857–64.
290. Moreno-González E, Loinaz Segurola C, Garcia Urena MA, et al. Liver transplantation for *Echinococcus granulosus* hydatid disease. Transplantation 1994; 58(7):797–800.
291. Loinaz C, Moreno-González E, Gómez R, et al. Liver transplantation in liver disease: Echinococcus granulosus. Transplant Proc 1998;30(7):3268–9.
292. Sobrino JM, Pulpon LA, Crespo MG, et al. Heart transplantation in a patient with liver hydatidosis. J Heart Lung Transplant 1993;12(3):531–3.
293. Bein T, Haerty W, Haller M, et al. Organ selection in intensive care: transplantation of a liver allograft, including calcified cyst of *Echinococcus granulosus*. Intensive Care Med 1993;19(3):182.
294. Koch S, Bresson-Hadni S, Miguet JP, et al. Experience of liver transplantation for incurable alveolar echinococcosis: a 45-case European collaborative report. Transplantation 2003;75(6):856–63.
295. Gupta RK, Jain M. Renal transplantation: potential source of microfilarial transmission. Transplant Proc 1998;30(8):4320–1.

Infections Transmitted by Transplantation

Michele I. Morris, MD[a], Staci A. Fischer, MD[b], Michael G. Ison, MD, MS[c,*]

KEYWORDS

• Organ transplant • Donor-derived infection • Transmission
• Donor screening

Infections are frequently transmitted through solid-organ and, to a lesser extent, stem cell transplantation. There are 2 major types of donor-derived infections that are transmitted: those that would be expected secondary to donor and recipient screening (ie, transmission of cytomegalovirus [CMV], Epstein-Barr virus [EBV], or toxoplasmosis from a seropositive donor to a seronegative recipient) and those that are unexpected despite routine donor screening (ie, human immunodeficiency virus (HIV) and hepatitis C virus [HCV] transmitted from a seronegative donor). Expected transmissions occur frequently and screening and prophylaxis strategies are applied to at-risk individuals in nearly all transplant centers globally. Several high profile donor-derived infectious disease transmissions have been recognized[1–9]; these reports have raised awareness of this rare complication of transplantation. Issues related to the epidemiology of, screening for, and management of proven or probable donor-derived infections are reviewed in this article.

EPIDEMIOLOGY AND SIGNIFICANCE OF INFECTIONS TRANSMITTED BY TRANSPLANTATION

Currently, the epidemiology of donor-derived infections has been extrapolated from reports made in the medical literature, to the Centers for Disease Control and Prevention, and to the Organ Procurement Transplantation Network (OPTN). OPTN Policy 4.7, which was enacted in November 2004, requires reporting by a transplant center of a confirmed or suspected donor-derived disease transmission to the organ

[a] Division of Infectious Diseases, University of Miami Miller School of Medicine, Miami, FL, USA
[b] Division of Infectious Diseases, The Warren Alpert Medical School of Brown University, Providence, RI, USA
[c] Divisions of Infectious Diseases & Organ Transplantation, Northwestern University Feinberg School of Medicine, Chicago, IL, USA
* Corresponding author. 645 North Michigan Avenue, Suite 900, Chicago, IL 60611.
E-mail address: mgison@northwestern.edu

Infect Dis Clin N Am 24 (2010) 497–514
doi:10.1016/j.idc.2010.02.002
0891-5520/10/$ – see front matter © 2010 Elsevier Inc. All rights reserved.

procurement organization (OPO) who must then report the transmission to the OPTN. Since the policy was enacted, the number of reports of proven or potential donor-derived disease transmission has increased significantly from 7 reports in 2005 to 102 reports in 2008. From this exponential increase, it is clear that the current system is only capturing a fraction of the true donor-derived infections.

The methodology used by the OPTN, through its Ad Hoc Disease Transmission Advisory Committee, to identify, evaluate, and classify donor-derived disease transmissions has recently been published.[10] A wide range of infectious diseases have been reported to the OPTN (**Table 1**). From these data, it is clear that several key features can be summarized:

1. Unexpected donor-derived infectious disease transmissions are rare. Despite current limitations of the systems to recognize these transmissions, they likely occur in less than 1% of all transplant procedures.
2. Unexpected donor-derived infectious diseases transmissions cause significant morbidity and mortality.
3. Nonreproducible (ie, false-positive) molecular diagnostics for viral infectious diseases occur and may result in discarding of organs.
4. Bacterial contamination of organs or bacterial infections and colonization in the donor occurs frequently but rarely results in transmission of infection.[11]

Table 1
Potential donor-derived infectious disease transmissions reported to OPTN 2005 to 2008

Disease	No. of Donor Reports	No. of Recipients with Confirmed Transmission	No. of Recipient Deaths Attributable to Donor-Derived Disease
Bacteria[a]	21	8	4
Fungus[b]	12	4	1
Mycobacterium tuberculosis and non-TB *Mycobacteria*	16	1	0
Parasitic[c]	15	8	2
Syphilis	4	1	0
Viral[d]	54	14	6
Expected transmissions[e]	14	–	–

[a] *Acinetobacter, Enterococcus* (including VRE), *Ehrlichia* spp, gram-positive bacteria, *Klebsiella, Legionella, Listeria,* Lyme disease, *Pseudomonas,* Rickettsia, *Serratia, Staphylococcus aureus, Veillonella;* bacterial meningitis and bacterial emboli.

[b] *Aspergillus* spp, *Candida* spp, histoplasmosis, zygomycetes.

[c] Babesia, Chagas, schistosomiasis, strongyloides.

[d] This includes 4 patients with both HIV and HCV transmission. All but 3 reports represent nonreproducible nucleic acid test (NAT) results except for 1 report of HCV with 3 transmissions, 1 report of HCV/HIV with 4 transmissions and 1 death, and 1 patient with HIV infection acquired after transplant.

[e] 14 expected transmissions: CMV, toxoplasmosis, and EBV.

Data from Complete list of donor screening assays for infectious agents and HIV diagnostic assays. Available at: http://www.fda.gov/BiologicsBloodVaccines/BloodBloodProducts/ApprovedProducts/LicensedProductsBLAs/BloodDonorScreening/InfectiousDisease/ucm080466.htm. Accessed July 13, 2009.

Unfortunately, when a transmission occurs, there is usually significant associated organ loss, morbidity, and mortality.

5. Communication remains a significant hindrance to early identification of cases and may contribute to morbidity and mortality. This is clearly highlighted with the recent transmission of tuberculosis.[12] Although a potential solution to this system was piloted (the Transplantation Transmission Sentinel Network), it has not been funded or implemented fully.[13]

Interest in donor-derived disease transmission is growing globally. Although the US OPTN/United Network for Organ Sharing (UNOS) Disease transmission Advisory Committee (DTAC) is a national system for biovigilence of organ recipients, many other countries have nascent systems in place or have systems under development. A proposed system in Australia would have the advantage of combining a national prospective monitoring system with a biobank of specimens from all organ donors and recipients that would facilitate identification and evaluation of potential donor-derived disease transmissions. A group of global leaders has begun to meet to develop common definitions and evaluate plans to identify and manage proven donor-derived disease transmissions.

CURRENT SCREENING REQUIREMENTS AND LIMITATIONS

Organ donor screening in the United States is regulated by the OPTN to help ensure a uniform standard of testing through the activities of the nation's OPOs (**Table 2**). OPTN policy 2.0 outlines recommended donor screening tests to identify organisms that are potentially transmissible to transplant recipients; OPTN policy 4.0 documents what diseases, if known to be present in the donor, should be disclosed to the recipient centers.[14,15] Despite this minimum standard, testing practices vary among individual OPOs, depending in part on laboratory availability and geographic limitations. Screening requirements for human tissues and cellular products are regulated by the US Food and Drug Administration (FDA; see **Table 2**).

All potential donors are screened for transmissible infectious diseases using an FDA-licensed, -approved, or -cleared screening test if such a test is commercially

Table 2
Screening tests required for organ, tissue, and hematopoietic stem cell donors in the United States

Test	Organ	Tissue	Hematopoietic Stem Cells
HIV I/II antibody	X	X	X
HIV NAT		X	X
Syphilis	X	X	X
HTLV-1/-2 antibody		X[a]	X
CMV antibody	X	X[a]	X
EBV antibody	X	X	X
HBc antibody	X	X	X
HBs antigen	X	X	X
HCV antibody	X	X	X
HCV NAT		X	X

[a] Testing must be done only on human cellular tissue/products that are viable and leukocyte rich.

available (**Table 3**)[15]; the use of FDA-approved diagnostic tests is permitted if no screening test is commercially available by current policy. There are important differences between the sensitivity and specificity of diagnostic and screening tests. Diagnostic tests are designed for maximum specificity, to be used to evaluate a patient with some pretest probability of infection. There is no requirement that diagnostic tests be performed according to the test manufacturer's instructions; modifications of the test are allowed if the testing laboratory validates any changes they make. Such flexibility is not permitted with donor screening tests, which are standardized for maximum sensitivity to be used in testing a low-prevalence population. Screening tests optimized for sensitivity may have a higher incidence of false-positive results relative to diagnostic tests, but this has been acceptable to applications such as blood bank screening, although it might be problematic in a clinical setting in which such results might lead to an incorrect patient diagnosis. Differences also exist between tests approved for use in living versus cadaveric donors. The FDA defines cadaveric donors as those whose heartbeat has ceased; all organ donors have a heartbeat when screening tests are collected, so FDA-licensed living donor screening tests must be used.

Although testing for HIV, hepatitis B virus (HBV), and HCV is currently required for all donors, transmission may occur despite negative serology. The dynamics of viremia during primary infection with HIV, HCV, and HBV share some basic commonalities, although they differ in predictable virus-specific detection capability because of variations in the pattern of host response to each pathogen. All 3 viruses share a sequence of initial infection followed by a pre–ramp-up phase of early viremia. Circulating virus is currently not measurable during this pre–ramp-up phase using any of the available assays. The limit of detectability for most viruses is approximately 1 copy per 20 mL or 0.05 copies per mL, the viral concentration that might be present in a unit of red blood cells (RBC) containing a single HCV copy.[16] Viral replication proceeds logarithmically during the ramp-up phase until it reaches a plateau level. Ramp-up and plateau phases for each virus have been studied and can be characterized relative to the typical appearance of clinical symptoms (**Fig. 1**).[16–18]

Viral infections such as HIV, HCV, and HBV are potentially infectious to others exposed to the initial host through sharing of blood and body fluids or organs. Once primary infection occurs, there is a period of time, known as the eclipse phase, during which virus is replicating within the host in a localized fashion such that the levels circulating in the bloodstream are neither measurable by current methods nor transmissible by transfusion, but transmission through organ transplantation could occur. This is followed by a window period of viremia during which infection from bodily fluids can occur but detection by the most sensitive assays currently available is not possible. This results in a predictable residual risk of infection, the probability of infectious exposure despite laboratory screening. Newer screening assays are evaluated for their infection yield, the number of new infections detected through the enhanced sensitivity provided by such tests in comparison to previous screening methods.[19] The incidence window period model was formulated to assess the residual risk of infection in a given population screened with a specific test for which the infection window period has been previously established.[20–22] Testing focused on the identification of early infection is particularly important for the organ transplant recipient, as viral replication may occur at higher levels in donor organs than in the bloodstream, as in the case of occult viral hepatitis in a potential liver donor.

Much of the recent effort in assay development for blood and organ donor screening has been targeted at methods that provide earlier detection of infection, narrowing the infectious window period to decrease the residual risk of donor infection. Most serologic tests can diagnose prevalent infection, donors with exposure to a pathogen at a time period in the past who have developed a predictable and complete host response. Additional work has focused on the diagnosis of incident infection, new cases recently exposed to virus in which previous screening assays would fail to detect virus. Mathematical modeling largely based on seroconversion rates in repeat blood donors has been used to help predict the rate of incident infection in a given population. Mandatory nucleic acid testing (NAT) for HIV and HCV in tissue donors has helped achieve a better understanding of incident infection rates in organ donors, many of whom are also tissue donors, but data specific to the organ donor population are still lacking.[23] The available literature does suggest a higher rate of incident infection in organ donors compared with blood donors.[24–27]

HIV Screening Tests

HIV serologic tests have been available since 1985 and current assays are more sensitive in early infection, as well as in the detection of HIV-2 and type O strains.[28,29] Fourth generation assays available outside the United States combine antibody and antigen screening to shorten the infectious window period.[30–32] Such tests are more sensitive than third-generation assays, but retain specificity and are significantly less expensive than NAT.

NAT for HIV requires sophisticated laboratory personnel, specialized equipment, and more time than serologic assays. It is the most sensitive assay for the detection of incident HIV infection, but is less specific. Individual donor NAT (ID-NAT) can be more sensitive in detecting very early seroconversion. Although ID-NAT is used by some OPOs for screening organ donors, specimens obtained from donors with low-level viremia may only intermittently contain detectable virus and likewise false-positive results have been described.[33]

Commercial testing platforms vary in sensitivity and specificity. Multiplex NAT assays exist that detect HIV-1 and HCV RNA simultaneously. When multiplex NAT results are positive, a discriminatory NAT must be used containing primers specific to HIV and HCV, to distinguish the type of RNA present in the donor specimen; if the assay for either virus is positive, a positive screen is reported. If the individual NATs are negative, typically the multiplex is repeated to help identify initial false-positive results. Test platforms are also available that test for single virus and have no FDA-approved method for detecting a false-positive result; no standardized testing algorithm exists for the purposes of organ donor screening.

HCV Screening Tests

Serologic testing for HCV has improved in sensitivity since first becoming available in 1990, resulting in a shorter window period for the newer assays. Combination antigen-antibody fourth generation assays are not yet licensed in the United States, although their sensitivity may approach that of HCV MP-NAT.[34] Because of the long window period inherent to infection with hepatitis C, NAT significantly improves the sensitivity of HCV screening compared with second- and third-generation serologic testing.[35]

HBV Screening Tests

Hepatitis B screening is slightly more complex because of the existence of multiple serologic tests that allow the identification of early and established infection by using HBsAg and HBcAb, total immunoglobulin, and IgM. It seems that currently available and highly sensitive testing for HBsAg is able to identify virtually all blood donors

Table 3
Licensed donor screening assays for infectious diseases

Test	Format	Approved Indications	Manufacturer
HBV			
Hepatitis B Surface Antigen Assays			
Genetic Systems HBsAg EIA 2.0	EIA	Living: S, P Cadaveric: S	Bio-Rad Laboratories
Auszyme Monoclonal	EIA	Living: S, P Cadaveric: S	Abbott Laboratories
Abbott Prism HBsAg Assay	ChLIA	Living: S, P Cadaveric: S	Abbott Laboratories
Ortho Antibody to HBsAg ELISA Test System 3	EIA	Living: S, P	Ortho-Clinical Diagnostics, Inc
Hepatitis B Core Antibody Assays			
Corzyme	EIA	Living: S, P	Abbott Laboratories
Ortho HBc ELISA Test System	EIA	Living: S, P	Ortho-Clinical Diagnostics, Inc
Abbott Prism HBcore	ChLIA	Living: S, P	Abbott Laboratories
Hepatitis B Viral NAT			
COBAS Ampliscreen HBV Test	PCR	Living: P Cadaveric: S, EP	Roche Molecular Systems, Inc
Procleix Ultrio	TMA	Living: P, S Cadaveric: S, EP	Gen-Probe, Inc
Cobas TaqScreen MPX	PCR	Living; P	Roche Molecular Systems Inc
HCV			
Anti-HCV Assays			
Abbott HCV EIA 2.0	EIA	Living: S, P Cadaveric: S	Abbott Laboratories
Abbott Prism HCV	ChLIA	Living: S, P Cadaveric: S	Abbott Laboratories
Ortho HCV Version 3.0 ELISA Test System	EIA	Living: S, P	Ortho-Clinical Diagnostics, Inc

HCV NAT			
Cobas Ampliscreen HCV Test Version 3.0	PCR	Living: P Cadaveric: S, EP	Roche Molecular Systems
Procleix HIV-1/HCV	TMA	Living: P Cadaveric: S, EP	Gen-Probe, Inc
Procleix Ultrio	TMA	Living: P, S Cadaveric: S, EP	Gen-Probe, Inc
HIV-1 and -2			
Anti-HIV-1/-2 Assays			
Genetic Systems HIV-1/HIV-2 Plus 0 EIA	EIA	Living: S, P Cadaveric: S	Bio-Rad Laboratories
HIVAB HIV-1/HIV-2 (rDNA) EIA	EIA	Living: S, P Cadaveric: S	Abbott Laboratories
Anti-HIV-1 Assay			
Genetic Systems rLAV EIA	EIA	Living: S,P	Bio-Rad Laboratories
HIV-1 (Western blot)	EIA	Living: S, P, U	Cambridge Biotech Corp
Anti-HIV-2 Assay			
Genetic Systems HIV-2 EIA	EIA	Living: S, P	Bio-Rad Laboratories
HIV-1 NAT			
Cobas AmpliScreen HIV-1 Test, version 1.5	PCR	Living: P Cadaveric: S, EP	Roche Molecular Systems
Procleix HIV-1/HCV	TMA	Living: P Cadaveric: S, EP	Gen-Probe, Inc
Procleix Ultrio	TMA	Living: P Cadaveric: S, EP	Gen-Probe, Inc

Abbreviations: ChLIA, chemiluminescent immunoassay; EIA, enzyme immunoassay; EP, EDTA plasma; NAT, nucleic acid test; P, plasma; PCR, polymerase chain reaction; S, serum; TMA, transcription-mediated amplification; U, urine.

Data from Testing HCT/P donors for relevant communicable disease agents and diseases. Available at: http://www.fda.gov/BiologicsBloodVaccines/SafetyAvailability/TissueSafety/ucm095440.htm#approved. Accessed July 30, 2009.

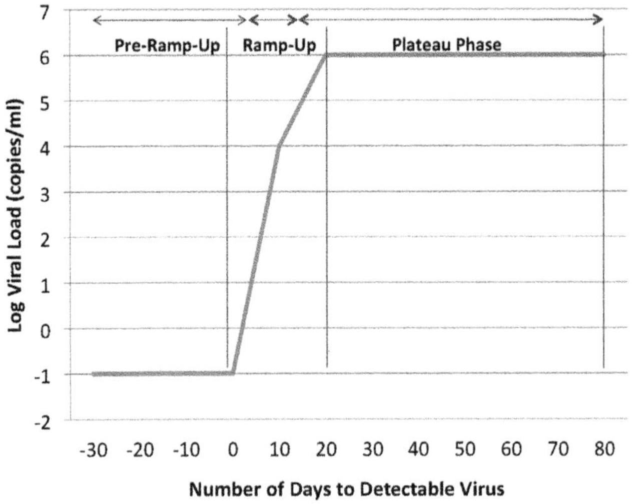

Fig. 1. Typical course of viral infections.

undergoing seroconversion at a time when the level of circulating virus is low, making serology a comparable screening tool to NAT for the detection of early HBV infection.[18,36]

HTLV-1/-2

Prospective testing for HTLV-1/-2 has been mandated for potential blood, organ, and tissue donors, but because of a change in the availability of the most commonly used FDA-licensed screening assay for individual organ donors, the requirement for screening all organ donors has been removed.[14] The only FDA-approved screening test available in the United States after December 31, 2009 will be the Abbott Prism HTLV I/HTLV II assay, a high-throughput and expensive testing system that is not optimized for use in screening organ donors.

THE CHALLENGES OF INFECTIOUS DISEASE TESTING IN THE ORGAN DONOR

Deceased organ donors often require intensive medical care before becoming organ donor candidates. Such care often includes the transfusion of large volumes of blood products and crystalloid, which can potentially result in plasma dilution significant enough to produce false-negative results. Careful evaluation of the total volume of fluid infused before specimen collection must occur to determine if the degree of plasma dilution has the potential to affect infection screening tests.[37]

Deceased organ donor infection screening is also challenged by timing constraints. Unstable donors must be supported medically while tests are being processed. Such medical care, if timing is prolonged, may be unsuccessful in maintaining organ perfusion and viability. This support may consume limited hospital resources and potentially increase the stress on the donor family facing the loss of a loved one. Specimens collected after cessation of blood flow may not provide accurate results on infection screen tests because of interference from products of decomposition. When organs are procured before the confirmation of final test results, maintaining such organs before implantation can result in increased cold ischemia time and poorer organ function after transplant.

Most of the newer assays developed for donor screening are high-throughput multiplex tests that were developed to conform to the needs of the blood-banking industry. Such assays require specialized equipment and personnel, and are best suited to scheduled runs during daytime hours. Most organ donor testing is done outside of the normal daytime hours.[38] The ideal testing platform for organ donor screening would permit individual donor testing for the major viral pathogens with a well-defined and rapid confirmatory test algorithm. Development of such assays for the relatively small transplant market may not be economically attractive to industry without financial or regulatory incentives from governmental agencies involved in safety monitoring and laboratory oversight. Until specialized transplant screening platforms are more widely available, organ procurement agencies will face the challenges of changing testing availability and limited alternative platforms designed for use in transplant screening.

With all of the challenges faced by organ recipients, transplant waiting lists continue to increase. In 2006, 95,000 patients were waiting for organs, and 6300 died while on the transplant waiting list.[39] Advances in transplantation have increased the demand for surgery, and improvements in medical care have allowed more people to survive with critical organ failure to become candidates. In this context, improving screening accuracy and timing is critically important to avoid further limiting access to organ transplant.

One of the major challenges of organ donor screening is the lack of availability of detailed historical information regarding the lifetime risk of pathogen exposure. Blood donor and population studies may allow the OPO to predict what optional screening tests might be most useful to optimize recipient safety, however additional testing increases the likelihood of false-positive results with the potential for unnecessary organ loss. Defining the at-risk population of donors for targeted testing remains a challenge as new assays become available and are incorporated into practice.

NEWER AND OPTIONAL ASSAYS FOR TARGETED USE IN ORGAN DONOR SCREENING

The decision to screen organ donors for specific pathogens must be based on the frequency of infection in the donor population, the availability of licensed screening tests, and the potential severity of donor-transmitted illness. Screening decisions may be modulated by the availability of therapeutic options if infection is found.

Chagas Disease

Case reports of Chagas disease transmission through solid-organ and stem cell transplantation seem to support screening. However prospective testing with results available before organ implantation may not be available at many centers.[40–44] Given the frequency of false-positive results of preliminary testing and the lack of access to preemptive therapy in the United States, management of test results remain a major challenge.[45] Follow-up monitoring after transplant is necessary and may require assistance from the Centers for Disease Control (CDC). Benznidazole and nifurtimox are not commercially available; these medications must be requested directly from the CDC when infection is confirmed. Chagas disease testing may be used in a more targeted fashion in organ donation if donor screening can be optimized; this is currently being done at several OPOs. It is estimated that more than 100,000 people in the United States are chronically infected with this parasite; occult parasitemia has been confirmed in a significant percentage of blood donors identified by the presence of antibody on serologic screening tests.[46,47] Efforts to predict infection risk with screening questionnaires have been validated in the blood donor population but may be impossible in deceased donor screening because of potential limitations in the historical information that can be obtained from living contacts.[48,49] Time spent living in the Central and South American countries where the disease is endemic seems to correlate best with positive serology results, predicting a higher incidence in some blood donor populations containing a large population of immigrants from these areas.[50–52] Testing in some areas of the country may not be useful, given the extremely low incidence of infection.[53] Even when screening indicates the possibility of infection, none of the currently available screening assays can provide 100% sensitivity in disease detection.[54]

West Nile Virus

Epidemiologic data are particularly important when screening is used to identify potential donors infected with West Nile virus (WNV). Although transmission through blood and organ donation has occurred[55–57] and blood donor screening is currently mandated in the United States,[58] no single test is sufficiently sensitive to capture many cases during early infection. Even NAT, generally regarded as the most sensitive assay for viral pathogens, may miss a substantial number of infections with low-level viremia.[59–61] NAT testing and sophisticated serologic assays may allow the identification of infectious donors.[5,62]

Mycobacterium Tuberculosis

Screening of potential transplant recipients using purified protein derivative skin testing has been a standard part of the pretransplant evaluation. Donor screening for *Mycobacterium tuberculosis* has been limited to historical data regarding risk factors, previous skin test findings, and exposure history. In lung donors, who are at highest risk for donor-derived mycobacterial infection, bronchoscopic sampling for acid-fast smear and culture can be used to supplement the required sputum Gram stain, but results from testing at the time of organ procurement may be delayed if traditional nonmolecular studies are used. A recent widely publicized case of donor-derived tuberculosis (TB) that resulted in the infection of 2 of the 3 transplant recipients and resulted in 1 death,[12] combined with the availability of new blood tests to measure for previous exposure to the TB bacillus, have led to discussions regarding donor TB screening in the organ procurement community.[63] Until such testing has been validated in other settings, including the organ recipient population,[64,65] OPOs will continue to rely on historical information and donor physical examination to guide TB risk assessment.

Strongyloides Stercoralis

Hyperinfection strongyloidiasis is a life-threatening infection that can present a diagnostic challenge after transplant. Subclinical infection may persist in an asymptomatic host for decades, reactivating in the face of immunosuppression. Most cases of hyperinfection syndrome stem from previous infection of the transplant recipient, however cases of probable donor origin have been reported.[66,67] Infection should be suspected in donors and recipients with a history of residence in tropical or subtropical areas, although infection can occur in more temperate areas with poor sanitation, including parts of the southeastern United States.[68] Although it is estimated that approximately 90 million people worldwide may be infected with *Strongyloides stercoralis*, screening of donors has a limited role, except possibly for intestinal donors from endemic areas at high risk.[69] Targeted antibody testing of recipients is more likely to be useful in preventing disease after transplant.[70]

Toxoplasma Gondii

Donor infection with *Toxoplasma gondii* can cause significant disease, which may be particularly severe in the nonimmune recipient.[71] Heart transplant patients are at highest risk because of the parasite's propensity to encyst in myocardial tissue. Disease can occur in noncardiac transplant as well, leading to a nonspecific presentation with multisystem organ failure that is often diagnosed at autopsy.[72–74] Routine prophylaxis with trimethoprim/sulfamethoxazole may decrease the incidence of severe disease, but screening to identify the seronegative recipient of a seropositive donor may help identify patients at risk for fulminant disease and promote early initiation of posttransplant prophylaxis.[75,76]

Coccidioides Immitis, Histoplasma Capsulatum, and Other Endemic Fungi

Identification of risk factors for exposure to endemic fungi is relatively straightforward, as infection is associated with previous residence in specific locations. Screening donors and recipients who are at risk for latent infection is more challenging, as serologic tests may be negative even with widespread organ involvement.[77] Awareness of risk factors present in a donor history may assist in the early recognition and successful diagnosis and treatment of infected recipients.[78] Well-documented cases of donor-transmitted coccidioidomycosis have been reported, although the risk of transmission from seropositive donors in endemic areas seems to be low.[79] This may be a result of the use of prolonged fluconazole prophylaxis after transplant, a practice that may decrease the incidence of donor-derived disease in addition to preventing reactivation or new infection in some recipients. Further study is needed to determine the best screening modality for donor-derived endemic fungal infection.

MANAGEMENT OF RECIPIENTS OF ORGANS FROM INCREASED RISK DONORS

Because of the shortage of donor organs, some recipients receive organs from donors with identified risk factors and/or screening tests that are positive for several infections. HIV infection in the donor remains a contraindication to transplantation, but many centers use donors with positive screening serology for hepatitis B or C in selected patient populations.

Hepatitis B may be transmitted from HBsAg-positive donors, with transmission rates as high as 80% to 100% without intervention, or HBsAg-negative, HBcAb-positive donors, with a significantly lower risk of transmission.[80–83] Pretransplant vaccination of the recipient helps to minimize the risk of transmission, although seroconversion may be limited in the patient with end-stage organ disease. Posttransplant prophylaxis with hepatitis B immune globulin (HBIg) and antiviral therapy may be helpful, but increasing viral resistance and the effect of immunosuppressive therapy on viral replication may limit the efficacy of posttransplant prophylaxis.[80,84] Some transplant programs decline HBsAg(+) or HBsAg(−)/HBcAb(+) donors although most use organs from these donors in previously vaccinated patients or in patients willing to take posttransplant prophylaxis. A recent trial demonstrated that kidneys from HBsAg(+) donors may be safely used in HBsAb(+) recipients, with posttransplant HBIg and lamivudine prophylaxis.[85]

The use of hepatitis C seropositive donors is more controversial. Organs from donors with active hepatitis C transmit infection at a high rate.[86,87] Several studies have demonstrated the short-term safety of transplantation of HCV(+) donor organs into HCV(+) recipients,[88,89] although use of HCV(+) organs in HCV(−) recipients is typically avoided because of the risk of liver disease and sepsis in such circumstances, as well as the risk of acute rejection in posttransplant treatment of hepatitis C with interferon-based therapies. The use of HCV(+) donor organs in life-threatening situations is commonplace, however, as there is a shortage of organ donors and mortality on the waiting list is often greater than that in patients with posttransplant hepatitis C.

Unfortunately, infections can be transmitted despite negative screening serology. Although there is significant controversy on how accurate the high-risk criteria are at identifying donors who have an infection that is missed using current serologic methods,[90] these criteria have been incorporated into OPTN policy, which requires that the transplant centers obtain consent from the potential recipients to use organs from high-risk donors.[15] The effect of the requirement to obtain special consent when using organs from increased risk donors has not been well studied and patients may inadvertently turndown an organ without understanding the potential higher risk of adverse outcomes by remaining on the waitlist. A recent consensus conference addressing testing methods for HIV, HBV and HCV in organ donors recommended that donors no longer be labeled high risk but instead be referred to as increased risk donors and that they should be tested by HIV and HCV NAT in an attempt to increase the safety and utilization of these organs (personal communication, Atul Humar, MD, 2009). Management of recipients of organs from increased risk donors is unclear, with no controlled trials available to dictate effective follow-up evaluation and care. The 1994 guidelines for preventing transmission of HIV through transplantation and the experts at this recent consensus conference recommended that recipients of organs from increased risk donors be tested for HIV, HCV, and HBV at periodic intervals after transplant (1, 3, and 12 months). Immunosuppressive therapy alters serologic responses to infection and as a result, infection can be transmitted and only detected by viral load assessments of the recipients. In most cases of donor-to-recipient HCV transmission, serology has remained negative after transplant despite active viral replication and increased liver function tests. Likewise, in the recent HIV/HCV cotransmission event, 1 of the 4 recipients had an indeterminant HIV serology but detectable virus 9 months after transplant.[1,91] Any posttransplant testing of recipients for viral infections should include serologic and NAT/viral load assessments.

MANAGEMENT OF RECIPIENTS WITH DONOR-DERIVED INFECTIONS

Guidelines for the management of expected donor-derived infections, such as CMV and toxoplasmosis, are well established and are frequently incorporated into routine posttransplant care at most transplant centers. Although unexpected donor-derived infections are rare, it is critical to consider the donor as the source of any posttransplant infection. Failure to consider that an infection is potentially donor-derived will undoubtedly result in missed recognition. Recipients are typically cared for in several hospitals which will, in turn, limit the recognition of the infection as there are no robust mechanisms to identify complications in multiple recipients of the same donor. The clearest example of this occurred with 1 of the recent lymphocytic choriomeningitis virus transmission in which all of the recipients developed altered mental status, sepsis, and hepatitis but recognition of the cluster was not made initially because the patients were cared for by 3 separate hospitals.[4] As soon as a single organ recipient presents with an atypical course or concern for an infection that may have been of donor origin, the local OPO should be contacted immediately. The OPO should have a mechanism in place to rapidly assess the status of all other recipients of organs, tissues, or vessels from the same donor and report the concern to the OPTN as required by current policy.[15] If a potential infection is considered, an infectious disease physician should be consulted to help guide antimicrobial treatment and microbiologic investigations.

SUMMARY AND FURTHER RESEARCH

Donor-derived infectious diseases are a rare but clinically significant complication of solid-organ transplantation. The actual incidence of unexpected donor-derived infectious diseases is not known but has been estimated to complicate about 1% of organ transplants. It is critical to consider donor origin for all early posttransplant infections as there are currently no standardized biovigilence systems to allow early recognition of a potential donor-derived disease transmission. Research is desperately needed to advance our understanding of the risk factors associated with disease transmission, optimal screening of donors for infectious diseases, and mechanisms to facilitate recognition and management of transmitted infections. Further, improved platforms for screening that are appropriate for the needs of the transplant community are needed, and sensitivity and specificity of existing testing needs to be improved to decrease the risk of disease transmission and minimize loss of organs through false-positive testing.

REFERENCES

1. Ahn J, Cohen SM. Transmission of human immunodeficiency virus and hepatitis C virus through liver transplantation. Liver Transpl 2008;14(11):1603–8.
2. Bowen PA 2nd, Lobel SA, Caruana RJ, et al. Transmission of human immunodeficiency virus (HIV) by transplantation: clinical aspects and time course analysis of viral antigenemia and antibody production. Ann Intern Med 1988;108(1):46–8.
3. Calabrese F, Angelini A, Cecchetto A, et al. HIV infection in the first heart transplantation in Italy: fatal outcome. Case report. APMIS 1998;106(4):470–4.
4. Fischer SA, Graham MB, Kuehnert MJ, et al. Transmission of lymphocytic choriomeningitis virus by organ transplantation. N Engl J Med 2006;354(21):2235–49.
5. Iwamoto M, Jernigan DB, Guasch A, et al. Transmission of West Nile virus from an organ donor to four transplant recipients. N Engl J Med 2003;348(22):2196–203.
6. Limaye AP, Connolly PA, Sagar M, et al. Transmission of *Histoplasma capsulatum* by organ transplantation. N Engl J Med 2000;343(16):1163–6.
7. Lumbreras C, Sanz F, Gonzalez A, et al. Clinical significance of donor-unrecognized bacteremia in the outcome of solid-organ transplant recipients. Clin Infect Dis 2001;33(5):722–6.
8. Palacios G, Druce J, Du L, et al. A new arenavirus in a cluster of fatal transplant-associated diseases. N Engl J Med 2008;358(10):991–8.
9. Srinivasan A, Burton EC, Kuehnert MJ, et al. Transmission of rabies virus from an organ donor to four transplant recipients. N Engl J Med 2005;352(11):1103–11.
10. Ison MG, Hager J, Blumberg E, et al. Donor-derived disease transmission events in the United States: data reviewed by the OPTN/UNOS Disease Transmission Advisory Committee. Am J Transplant 2009;9(8):1929–35.
11. Lumbreras C. Bacterial pathogens and donor transmission. 3rd International Transplant Infectious Diseases Conference. Prague (Czech Republic), 2007.
12. Transplantation-transmitted tuberculosis–Oklahoma and Texas, 2007. MMWR Morb Mortal Wkly Rep 2008;57(13):333–6.

13. Fishman JA, Strong DM, Kuehnert MJ. Organ and tissue safety workshop 2007: advances and challenges. Cell Tissue Bank 2009;10(3):271–80.
14. 2.0 Minimum procurement standards for an organ procurement organization (OPO). Available at: http://www.unos.org/PoliciesandBylaws2/policies/pdfs/policy_2.pdf. Accessed March 15, 2010.
15. 4.0 Acquired Immune Deficiency Syndrome (AIDS), human pituitary derived growth hormone (HPDGH), and reporting of potential recipient diseases or medical conditions, including malignancies, of donor origin. Available at: http://www.unos.org/PoliciesandBylaws2/policies/pdfs/policy_16.pdf. Accessed March 15, 2010.
16. Glynn SA, Wright DJ, Kleinman SH, et al. Dynamics of viremia in early hepatitis C virus infection. Transfusion 2005;45(6):994–1002.
17. Fiebig EW, Wright DJ, Rawal BD, et al. Dynamics of HIV viremia and antibody seroconversion in plasma donors: implications for diagnosis and staging of primary HIV infection. AIDS 2003;17(13):1871–9.
18. Biswas R, Tabor E, Hsia CC, et al. Comparative sensitivity of HBV NATs and HBSAG assays for detection of acute HBV infection. Transfusion 2003;43(6):788–98.
19. Busch MP, Glynn SA, Stramer SL, et al. A new strategy for estimating risks of transfusion-transmitted viral infections based on rates of detection of recently infected donors. Transfusion 2005;45(2):254–64.
20. Schreiber GB, Busch MP, Kleinman SH, et al. The risk of transfusion-transmitted viral infections. The Retrovirus Epidemiology Donor Study. N Engl J Med 1996;334(26):1685–90.
21. Kleinman S, Busch MP, Korelitz JJ, et al. The incidence/window period model and its use to assess the risk of transfusion-transmitted human immunodeficiency virus and hepatitis C virus infection. Transfus Med Rev 1997;11(3):155–72.
22. Dodd RY, Notari EPt, Stramer SL. Current prevalence and incidence of infectious disease markers and estimated window-period risk in the American Red Cross blood donor population. Transfusion 2002;42(8):975–9.
23. Nucleic acid testing (NAT) for human immunodeficiency virus type 1 (HIV-1) and hepatitis C (HCV): testing, product disposition, and donor deferral and reentry. Available at: http://www.fda.gov/downloads/BiologicsBloodVaccines/GuidanceComplianceRegulatoryInformation/Guidances/Blood/ucm080278.pdf. Accessed March 15, 2010.
24. Challine D, Pellegrin B, Bouvier-Alias M, et al. HIV and hepatitis C virus RNA in seronegative organ and tissue donors. Lancet 2004;364(9445):1611–2.
25. Yao F, Seed C, Farrugia A, et al. Comparison of the risk of viral infection between the living and nonliving musculoskeletal tissue donors in Australia. Transpl Int 2008;21(10):936–41.
26. Zou S, Dodd RY, Stramer SL, et al. Probability of viremia with HBV, HCV, HIV, and HTLV among tissue donors in the United States. N Engl J Med 2004;351(8):751–9.
27. Lefrere JJ, Sellami F, Larderie P, et al. Six years' experience testing organ donors for viral markers in France. Transfusion 1997;37(5):565–6.
28. Yeom JS, Lee JB, Ryu SH, et al. Evaluation of a new third-generation ELISA for the detection of HIV infection. Ann Clin Lab Sci 2006;36(1):73–8.
29. Louie B, Pandori MW, Wong E, et al. Use of an acute seroconversion panel to evaluate a third-generation enzyme-linked immunoassay for detection of human

immunodeficiency virus-specific antibodies relative to multiple other assays. J Clin Microbiol 2006;44(5):1856–8.
30. Yilmaz G. Diagnosis of HIV infection and laboratory monitoring of its therapy. J Clin Virol 2001;21(3):187–96.
31. Yeom JS, Jun G, Chang Y, et al. Evaluation of a new fourth generation enzyme-linked immunosorbent assay, the Ig HIV Ag-Ab plus, with a combined HIV p24 antigen and anti-HIV-1/2/o screening test. J Virol Methods 2006; 137(2):292–7.
32. Kwon JA, Yoon SY, Lee CK, et al. Performance evaluation of three automated human immunodeficiency virus antigen-antibody combination immunoassays. J Virol Methods 2006;133(1):20–6.
33. Kleinman S. Blood donor screening with nucleic acid amplification tests for human immunodeficiency virus, hepatitis C virus, and hepatitis B virus. ISBT Sci Series 2008;3:191–5.
34. Tobler LH, Stramer SL, Lee SR, et al. Performance of ortho HCV core antigen and TRAK-c assays for detection of viraemia in pre-seroconversion plasma and whole blood donors. Vox Sang 2005;89(4):201–7.
35. Simone AG, David JW, Steven HK, et al. Dynamics of viremia in early hepatitis C virus infection. Transfusion 2005;45(6):994–1002.
36. Stramer SL. Current risks of transfusion-transmitted agents: a review. Arch Pathol Lab Med 2007;131(5):702–7.
37. Part 1270. Human tissue intended for transplantation. Available at: http://www.accessdata.fda.gov/scripts/cdrh/cfdocs/cfcfr/CFRSearch.cfm?CFRPart=1270. Accessed March 15, 2010.
38. Caliendo A. HIV, HCV, HBC NAT for organ donors. Chicago: Laboratory Issues; 2009.
39. Abouna GM. Organ shortage crisis: problems and possible solutions. Transplant Proc 2008;40(1):34–8.
40. Chagas disease after organ transplantation–United States, 2001. MMWR Morb Mortal Wkly Rep 2002;51(10):210–2.
41. Chagas disease after organ transplantation–Los Angeles, California, 2006. MMWR Morb Mortal Wkly Rep 2006;55(29):798–800.
42. Pasternak J, Amato Neto V, Hammerschlack N. Chagas' disease after bone marrow transplantation. Bone Marrow Transplant 1997;19(9):958.
43. Villalba R, Fornes G, Alvarez MA, et al. Acute Chagas' disease in a recipient of a bone marrow transplant in Spain: case report. Clin Infect Dis 1992;14(2): 594–5.
44. Kun H, Moore A, Mascola L, et al. Transmission of *Trypanosoma cruzi* by heart transplantation. Clin Infect Dis 2009;48(11):1534–40.
45. Altclas J, Sinagra A, Dictar M, et al. Chagas disease in bone marrow transplantation: an approach to preemptive therapy. Bone Marrow Transplant 2005;36(2):123–9.
46. Bern C, Montgomery SP, Herwaldt BL, et al. Evaluation and treatment of Chagas disease in the United States: a systematic review. JAMA 2007;298(18): 2171–81.
47. Leiby DA, Herron RM Jr, Garratty G, et al. *Trypanosoma cruzi* parasitemia in US blood donors with serologic evidence of infection. J Infect Dis 2008;198(4): 609–13.
48. Appleman MD, Shulman IA, Saxena S, et al. Use of a questionnaire to identify potential blood donors at risk for infection with *Trypanosoma cruzi*. Transfusion 1993;33(1):61–4.

49. O'Brien SF, Chiavetta JA, Fan W, et al. Assessment of a travel question to identify donors with risk of *Trypanosoma cruzi*: operational validity and field testing. Transfusion 2008;48(4):755–61.
50. Leiby DA, Read EJ, Lenes BA, et al. Seroepidemiology of *Trypanosoma cruzi*, etiologic agent of Chagas' disease, in US blood donors. J Infect Dis 1997; 176(4):1047–52.
51. Nowicki MJ, Chinchilla C, Corado L, et al. Prevalence of antibodies to *Trypanosoma cruzi* among solid organ donors in southern California: a population at risk. Transplantation 2006;81(3):477–9.
52. Leiby DA, Herron RM Jr, Read EJ, et al. *Trypanosoma cruzi* in Los Angeles and Miami blood donors: impact of evolving donor demographics on seroprevalence and implications for transfusion transmission. Transfusion 2002;42(5): 549–55.
53. Bryan CF, Tegtmeier GE, Rafik N, et al. The risk for Chagas' disease in the midwestern United States organ donor population is low. Clin Transplant 2004; 18(Suppl 12):12–5.
54. Souza FF, Castro ESO, Marin Neto JA, et al. Acute chagasic myocardiopathy after orthotopic liver transplantation with donor and recipient serologically negative for *Trypanosoma cruzi*: a case report. Transplant Proc 2008;40(3): 875–8.
55. West Nile virus infection in organ donor and transplant recipients–Georgia and Florida, 2002. MMWR Morb Mortal Wkly Rep 2002;51(35):790.
56. West Nile virus infections in organ transplant recipients–New York and Pennsylvania, August–September, 2005. MMWR Morb Mortal Wkly Rep 2005;54(40): 1021–3.
57. Detection of West Nile virus in blood donations–Puerto Rico, 2007. MMWR Morb Mortal Wkly Rep 2008;57(21):577–80.
58. Use of nucleic acid tests to reduce the risk of transmission of West Nile virus from donors of whole blood and blood components intended for transfusion and donors of human cells, tissues, and cellular and tissue-based products (HCT-Ps). Available at: http://www.fda.gov/downloads/BiologicsBloodVaccines/GuidanceComplianceRegulatoryInformation/Guidances/Blood/ucm078614.pdf. Accessed March 15, 2010.
59. Macedo de Oliveira A, Beecham BD, Montgomery SP, et al. West Nile virus blood transfusion-related infection despite nucleic acid testing. Transfusion 2004; 44(12):1695–9.
60. Update: West Nile virus screening of blood donations and transfusion-associated transmission–United States, 2003. MMWR Morb Mortal Wkly Rep 2004;53(13): 281–4.
61. West Nile virus transmission through blood transfusion–South Dakota, 2006. MMWR Morb Mortal Wkly Rep 2007;56(4):76–9.
62. Zhang W, Wu J, Li Y, et al. Rapid and accurate in vitro assays for detection of West Nile virus in blood and tissues. Transfus Med Rev 2009;23(2):146–54.
63. Jazrawi A, Jones M, Kfoury AG, et al. Tuberculosis in a solid-organ transplant recipient: modern-day implications. J Heart Lung Transplant 2009;28(2): 191–3.
64. Manuel O, Humar A, Preiksaitis J, et al. Comparison of quantiferon-TB gold with tuberculin skin test for detecting latent tuberculosis infection prior to liver transplantation. Am J Transplant 2007;7(12):2797–801.
65. Lindemann M, Dioury Y, Beckebaum S, et al. Diagnosis of tuberculosis infection in patients awaiting liver transplantation. Hum Immunol 2009;70(1):24–8.

66. Patel G, Arvelakis A, Sauter BV, et al. Strongyloides hyperinfection syndrome after intestinal transplantation. Transpl Infect Dis 2008;10(2):137–41.
67. Lichtenberger P, Rosa-Cunha I, Morris M, et al. Hyperinfection strongyloidiasis in a liver transplant recipient treated with parenteral ivermectin. Transpl Infect Dis 2009;11(2):137–42.
68. Stone WJ, Schaffner W. Strongyloides infections in transplant recipients. Semin Respir Infect 1990;5(1):58–64.
69. Martin-Davila P, Fortun J, Lopez-Velez R, et al. Transmission of tropical and geographically restricted infections during solid-organ transplantation. Clin Microbiol Rev 2008;21(1):60–96.
70. Avery RK. Recipient screening prior to solid-organ transplantation. Clin Infect Dis 2002;35(12):1513–9.
71. Derouin F, Pelloux H. Prevention of toxoplasmosis in transplant patients. Clin Microbiol Infect 2008;14(12):1089–101.
72. Campbell AL, Goldberg CL, Magid MS, et al. First case of toxoplasmosis following small bowel transplantation and systematic review of tissue-invasive toxoplasmosis following noncardiac solid organ transplantation. Transplantation 2006;81(3):408–17.
73. Mayes JT, O'Connor BJ, Avery R, et al. Transmission of *Toxoplasma gondii* infection by liver transplantation. Clin Infect Dis 1995;21(3):511–5.
74. Barcan LA, Dallurzo ML, Clara LO, et al. *Toxoplasma gondii* pneumonia in liver transplantation: survival after a severe case of reactivation. Transpl Infect Dis 2002;4(2):93–6.
75. Gourishankar S, Doucette K, Fenton J, et al. The use of donor and recipient screening for *Toxoplasma* in the era of universal trimethoprim sulfamethoxazole prophylaxis. Transplantation 2008;85(7):980–5.
76. Hermanns B, Brunn A, Schwarz ER, et al. Fulminant toxoplasmosis in a heart transplant recipient. Pathol Res Pract 2001;197(3):211–5.
77. Blair JE, Mulligan DC. Coccidioidomycosis in healthy persons evaluated for liver or kidney donation. Transpl Infect Dis 2007;9(1):78–82.
78. Blair JE. Approach to the solid organ transplant patient with latent infection and disease caused by Coccidioides species. Curr Opin Infect Dis 2008;21(4):415–20.
79. Braddy CM, Heilman RL, Blair JE. Coccidioidomycosis after renal transplantation in an endemic area. Am J Transplant 2006;6(2):340–5.
80. Chung RT, Feng S, Delmonico FL. Approach to the management of allograft recipients following the detection of hepatitis B virus in the prospective organ donor. Am J Transplant 2001;1(2):185–91.
81. Wolf JL, Perkins HA, Schreeder MT, et al. The transplanted kidney as a source of hepatitis B infection. Ann Intern Med 1979;91(3):412–3.
82. Wachs ME, Amend WJ, Ascher NL, et al. The risk of transmission of hepatitis B from HBsAg(-), HBcAb(+), HBIgM(-) organ donors. Transplantation 1995;59(2):230–4.
83. Fong TL, Bunnapradist S, Jordan SC, et al. Impact of hepatitis B core antibody status on outcomes of cadaveric renal transplantation: analysis of United Network of Organ Sharing database between 1994 and 1999. Transplantation 2002;73(1):85–9.
84. Tur-Kaspa R, Burk RD, Shaul Y, et al. Hepatitis B virus DNA contains a glucocorticoid-responsive element. Proc Natl Acad Sci U S A 1986;83(6):1627–31.
85. Jiang H, Wu J, Zhang X, et al. Kidney transplantation from hepatitis B surface antigen positive donors into hepatitis B surface antibody positive recipients: a prospective nonrandomized controlled study from a single center. Am J Transplant 2009;9(8):1853–8.

86. Fishman JA, Rubin RH, Koziel MJ, et al. Hepatitis C virus and organ transplantation. Transplantation 1996;62(2):147–54.
87. Candinas D, Joller-Jemelka HI, Schlumpf R, et al. Hepatitis C RNA prevalence in a western European organ donor pool and virus transmission by organ transplantation. J Med Microbiol 1994;41(4):220–3.
88. Vargas HE, Laskus T, Wang LF, et al. The influence of hepatitis C virus genotypes on the outcome of liver transplantation. Liver Transpl Surg 1998;4(1):22–7.
89. Ali MK, Light JA, Barhyte DY, et al. Donor hepatitis C virus status does not adversely affect short-term outcomes in HCV+ recipients in renal transplantation. Transplantation 1998;66(12):1694–7.
90. Guidelines for preventing transmission of human immunodeficiency virus through transplantation of human tissue and organs. MMWR Recomm Rep 1994;43(RR-8):1–17.
91. Ison MG, Friedewald JJ. Transmission of human immunodeficiency virus and hepatitis C virus through liver transplantation. Liver Transpl 2009;15(5):561 [author reply: 62].

Immunotherapy and Vaccination After Transplant: The Present, the Future

Vincent C. Emery, PhD[a,*], Hermann Einsele, PhD[b],
Sowsan Atabani, PhD[a,c], Tanzina Haque, PhD[c]

KEYWORDS

• Cytomegalovirus • Papillomavirus • Epstein-Barr virus
• Varicella-zoster virus

Despite the progress in immunosuppressive drugs to manage and minimize organ rejection after transplantation, infectious complications remain a major cause of morbidity.[1] Infections such as herpes simplex virus 1 (HSV-1) and varicella-zoster virus (VZV) have been successfully controlled through the deployment of prophylactic acyclovir or its prodrug valaciclovir,[2,3] whereas prophylactic and preemptive therapy with valganciclovir has been instrumental in managing human cytomegalovirus (HCMV) infections.[4,5] However, the management of Epstein-Barr virus (EBV), human herpes virus-6 (HHV-6), adenovirus, hepatitis C virus (HCV), hepatitis B virus (HBV), papillomavirus, and BK virus infections remains challenging. In addition, the side effect profile of ganciclovir and the possibility that drug resistance may develop with long-term prophylactic use in high-risk patients, such as those needing lung transplants, have stimulated interest in other management strategies.[6] This article focuses on advances in the area of vaccinology for some of these infections and in the use of adoptive immunotherapy. At present, many of these approaches in transplant recipients have focused on infections such as HCMV, but the opportunity to using these examples as proof of concept for other infections is discussed.

[a] Department of Infection (Royal Free Campus), University College London, Rowland Hill Street, Hampstead, London, NW3 2QG, UK
[b] Department of Medicine, University of Wuerzburg, Klinikstrasse 6 97070, Wuerzburg, Germany
[c] Department of Virology, Royal Free Hampstead NHS Trust, London Street, Hampstead, London, NW3 2QG, UK
* Corresponding author.
E-mail address: v.emery@ucl.ac.uk

Infect Dis Clin N Am 24 (2010) 515–529
doi:10.1016/j.idc.2010.01.004
id.theclinics.com
0891-5520/10/$ – see front matter © 2010 Elsevier Inc. All rights reserved.

VACCINATION

HCMV Vaccines

The earliest vaccine deployed for HCMV infections was the low-passage, live, attenuated Towne strain of HCMV by Plotkin and colleagues.[7,8] The results of a trial in kidney transplant recipients showed that immunization was unable to prevent infection but was associated with a reduction in the severity of HCMV disease.[9] Despite these encouraging findings, progress on an HCMV vaccine has been slow in the intervening years, with several vaccine preparations being formulated but, until recently, few showing sufficient protection to warrant further study.[10–13] These vaccine preparations are summarized in **Table 1**. A fundamental question relating to the use of vaccination to control and potentially eradicate HCMV infection is the level of vaccine coverage required to induce herd immunity in the general population, and of the vaccine efficacy required to control replication and disease after transplantation. A key study by Griffiths and colleagues[14] showed that, in high resource countries such as the United Kingdom and United States where HCMV seroprevalence rates are approximately 60%, the basic reproductive number (Ro; the number of new infections arising from 1 infected individual) for HCMV in women of child-bearing age was approximately 2.4. Thus, a vaccine coverage of around 62% would be sufficient to lead to herd immunity and eradication of HCMV without a significant effect on the incidence of congenital HCMV infection/disease. In the transplant setting, vaccination could be deployed in high-risk patients who are seronegative or as a prophylactic vaccine in patients who are already seropositive for HCMV. One study provided an estimate of the basic reproductive number for HCMV in these 2 clinical settings for liver transplant recipients.[15] These data indicate that in the D+R− setting, the Ro for HCMV is approximately 15, meaning that a vaccine would need to have an efficacy against replication of approximately 93% if it was to fully control replication. In contrast, the Ro for HCMV in the D+R+ group was reduced to 2.4, indicating that an HCMV vaccine deployed as an immunotherapeutic in these patients would only need to achieve an efficacy of about 60% to successfully control HCMV replication. The ability to affect the probability of HCMV disease is intimately linked to the relationship between viral load and disease. In all cases to date, viral load and probability of HCMV disease follow a sigmoidal pattern whereby the risk of HCMV disease increases substantially at certain viral-load thresholds.[16] In the context of vaccination, a vaccine that did not eradicate infection/replication but which induced a sufficient level of immunity to partially control HCMV replication could still have a profound effect on

Table 1
HCMV vaccines currently undergoing human trials

Vaccine	Description	Status
Towne	Live attenuated	Being used in prime boost with DNA vaccines
gB	Recombinant, soluble	Phase II studies complete in healthy; undergoing phase I in solid-organ transplant recipients
Canarypox pp65	Live single-cycle expression	Phase I
pp65, gB	DNA plasmid	Phase I
AlphaVax	Alphavirus expressing gB and pp65-IE1 fusion protein Single-cycle expression	Phase I

the incidence and severity of HCMV disease. This concept is summarized in **Fig. 1** and is consistent with the findings of the Towne vaccine study described earlier.

At present, the most encouraging results for an HCMV vaccine have come from the recombinant glycoprotein B (gB) vaccine. gB is a major site for neutralizing antibodies and can adsorb up to 80% of the serum-neutralizing antibodies in healthy seropositive individuals.[17] In addition, purified and recombinant gB has been shown to elicit high-level humoral immunity in animal models and protect against fetal loss in a guinea pig model.[18,19] Recombinant gB consisting of the extracellular domain and the intracellular domain, but with a truncated transmembraneous domain, has been expressed in mammalian cell culture and subjected to phase I and II clinical trials.[20–22] The vaccine is highly immunogenic when administered with the adjuvant MF59 (3 doses at months 0, 1, and 6) yielding neutralizing titers in seronegative volunteers that were in excess of those found with natural immunity. In addition, the vaccine boosted neutralizing titers when given to seropositive individuals. The results of a randomized double-blind, placebo-controlled, phase II study in 464 seronegative women within 1 year of them giving birth have recently been reported.[23] The vaccine efficacy was 50%, reducing the number of seroconversions from 31 in the placebo group to 18 in the vaccine group. These results are encouraging and have rekindled interest in the HCMV vaccine area by small and large pharma.

Do these results have any effect on the vaccination of transplant patients against HCMV? One of the challenges in the transplant setting is the need for the gB vaccine to be given as 3 doses over a period of 6 months. Many patients proceed to transplant before the full course of vaccination can be given, and so the likelihood of protection may be reduced. Nevertheless, one study ongoing at the Royal Free Hospital, London, and coordinated by scientists at University College London, has recruited renal and liver transplant patients (seropositive and seronegative before transplant) into a placebo-controlled trial of the gB-MF59 vaccine with an end point of viral replication (incidence and kinetics) after transplantation. At the time of writing, this trial has not reported its results, but these should be available in 2010.

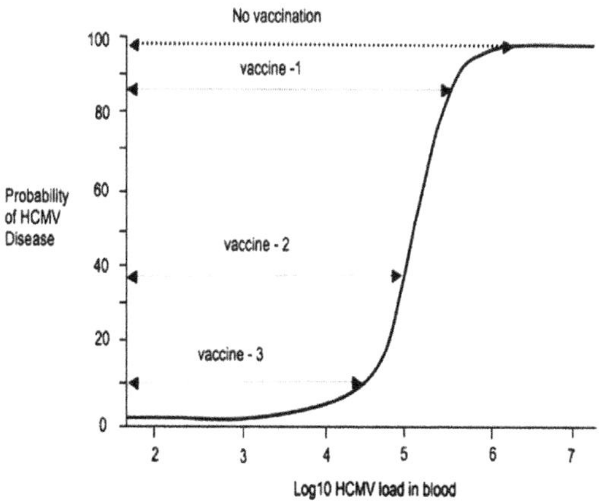

Fig. 1. The relationship between HCMV load and probability of disease and the potential effects of vaccination. In the scenario shown, in the absence of vaccination the patient would reach a viral load of $6\log_{10}$ genomes/mL of blood with an associated disease probability of 97%. The 3 vaccines 1, 2 and 3 have increasing efficacy by reducing viral load in blood by 0.5, 1.0, and $1.5\log_{10}$, which reduces disease probability to 86%, 37%, and 10% respectively. Comparable reductions can be modeled if the patient was destined to experience a maximum viral load of $5\log_{10}$ genomes/mL blood.

Human Papillomavirus Vaccines

Papillomavirus infections remain an important pathogen in immunocompromised men and women with HIV or in transplant recipients, for whom the risks for common warts and anogenital lesions attributable to human papillomavirus (HPV) are substantially increased compared with healthy individuals.[24] In particular, female renal transplant recipients have a substantially increased risk for HPV-associated anogenital cancers and cervical intraepithelial neoplasia. The development of HPV-related anal tumors has also been documented after liver transplantation in a retrospective analysis.[25] Anal HPV-DNA was detectable in 23% of men and women before the induction of immunosuppression for a liver or kidney transplant.[26] The recent licensing of recombinant HPV vaccines based on the L1 protein of HPV types 6, 11, 16, and 18 for the prevention of genital warts, cervical dysplasia, and cervical cancer[27,28] has now provided opportunities to deploy such vaccines in the transplant setting. Because these vaccines work best in individuals before HPV exposure, it is likely that the first deployment may occur in the pediatric transplant setting. In the setting of immunosuppression, the safety of HPV vaccines has yet to be determined. However, extrapolation from the use of other nonlive vaccines suggests that HPV vaccine would be safe and induce effective, if diminished, immune responses, with no associated graft rejection or other serious adverse effects. In addition, given the risks of anogenital lesions, the ability to boost preexisting immunity to reduce or prevent anogenital lesions is also likely to be an important consideration in adult populations, especially in women receiving renal transplants. However, it is interesting that a recent cost-effectiveness analysis suggests that a program of HPV vaccination before transplantation is unlikely to be cost-effective.[29] Nothwithstanding this, clinical trials of HPV vaccines are underway in centers in North America.[30]

VZV Vaccine

To date, a prophylactic vaccine against VZV is the only live, attenuated herpes virus vaccine to be licensed in any country. It was initially tested, and has been widely used for the past few decades, in Japan. The currently available vaccine consists of attenuated virus from the Oka strain of VZV and has been in use safely and successfully in healthy children and adults in many other parts of the world.[31]

Among immunocompromised patients, including transplant recipients, varicella infections may be severe and even fatal. The clinical presentation may be atypical in immunocompromised patients, in whom the rash may be nonvesicular or even absent. Immunocompromised children and adults may present with abdominal zoster, characterized by abdominal and back pain, which may precede or occur in the absence of skin lesions,[32,33] posing a diagnostic challenge. VZV-associated cerebral vasculitis has also been described in the setting of immunocompromised patients.[34] In addition, recovery from VZV infection may be slow, with individuals remaining infectious for up to several weeks following initial clinical presentation. It is therefore important to consider protection of these susceptible populations with the use of the VZV vaccine, 2 doses of which provide 75% protection against any disease and at least 95% protection against severe disease and its complications among immunocompetent adults.[35]

The use of the live, attenuated varicella vaccine has been most extensively studied in children with acute lymphoblastic leukemia (ALL), but studies involving other immunocompromised populations are limited.[36] In a multicenter trial, the vaccine was shown to be safe and immunogenic when administered to children with ALL who had suspended maintenance chemotherapy for at least 1 week before and 1 week after vaccination.[37] Seroconversion rates varied from 42% to 96% and were, on average, lower than in healthy children. Incidence of recurrent varicella (herpes zoster) was also found to be less in immunocompromised vaccine recipients compared with that observed following natural infection.[38] In children with asymptomatic or mild symptoms of HIV infection, the VZV vaccine was found to be safe but less immunogenic than in healthy children, with seroconversion rates of approximately 60%.[39] A recent phase II trial determined the VZV vaccine to be safe and immunogenic among HIV-infected children with a history of varicella,[40] and no child had developed herpes zoster 2 years later. Fewer vaccine efficacy studies have been performed among HIV-infected adults: a boost in VZV-specific immunoglobulin G (IgG) was observed in HIV-infected patients on stable antiretroviral therapy for at least 3 months, with a nadir CD4 count greater than 400 cells/mL.[41]

Among children who have received liver and intestine transplants and are on maximum dosages of 0.3 mg/kg prednisolone on alternate days and trough tacrolimus levels of less than 10 ng/mL for more than 1 month, the varicella vaccine was found to be safe, immunogenic, and protective.[42] In the latter study, 16 children who were VZV IgG seronegative and aged between 13 and 76 months were immunized, and 87% and 86% of children developed humoral and cellular immunity, respectively. Five of the children developed a mild pain and erythema at the site of the injection, and another 4 developed fever and disseminated rash. Among 11 children with follow-up of 6 months or more after vaccination, there were 5 subsequent reported exposures to chickenpox (1 child with 2 exposures), none of which resulted in chickenpox.

A severe but nonfatal vaccine-associated disease has been reported in some children with an undiagnosed immunodeficiency.[43] However, no fatalities have been observed in this group, in whom mortality associated with natural infection is known to occur. Hence, overall, it is believed that the potential benefits of vaccination against VZV in the immunocompromised host far outweigh the risks.

Other Viral Vaccines

Although HBV vaccination has been available for many years it has not been widely deployed in the setting of HBV infection in patients transplanted for chronic HBV. However, in the context of dialysis patients, HBV vaccination is recommended, although the immune response to vaccination can be suboptimal, especially if given intramuscularly.[44] Recently, the use of the adjuvant 3-*O*-desacyl-4′-monophosphoryl lipid A (AS04) in conjunction with standard hepatitis B recombinant vaccine has led to enhanced immunogenicity (earlier and higher antibody titers) in dialysis patients.[45]

At the time of writing, the prospects for viral vaccines against adenoviruses, BK virus, and HCV remain poor. It is therefore unlikely that prototype vaccines will be forthcoming for these infectious complications in transplant and oncology patients. Nevertheless, the experience and data generated from studies of HCMV and papillomavirus vaccines should provide important information concerning the likely immunogenicity of new vaccines in the context of dialysis and the immunocompromised state following transplantation.

ADOPTIVE IMMUNOTHERAPY

Cytomegalovirus Immunotherapy

Antigen-specific T cells are essential for control of cytomegalovirus infection,[46] and HCMV has evolved several mechanisms to overcome this component of the immune response.[47] Immunotherapy offers an attractive way to improve immune reconstitution in transplanted patients, leading to control of viral replication without major side effects. As a consequence, this approach may reduce the use of antiviral chemotherapy and hence the adverse effects such as myelo- or nephrotoxicity and, furthermore, the evolutionary pressure on HCMV to develop drug resistance.

Various strategies to generate HCMV-specific T lymphocytes have been developed (these are reviewed in Ref.[48]). One of the most effective approaches for the ex vivo induction of HCMV-specific T cells is using CMV-infected fibroblasts, but the potential biologic risk that results from the use of live virus particles does not permit the use of infected antigen-presenting cells (APCs) for T cell stimulation under current good management practice (GMP) standards. Other approaches used to generate HCMV-specific T cells include HCMV peptide-pulsed dendritic cells (DCs),[49] HCMV antigen–pulsed DCs,[50] or using genetically modified APCs.[51] All of these methods are effective in producing HCMV-specific T cells in high yield, but the process is expensive and time consuming to produce a product that can be deployed clinically.

Riddell and colleagues[52] and Walter and colleagues[53] were the first to show that adoptive immunotherapy for HCMV-specific CD8+ T cell clones into patients at risk of HCMV disease protected them from CMV-related complications. In these studies, 1×10^9 to 2×10^9 CMV-specific CD8+ T cells were administered and these cells persisted in patients' blood for at least 8 weeks. HCMV prophylaxis was effective despite the progressive decline of these HCMV CD8 T cells in patients who did not develop a concomitant HCMV-specific CD4+ T_{Helper} response. Although these results were groundbreaking, they suffered from the use of historical controls.

In an alternative study, patients lacking HCMV immunity were reconstituted by the adoptive transfer of HCMV-specific T cell lines which were generated by 4 repetitive weekly stimulations with HCMV lysate in vitro.[54] These cells could be infused without any side effects, even in patients receiving their graft from a donor mismatched in 1 to 3 HLA antigens, implicating a potential use of this strategy even after haploidentical transplantation. This approach has advantages in the context of time compared with the generation of the CD8+ CMV–specific clones described earlier, and provides a more flexible application of the technique in patients with HCMV DNAemia at high risk for HCMV disease, without a loss of specificity and safety. These findings show that HCMV-specific adoptive immune transfer is a therapeutic option in patients who are DNAemic after stem cell transplantation and can be achieved by infusion of low numbers of CD4+ HCMV–specific T cell lines.

To facilitate the enrichment of virus-specific T cells, novel selection using the IFN-γ secretion assay conforming to current GMP regulations can be deployed.[55] HCMV-Ag can also be used to elicit a combined HCMV-specific CD4+ and CD8+ T cell response. Stimulation of HCMV-specific CD4+ and CD8+ T cells was similarly effective when using HCMV antigen compared with the costimulation with HCMV antigen and HCMV peptides.[56] As a result, an average of 1.3×10^8 CMV-specific stimulated, selected, and expanded T cells from 8/8 randomly selected HCMV-seropositive donors were generated in 10 days from a single 500-mL blood donation using only autologous cellular and humoral components compatible with current GMP regulations. The adoptively transferred T cells may then undergo further expansion in vivo if they are stimulated by HCMV-Ag–presenting cells providing an in vivo amplification step rather than relying on in vitro expansion.

Important questions remain with respect to the number of HCMV-specific T cells required for an effective adoptive transfer and their composition in respect to CD4+/CD8+ ratio and antigen specificity required for prevention or treatment of HCMV DNAemia after allogeneic stem cell transplantation. Further work is needed to define these parameters. However, improvements in immunologic assays have enabled direct quantification of HCMV-specific T cells. Analysis of phenotype and activity of antigen-specific T cells have contributed to a substantial improvement in understanding of the role and function of immune responses in vivo.[57–59] Thus, phenotypic analysis with HLA-peptide multimers and functional assays can now be used in the setting of adoptive T cell therapy. Peptide-HLA multimers allow an easy visualization and isolation of antigen-specific cytotoxic T lymphocytes (CTLs). T cells that bind multimeric HLA complexes can be isolated to high purity using magnetic beads or fluorescent antibody cell separation (FACS) sorting.[60] There are several reasons why the adoptive transfer of HCMV-specific CTLs freshly isolated from peripheral blood might be more efficient than the infusion of in vitro expanded and manipulated T cells. The process of in vitro expansion may increase the expression of the proapoptotic FAS molecule (CD95) and reduce telomere length of specific T cells, leading to a shorter survival of the adoptive transferred T cells[61] similar to that observed in aging human populations.[62] Various methods of cell generation result in different stages of T cell senescence. Freshly isolated and specifically selected T cells have greater expansion potential in vivo compared with repetitive in vitro stimulated T cells. However, specific stimulation ex vivo might reduce the risk for alloreactivity. In addition, the in vitro cell culture process increases not only the risk for contamination of the CTL preparation but also the costs for adoptive immunotherapy.

Although the availability of clinical-grade reagents for the selection of antigen-specific T cells has improved greatly in the last few years, not enough is known about the ideal composition of a cellular product that will be highly effective in use for adoptive transfer. The optimal targets for HCMV-specific T cell control have not been defined precisely despite evidence suggesting that the host makes a broad CD4 and CD8 response to most proteins in the HCMV proteome.[63] However, there is still controversy about the benefit of transferring different T cell subsets for adoptive immunotherapy: namely, should only CD4+ T cells or CD8+ T cells be transferred, or a combination of both?

In view of the many different methods of generating T cells, future studies must address the following questions, preferably in placebo-controlled studies: (1) which are the best T cell subpopulations to be used for antiviral T cell therapy; (2) what differentiation/activation stage or stages are associated with efficient expansion and antiviral control; (3) what is the ideal range of antigen specificities of the T cells; and (4) what is the optimal cell dose required to control replication, and does it depend on the viral load and net state of immunosuppression of the patient?

EBV Immunotherapy

EBV is associated with posttransplant lymphoproliferative disease (PTLD), a common complication after hematopoietic stem cell and solid-organ transplantations.[64] PTLD occurs in up to 15% of patients depending on the transplant type, age of the recipient, and the intensity of immunosuppression. With conventional treatments (reduction of immunosuppression, rituximab, radiotherapy, chemotherapy, surgery),[65–67] relapses are common and the overall mortality remains high (around 50%).[68]

The search for an optimum treatment has led to recent trials of adoptive transfer of T cell immunity directed against EBV. These studies should be compared with those on HCMV discussed in the previous section. More than 90% of PTLD are EBV positive and most tumor cells express full latent cycle proteins (EB nuclear antigens [EBNAs] 1, 2, 3a, 3b, 3c, and leader protein [LP]; latent membrane proteins [LMPs] 1, 2), with a few cells expressing lytic cycle proteins.[69] Some of these proteins, particularly the EBNA 3 family, are immunodominant targets for virus-specific CTL, thus making PTLD an ideal candidate for adoptive immunotherapy.[70] EBV readily infects and transforms B lymphocytes in vitro giving rise to a continually growing lymphoblastoid cell line (LCL) in which each cell expresses all EBV latent antigens. Irradiated LCL cells can then be used as APCs to stimulate and expand autologous peripheral blood mononuclear cells (PBMCs) into an EBV-specific CTL line.[71] Using this method, CTLs were grown ex vivo from HLA-matched hematopoietic stem cell donors and were used successfully to prevent and treat PTLD in respective stem cell recipients.[71,72] However, this approach is not feasible in solid-organ transplantation because the organ donor is not generally available to provide blood, and the donor and the recipients are not closely HLA matched. Attempts have been made to generate autologous CTL from patients before transplantation and from patients with PTLD.[73–75] However, the approach of generating autologous CTL from each transplant patient is prohibitively labor intensive and expensive for wide-scale use, and often there is not sufficient time to generate CTLs once PTLD has been diagnosed. An alternative strategy is to establish a bank of well-characterized EBV-specific CTL grown from EBV-seropositive healthy blood donors and provide these off-the-shelf CTLs to PTLD patients on a best HLA match basis (**Fig. 2**).[76] This third-party CTL strategy has several advantages: fully characterized CTLs are available for immediate use; 1 CTL line can be used for more than 1 PTLD patient, making it cost-effective; and these cells can be used to treat EBV-driven lymphomas in nontransplant immunosuppressed patients. A research team in Edinburgh University, Scotland, established a frozen bank of 100 EBV-specific CTL lines generated from Scottish blood donors selected to cover more than 99% of the HLA types of the UK population.[77] In a pilot study, the first of its kind in the United Kingdom, 8 patients with progressive PTLD were infused with these allogeneic CTLs, selected on the basis of best HLA matches between the CTL donor and PTLD patient, with 3 patients achieving a complete remission.[78] This CTL bank was then used in a multicenter phase II clinical trial to treat 33 PTLD patients (31 solid-organ and 2

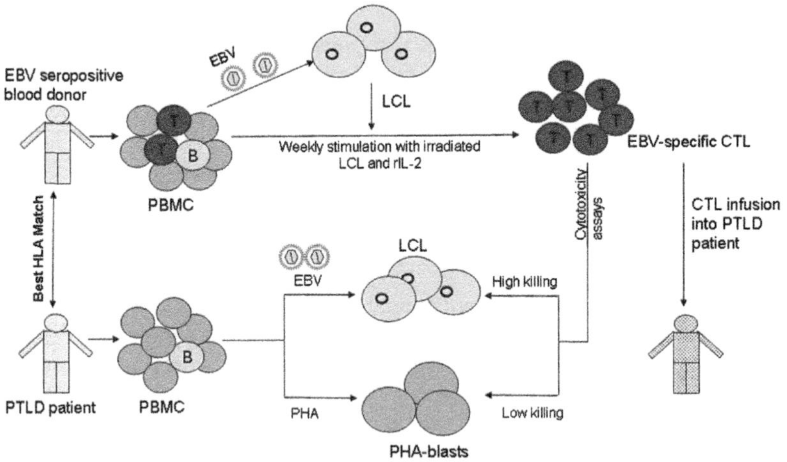

Fig. 2. Study design for the selection of partially HLA-matched third-party CTL for the treatment of PTLD. EBV-seropositive healthy blood donors were selected to cover most HLA types in the United Kingdom. PBMCs from blood donors were infected with EBV to obtain a LCL and irradiated LCL were used as APCs to stimulate and expand EBV-specific CTL from autologous PBMC in the presence of recombinant interleukin 2 (rIL2). PBMC from PTLD patients were collected to generate LCL and phytohemagglutinin blasts. Available CTL lines with the best HLA matches between the CTL donor and the PTLD patient were tested with in vitro cytotoxicity assays, and the CTL line showing the highest lysis of patient's LCL (EBV targets) and the lowest lysis of patient's PHA-blasts (non-EBV targets) was selected for infusion into the patient.

stem cell transplant recipients in the United Kingdom, Sweden, France, and Australia) who had failed to respond to conventional treatments.[79] At 6 months after treatment, 52% of patients had responded to the CTL infusions, with 14 achieving complete remission. A significantly better response was noted in patients receiving CTL with higher HLA matching (P = .001) and with higher numbers of CD4+ T cells (P = .001). No infusion-related toxicity or features of CTL-versus-host disease occurred in any of the infused patients and the third-party allogeneic CTL was considered a safe and effective form of treatment of PTLD.

A wide range of protocols have been used to generate CTL with specificities against individual EBV antigens (eg, LMP-1, LMP-2) by using APCs loaded with EBV peptides, or transfected with vaccinia or adenoviral vectors expressing selected EBV proteins.[80–82] An alternate approach is to redirect T cells to antigens on tumor cells using the recently developed chimeric T cell receptor (TCR) technology.[83] T cells expressing chimeric receptors with the antigen-binding domains of monoclonal antibodies fused to the downstream signal transducing elements of TCR can effectively target any tumor expressing that particular antigen without the need of major histocompatibility complex restriction.[84] Research is ongoing to generate T cells expressing the chimeric TCR containing the single variable chains of monoclonal antibodies against EBV latent membrane antigen, LMP-1 and LMP-2, fused to the CD3ζ chain, and to explore the possibility of their future use in clinical trials of targeting LMP-1 and LMP-2 expressing EBV-driven malignancies without the requirement of HLA restriction.

Adenovirus Immunotherapy

Although adoptive immunotherapy has been predominantly directed against HCMV and EBV infection, the lack of effective antiviral chemotherapy against adenovirus and the high morbidity and mortality associated with disseminated infection have resulted in interest in using T cells to control infection. Effective T cell function seems to be crucial in the control of adenovirus replication and reduction of immunosuppression and donor lymphocyte infusions have been shown to lead to a reduction in viral replication.[85,86] At present, one trial in pediatric stem cell transplant recipients has been reported using ex vivo isolated IFN-γ–producing T cells.[87] Infusions of between 1.2×10^3 and 50×10^3 T cells/kg were well tolerated in most patients, and in 5/6 patients, adenovirus loads decreased and replication resolved. Further controlled trials will be needed to judge the effectiveness of adoptive transfer of T cells against adenovirus and to optimize the initiation of therapy. The identification of several other potential T cell targets within the adenovirus proteome will also allow more complex T cell specificities to be generated, which should also allow more effective control of replication.[88] The ongoing experience with HCMV and EBV immunotherapy will be invaluable in the context of adoptive immunotherapy for adenovirus.

Researchers have also generated a multivirus-specific CTL line containing a mixture of cells that are capable of killing HCMV, adenovirus, and EBV target cells in in vitro cytotoxicity assays.[89,90] DCs and LCL, transduced with a clinical-grade recombinant adenovirus type 5 vector pseudotyped with an adenovirus type 35 fiber encoding CMVpp65 (Ad5f35CMVpp65), were used as APCs. These multivirus-specific CTL lines may be beneficial in treating transplant patients with combined HCMV, EBV, and adenoviral diseases.

SUMMARY

Vaccination and adoptive immunotherapy for herpes virus infections has become an attractive option for the control of a virus family that negatively affects transplantation.

In the future, enhanced ability to select antigen-specific T cells without significant in vitro manipulation should provide new opportunities for refining and enhancing adoptive immunotherapeutic approaches. In addition, the trials of HCMV vaccine that are currently underway provide significant hope that these and other viral vaccines will soon be deployed in the transplant population.

REFERENCES

1. Fischer SA. Emerging viruses in transplantation: there is more to infection after transplant than CMV and EBV. Transplantation 2008;86(10):1327–39.
2. Saral R, Burns WH, Laskin OL, et al. Acyclovir prophylaxis of herpes-simplex-virus infections. N Engl J Med 1981;305(2):63–7.
3. Sempere A, Sanz GF, Senent L, et al. Long-term acyclovir prophylaxis for prevention of varicella zoster virus infection after autologous blood stem cell transplantation in patients with acute leukemia. Bone Marrow Transplant 1992;10(6):495–8.
4. Khoury JA, Storch GA, Bohl DL, et al. Prophylactic versus preemptive oral valganciclovir for the management of cytomegalovirus infection in adult renal transplant recipients. Am J Transplant 2006;6(9):2134–43.
5. Paya C, Humar A, Dominguez E, et al. Efficacy and safety of valganciclovir vs. oral ganciclovir for prevention of cytomegalovirus disease in solid organ transplant recipients. Am J Transplant 2004;4(4):611–20.
6. Boivin G, Goyette N, Rollag H, et al. Cytomegalovirus resistance in solid organ transplant recipients treated with intravenous ganciclovir or oral valganciclovir. Antivir Ther 2009;14(5):697–704.
7. Plotkin SA, Huygelen C. Cytomegalovirus vaccine prepared in WI-38. Dev Biol Stand 1976;37:301–5.
8. Glazer JP, Friedman HM, Grossman RA, et al. Live cytomegalovirus vaccination of renal transplant candidates. A preliminary trial. Ann Intern Med 1979;91(5):676–83.
9. Plotkin SA, Smiley ML, Friedman HM, et al. Towne-vaccine-induced prevention of cytomegalovirus disease after renal transplants. Lancet 1984;1(8376):528–30.
10. Pass RF, Duliege AM, Boppana S, et al. A subunit cytomegalovirus vaccine based on recombinant envelope glycoprotein B and a new adjuvant. J Infect Dis 1999;180(4):970–5.
11. Adler SP, Plotkin SA, Gonczol E, et al. A canarypox vector expressing cytomegalovirus (CMV) glycoprotein B primes for antibody responses to a live attenuated CMV vaccine (Towne). J Infect Dis 1999;180(3):843–6.
12. Reap EA, Dryga SA, Morris J, et al. Cellular and humoral immune responses to alphavirus replicon vaccines expressing cytomegalovirus pp65, IE1, and gB proteins. Clin Vaccine Immunol 2007;14(6):748–55.
13. Temperton NJ. DNA vaccines against cytomegalovirus: current progress. Int J Antimicrob Agents 2002;19(3):169–72.
14. Griffiths PD, McLean A, Emery VC. Encouraging prospects for immunisation against primary cytomegalovirus infection. Vaccine 2001;19(11-12):1356–62.
15. Emery VC, Hassan-Walker AF, Burroughs AK, et al. Human cytomegalovirus (HCMV) replication dynamics in HCMV-naive and -experienced immunocompromised hosts. J Infect Dis 2002;185(12):1723–8.
16. Emery VC. Viral dynamics during active cytomegalovirus infection and pathology. Intervirology 1999;42(5-6):405–11.
17. Wagner B, Kropff B, Kalbacher H, et al. A continuous sequence of more than 70 amino acids is essential for antibody binding to the dominant antigenic site of glycoprotein gp58 of human cytomegalovirus. J Virol 1992;66(9):5290–7.

18. Marshall GS, Li M, Stout GG, et al. Antibodies to the major linear neutralizing domains of cytomegalovirus glycoprotein B among natural seropositives and CMV subunit vaccine recipients. Viral Immunol 2000;13(3):329–41.
19. Schleiss MR, Bourne N, Stroup G, et al. Protection against congenital cytomegalovirus infection and disease in guinea pigs, conferred by a purified recombinant glycoprotein B vaccine. J Infect Dis 2004;189(8):1374–81.
20. Pass RF, Burke RL. Development of cytomegalovirus vaccines: prospects for prevention of congenital CMV infection. Semin Pediatr Infect Dis 2002;13(3):196–204.
21. Mitchell DK, Holmes SJ, Burke RL, et al. Immunogenicity of a recombinant human cytomegalovirus gB vaccine in seronegative toddlers. Pediatr Infect Dis J 2002;21(2):133–8.
22. Pass RF. Development and evidence for efficacy of CMV glycoprotein B vaccine with MF59 adjuvant. J Clin Virol 2009;46:S73–6.
23. Pass RF, Zhang C, Evans A, et al. Vaccine prevention of maternal cytomegalovirus infection. N Engl J Med 2009;360(12):1191–9.
24. Tan HH, Goh CL. Viral infections affecting the skin in organ transplant recipients: epidemiology and current management strategies. Am J Clin Dermatol 2006;7(1):13–29.
25. Albright JB, Bonatti H, Stauffer J, et al. Colorectal and anal neoplasms following liver transplantation. Colorectal Dis 2009. [Epub ahead of print].
26. Roka S, Rasoul-Rockenschaub S, Roka J, et al. Prevalence of anal HPV infection in solid-organ transplant patients prior to immunosuppression. Transpl Int 2004;17:366–9.
27. Harper DM, Franco EL, Wheeler CM, et al. Sustained efficacy up to 4.5 years of a bivalent L1 virus-like particle vaccine against human papillomavirus types 16 and 18: follow-up from a randomised control trial. Lancet 2006;367(9518):1247–55.
28. FUTURE II Study Group. Quadrivalent vaccine against human papillomavirus to prevent high-grade cervical lesions. N Engl J Med 2007;356(19):1915–27.
29. Wong G, Howard K, Webster A, et al. The health and economic impact of cervical cancer screening and human papillomavirus vaccination in kidney transplant recipients. Transplantation 2009;87(7):1078–91.
30. Safety and immunogenicity of human papillomavirus (HPV) vaccine in solid organ transplant recipients; 2009. Available at: www.clinicaltrials.gov/ct2/show/NCT00677677. Accessed January 26, 2010.
31. Gershon AA, Katz SL. Perspective on live varicella vaccine. J Infect Dis 2008;197(Suppl 2):242–5.
32. Milone G, Di Raimondo F, Russo M, et al. Unusual onset of severe varicella in adult immunocompromised patients. Ann Hematol 1992;64:155–6.
33. Yagi T, Karasumo T, Hasegawa T, et al. Acute abdomen without cutaneous signs of varicella zoster virus infection as a late complication of allogeneic bone marrow transplantation: importance of empiric therapy with aciclovir. Bone Marrow Transplant 2000;25:1003–5.
34. Hovens MMC, Vaessen N, Sijpkens YWJ, et al. Unusual presentation of central nervous system manifestations of varicella zoster virus vasculopathy in renal transplant recipients. Transpl Infect Dis 2007;9:237–40.
35. Varicella. In: The green book: immunization against infectious disease. London (UK): Department of Health 2006, chapter 34.
36. Sartori AMC. A review of the varicella vaccine in immunocompromised individuals. Int J Infect Dis 2004;8:259–70.
37. Gershon AA, Steinbert SP, Gelb L, et al. Live attenuated varicella vaccine, efficacy for children with leukemia in remission. The national institute of allergy

and infectious diseases varicella vaccine collaborative study group. JAMA 1984; 252:355–62.
38. Hardy IB, Gershon A, Steinberg S, et al. The incidence of zoster after immunization with live attenuated varicella vaccine: a study in children with leukemia. N Engl J Med 1991;325:1545–50.
39. Levin MJ, Gershon AA, Weingberg A, et al. Immunization of HIV-infected children with varicella vaccine. J Pediatr 2001;139:305–10.
40. Gershon AA, Levin MJ, Weinberg A, et al. A phase II study of live attenuated varicella-zoster virus vaccine to boost immunity in human immunodeficiency virus infected children with previous varicella. Pediatr Infect Dis J 2009;28:653–5.
41. Geretti AM, BHIVA Immunization Writing Committee. British HIV Association guidelines for immunization of HIV-infected adults in 2008. HIV Med 2008;9: 795–848.
42. Weinberg A, Horslen SP, Kaufmann SS, et al. Safety and immunogenicity of varicella-zoster virus vaccine in pediatric liver and intestine transplant recipients. Am J Transplant 2006;6:565–8.
43. Gershon AA. Varicella vaccine: rare serious problems: but the benefits still outweigh the risks. J Infect Dis 2003;188:945–7.
44. Barraclough KA, Wiggins KJ, Hawley CM, et al. Intradermal versus intramuscular hepatitis B vaccination in hemodialysis patients: a prospective open-label randomized controlled trial in nonresponders to primary vaccination. Am J Kidney Dis 2009;54(1):95–103.
45. Beran J. Safety and immunogenicity of a new hepatitis B vaccine for the protection of patients with renal insufficiency including pre-haemodialysis and haemodialysis patients. Expert Opin Biol Ther 2008;8(2):235–47.
46. Gandhi MK, Khanna R. Human cytomegalovirus: clinical aspects, immune regulation, and emerging treatments. Lancet Infect Dis 2004;4(12):725–38.
47. Lilley BN, Ploegh HL. Viral modulation of antigen presentation: manipulation of cellular targets in the ER and beyond. Immunol Rev 2005;207:126–44.
48. Peggs KS. Adoptive T cell immunotherapy for cytomegalovirus. Expert Opin Biol Ther 2009;9(6):725–36.
49. Einsele H, Rauser G, Grigoleit U, et al. Induction of CMV-specific T-cell lines using Ag-presenting cells pulsed with CMV protein or peptide. Cytotherapy 2002;4(1): 49–54.
50. Peggs K, Verfuerth S, Mackinnon S. Induction of cytomegalovirus (CMV)-specific T-cell responses using dendritic cells pulsed with CMV antigen: a novel culture system free of live CMV virions. Blood 2001;97(4):994–1000.
51. Koehne G, Gallardo HF, Sadelain M, et al. Rapid selection of antigen-specific T lymphocytes by retroviral transduction. Blood 2000;96(1):109–17.
52. Riddell SR, Watanabe KS, Goodrich JM, et al. Restoration of viral immunity in immunodeficient humans by the adoptive transfer of T cell clones. Science 1992;257(5067):238–41.
53. Walter EA, Greenberg PD, Gilbert MJ, et al. Reconstitution of cellular immunity against cytomegalovirus in recipients of allogeneic bone marrow by transfer of T-cell clones from the donor. N Engl J Med 1995;333(16):1038–44.
54. Einsele H, Roosnek E, Rufer N, et al. Infusion of cytomegalovirus (CMV)-specific T cells for the treatment of CMV infection not responding to antiviral chemotherapy. Blood 2002;99(11):3916–22.
55. Cobbold M, Khan N, Pourgheysari B, et al. Adoptive transfer of cytomegalovirus-specific CTL to stem cell transplant patients after selection by HLA-peptide tetramers. J Exp Med 2005;202(3):379–86.

56. Fujita Y, Leen AM, Sun J, et al. Exploiting cytokine secretion to rapidly produce multivirus-specific T cells for adoptive immunotherapy. J Immunother 2008; 31(7):665–74.
57. Nebbia G, Mattes FM, Smith C, et al. Polyfunctional cytomegalovirus-specific CD4+ and pp65 CD8+ T cells protect against high-level replication after liver transplantation. Am J Transplant 2008;8:2590–9.
58. La RC, Krishnan A, Longmate J, et al. Programmed death-1 expression in liver transplant recipients as a prognostic indicator of cytomegalovirus disease. J Infect Dis 2008;197(1):25–33.
59. Egli A, Binet I, Binggeli S, et al. Cytomegalovirus-specific T-cell responses and viral replication in kidney transplant recipients. J Transl Med 2008;6:29.
60. Szmania S, Galloway A, Bruorton M, et al. Isolation and expansion of cytomegalovirus-specific cytotoxic T lymphocytes to clinical scale from a single blood draw using dendritic cells and HLA-tetramers. Blood 2001;98(3): 505–12.
61. Tan R, Xu X, Ogg GS, et al. Rapid death of adoptively transferred T cells in acquired immunodeficiency syndrome. Blood 1999;93(5):1506–10.
62. Fletcher JM, Vukmanovic-Stejic M, Dunne PJ, et al. Cytomegalovirus-specific CD4+ T cells in healthy carriers are continuously driven to replicative exhaustion. J Immunol 2005;175(12):8218–25.
63. Sylwester AW, Mitchell BL, Edgar JB, et al. Broadly targeted human cytomegalovirus-specific CD4+ and CD8+ T cells dominate the memory compartments of exposed subjects. J Exp Med 2005;202(5):673–85.
64. Burns DM, Crawford DH. Epstein-Barr virus-specific cytotoxic T-lymphocytes for adoptive immunotherapy of post-transplant lymphoproliferative disease. Blood Rev 2004;18(3):193–209.
65. Starzl TE, Nalesnik MA, Porter KA, et al. Reversibility of lymphomas and lymphoproliferative lesions developing under cyclosporin-steroid therapy. Lancet 1984; 1(8377):583–7.
66. Swinnen LJ, Mullen GM, Carr TJ, et al. Aggressive treatment for postcardiac transplant lymphoproliferation. Blood 1995;86(9):3333–40.
67. Choquet S, Leblond V, Herbrecht R, et al. Efficacy and safety of rituximab in B-cell post-transplantation lymphoproliferative disorders: results of a prospective multicenter phase 2 study. Blood 2006;107(8):3053–7.
68. Opelz G, Dohler B. Lymphomas after solid organ transplantation: a collaborative transplant study report. Am J Transplant 2004;4(2):222–30.
69. Timms JM, Bell A, Flavell JR, et al. Target cells of Epstein-Barr-virus (EBV)-positive post-transplant lymphoproliferative disease: similarities to EBV-positive Hodgkin's lymphoma. Lancet 2003;361(9353):217–23.
70. Khanna R, Burrows SR. Role of cytotoxic T lymphocytes in Epstein-Barr virus-associated diseases. Annu Rev Microbiol 2000;54:19–48.
71. Rooney CM, Smith CA, Ng CY, et al. Use of gene-modified virus-specific T lymphocytes to control Epstein-Barr-virus-related lymphoproliferation. Lancet 1995;345(8941):9–13.
72. Rooney CM, Smith CA, Ng CY, et al. Infusion of cytotoxic T cells for the prevention and treatment of Epstein-Barr virus-induced lymphoma in allogeneic transplant recipients. Blood 1998;92(5):1549–55.
73. Haque T, Amlot PL, Helling N, et al. Reconstitution of EBV-specific T cell immunity in solid organ transplant recipients. J Immunol 1998;160(12):6204–9.
74. Khanna R, Bell S, Sherritt M, et al. Activation and adoptive transfer of Epstein-Barr virus-specific cytotoxic T cells in solid organ transplant patients with

posttransplant lymphoproliferative disease. Proc Natl Acad Sci U S A 1999; 96(18):10391–6.
75. Savoldo B, Huls MH, Liu Z, et al. Autologous Epstein-Barr virus (EBV)-specific cytotoxic T cells for the treatment of persistent active EBV infection. Blood 2002;100(12):4059–66.
76. Haque T, Taylor C, Wilkie GM, et al. Complete regression of posttransplant lymphoproliferative disease using partially HLA-matched Epstein Barr virus-specific cytotoxic T cells. Transplantation 2001;72(8):1399–402.
77. Wilkie GM, Taylor C, Jones MM, et al. Establishment and characterization of a bank of cytotoxic T lymphocytes for immunotherapy of Epstein-Barr virus-associated diseases. J Immunother 1997;27(4):309–16.
78. Haque T, Wilkie GM, Taylor C, et al. Treatment of Epstein-Barr-virus-positive post-transplantation lymphoproliferative disease with partly HLA-matched allogeneic cytotoxic T cells. Lancet 2002;360(9331):436–42.
79. Haque T, Wilkie GM, Jones MM, et al. Allogeneic cytotoxic T-cell therapy for EBV-positive posttransplantation lymphoproliferative disease: results of a phase 2 multicenter clinical trial. Blood 2007;110(4):1123–31.
80. Khanna R, Burrows SR, Nicholls J, et al. Identification of cytotoxic T cell epitopes within Epstein-Barr virus (EBV) oncogene latent membrane protein 1 (LMP1): evidence for HLA A2 supertype-restricted immune recognition of EBV-infected cells by LMP1-specific cytotoxic T lymphocytes. Eur J Immunol 1998;28(2): 451–8.
81. Gottschalk S, Edwards OL, Sili U, et al. Generating CTLs against the subdominant Epstein-Barr virus LMP1 antigen for the adoptive immunotherapy of EBV-associated malignancies. Blood 2003;101(5):1905–12.
82. Sing AP, Ambinder RF, Hong DJ, et al. Isolation of Epstein-Barr virus (EBV)-specific cytotoxic T lymphocytes that lyse Reed-Sternberg cells: implications for immune-mediated therapy of EBV+ Hodgkin's disease. Blood 1997;89(6): 1978–86.
83. Eshhar Z, Waks T, Gross G, et al. Specific activation and targeting of cytotoxic lymphocytes through chimeric single chains consisting of antibody-binding domains and the gamma or zeta subunits of the immunoglobulin and T-cell receptors. Proc Natl Acad Sci U S A 1993;90(2):720–4.
84. Sadelain M, Brentjens R, Riviere I. The promise and potential pitfalls of chimeric antigen receptors. Curr Opin Immunol 2009;21(2):215–23.
85. Chakrabarti S, Mautner V, Osman H, et al. Adenovirus infections following allogeneic stem cell transplantation: incidence and outcome in relation to graft manipulation, immunosuppression, and immune recovery. Blood 2002;100(5): 1619–27.
86. Bordigoni P, Carret AS, Venard V, et al. Treatment of adenovirus infections in patients undergoing allogeneic hematopoietic stem cell transplantation. Clin Infect Dis 2001;32(9):1290–7.
87. Feuchtinger T, Matthes-Martin S, Richard C, et al. Safe adoptive transfer of virus-specific T-cell immunity for the treatment of systemic adenovirus infection after allogeneic stem cell transplantation. Br J Haematol 2006;134(1):64–76.
88. Feuchtinger T, Richard C, Joachim S, et al. Clinical grade generation of hexon-specific T cells for adoptive T-cell transfer as a treatment of adenovirus infection after allogeneic stem cell transplantation. J Immunother 2008;31(2): 199–206.
89. Karlsson H, Brewin J, Kinnon C, et al. Generation of trispecific cytotoxic T cells recognizing cytomegalovirus, adenovirus, and Epstein-Barr virus: an approach

for adoptive immunotherapy of multiple pathogens. J Immunother 2007;30(5): 544–56.
90. Hanley PJ, Cruz CR, Savoldo B, et al. Functionally active virus-specific T cells that target CMV, adenovirus, and EBV can be expanded from naive T-cell populations in cord blood and will target a range of viral epitopes. Blood 2009;114(9): 1958–67.

Index

Note: Page numbers of article titles are in **boldface** type.

Infect Dis Clin N Am 24 (2010) 531–540
doi:10.1016/S0891-5520(10)00024-3

0891-5520/10/$ – see front matter © 2010 Elsevier Inc. All rights reserved.

id.theclinics.com

E

F

G

H

S

T

V

Moving?

Make sure your subscription moves with you!

To notify us of your new address, find your **Clinics Account Number** (located on your mailing label above your name), and contact customer service at:

Email: journalscustomerservice-usa@elsevier.com

800-654-2452 **(subscribers in the U.S. & Canada)**
314-447-8871 **(subscribers outside of the U.S. & Canada)**

Fax number: 314-447-8029

Elsevier Health Sciences Division
Subscription Customer Service
3251 Riverport Lane
Maryland Heights, MO 63043

*To ensure uninterrupted delivery of your subscription, please notify us at least 4 weeks in advance of move.

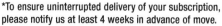

ELSEVIER

Printed and bound by CPI Group (UK) Ltd, Croydon, CR0 4YY
03/10/2024
01040445-0009